Fascial Distortion Model in Clinical Practice

Stefan Anker

Fascial Distortion Model in Clinical Practice

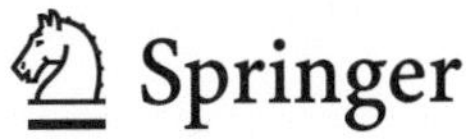 Springer

Stefan Anker
Vienna, Austria

ISBN 978-3-662-72080-6   ISBN 978-3-662-72081-3   (eBook)
https://doi.org/10.1007/978-3-662-72081-3

Foreword 1 for the English Edition

It has been said the Fascial Distortion Model (FDM) is easy to learn but difficult to master. Learning and using the FDM is a journey that will extend throughout one's career when a practitioner is inspired by success. The inspiration to embrace FDM often comes from personal experience with the FDM, either performing or receiving successful treatment. How a person is introduced to the FDM is important to their long-term successful use of the model. Clear and concise foundational content is critical to the development of a solid knowledge base. Thoroughly understanding the basic concepts of the FDM provides the basis for their own intellectual and practical growth in the model. Every patient evaluated and treatment provided in the FDM builds an FDM framework that allows a practitioner to grow and understand the model. Growth in the model is a lifelong process.

Stefan Anker's mastery of the model is evident in the clarity of his presentation of the FDM basics. His years of teaching courses in many countries and several languages have provided him with a voice to clearly express the concepts of the FDM. This content is valuable to the beginning and experienced practitioner alike. This text will be a very valuable tool for anyone interested in learning the core concepts of the FDM.

Stefan Anker's expertise as a practitioner of the FDM is also evident in the knowledge he shares throughout the textbook. Beautiful illustrations accompany excellent insights into the finer details of the model and can be found throughout. It is these details that will make this book a valuable addition to the library of every practitioner. Thorough study and review of this text will help the experienced practitioner dive more deeply into the concepts of the model and uncover a better understanding of the FDM.

I have had the pleasure of working and teaching alongside Stefan Anker as he has served the FDM community through service to the EFDMA (European FDM Association) and the FDMGO (FDM Global Organization). I have been inspired by his integrity and commitment to the work of Dr. Stephen Typaldos and his efforts to make that knowledge available to others around the world. Stefan Anker's passion for helping people and spreading the FDM is clearly demonstrated in this excellent work. I look forward to rereading the text time and again in an attempt to uncover and incorporate his wisdom on the journey to FDM mastery.

Todd Capistrant DO, MHA, CS FAFDMA
FDM Instructor (AFDMA)
Owner FDM Academy, LLC

Foreword 2 for the English Edition

Having collaborated extensively in various committees such as the EFDMA, the FDM-GO and the Organizing Committee of the FDM World Congress 2011 in Vienna for more than two decades, I have come to know Stefan Anker as a calm, structured and persistent thinker.

While I've personally met Stephen Typaldos and was certified by him as an FDM instructor, Stefan Anker's enthusiasm for FDM arose from studying his writings, teachings from Typaldos-certified instructors and colleagues, and successes in clinical implementation in practice, but without ever having met him. Due to Typaldos' sudden and early death, Stefan Anker was denied a meeting by a mere few months. This proves good-quality literature to be a valid substitute for personal contact.

This book is particularly exciting due to its consistent and orderly structure. All aspects of FDM are dealt with in sequence—philosophical, physiological, and practical – and I find the excellent illustrations especially impressive. As a contributor to several books and co-author of a textbook on FDM, I know how difficult it is to convey a clear picture of one's own ideas using illustrations. Conventional medical illustrations cannot be relied on in the field of FDM, as the model of traditional anatomy fundamentally differs from the model of fascial distortion. The images created by the author are clear and understandable. This leads to a vivid depiction of fascial distortions, an important prerequisite for success in practice.

Stefan Anker is also a pioneer in the nomenclature of techniques used in the Typaldos method. Similar to chemistry, clear, comprehensive terms are a basic prerequisite for meaningful discourse. Innovations within the model and method also require a uniform nomenclature and clear terminology in the teaching of FDM, something that Dr. Typaldos emphasized on numerous occasions.

Another aspect that I particularly like about this book is the decreased priority of arbitrarily delineated body parts, such as "knee joint" or "cervical spine". These are all terms from traditional orthopedic models based on an anatomy of discontinuity. In FDM, such terms are meaningless, as the fascia in its continuity dissolves these boundaries.

This book represents a solid textbook for the reader, covering all areas from practical guidance to a review of fine details of the model, and will provide an excellent basis for clinical success.

Dr. med. Georg Harrer
FDM Instructor
Founding President European
FDM Association (EFDMA)

Medical Disclaimer

The content presented in this textbook is intended solely for information and continuing education purposes. It does not constitute a recommendation or endorsement of the diagnostic methods, treatments, or medications described or mentioned. The text does not claim to be comprehensive, nor can the timeliness, accuracy, or balance of the information provided be guaranteed. Under no circumstances does the text replace professional advice from physicians or therapists. The text must not be used by individuals without professional training as a basis for independent diagnosis or as justification for the initiation, modification, or discontinuation of the treatment of illnesses. Always consult physicians or therapists you trust if you have any health-related questions or concerns.

Gender-Inclusive Language

This textbook implements gender-inclusive language by alternating and combining different genders for singular terms referring to people in each chapter. In the plural, the wording in all chapters equally includes all genders.

Acknowledgment

The decision to write a textbook on the Fascial Distortion Model and the Typaldos method was made in 2020 at the onset of the coronavirus pandemic. This event provided me with the necessary time to reflect on my experience as an FDM instructor and therapist. After two years of intensive work, it is time to thank all those who contributed to the success of this book.

Thanks to

Melinda, for her support in all phases of this project, from clarifying content-related questions to image design and beyond,
Keisuke Tanaka FDM.O, Christoph Rossmy D.O, Marjorie Kasten, and Dr. med. Georg Harrer, who, as companions of Stephen Typaldos, conveyed his concepts to me in all their facets,
Andreas Görg for the editing and the refreshing collaboration,
Jan Maan for his contribution to the illustrations in the book,
Herbert Flieder for the production of the photographs,
Angelika, Magdalena, and Christoph, who have given a face to the treatment of distortion,
Petra Fraberger and Dr. med. Lukas Trimmel for their professional feedback and
all my patients, course participants, and colleagues, through whom I was able to deepen my knowledge over the years.

As you work with this book and apply the Fascial Distortion Model and the Typaldos method, I wish you much enjoyment and plenty of positive feedback from your patients.

Vienna, March 2022   Stefan Anker

Contents

The Fascial Distortion Model: The Theoretical Foundations of the Typaldos Method

Therapy-resistant symptoms following physical trauma, symptoms that cannot be explained or resolved using conventional medical concepts, or acute pain and persistent movement restrictions—when faced with these challenges, physicians and therapists in clinical practice repeatedly reach their limits.

Stephen Typaldos (1957–2006) was also familiar with this situation from his daily work as a physician. However, instead of accepting the limitations of conventional therapeutic approaches, he sought possible solutions. The result of his research was the Fascial Distortion Model (FDM), an independent etiology for a wide variety of clinical presentations. In doing so, he advocated for a shift in perspective in medicine: when pain and functional limitations are viewed as consequences of fascial distortions, it opens the door to new and effective therapeutic approaches.

Typaldos was a Doctor of Osteopathic Medicine (DO) and, as such, was authorized to practice medicine in the United States without restriction. In his medical practice, he treated patients with musculoskeletal complaints, as well as internal and neurological diseases, according to the principles of the Fascial Distortion Model. To implement his concepts in clinical practice, he primarily used a manual therapy approach. This is known as the "Typaldos method" (also called "Typaldos manual therapy") and is the focus of this textbook.

The Typaldos method is the best-known way to apply the Fascial Distortion Model in clinical practice. However, it would be a misinterpretation to view Typaldos' concepts primarily as a form of manual therapy. Typaldos used the FDM to consider better treatment options across a wide range of medical specialties. He wanted to integrate his perspective into medicine, not position it apart from it. His goal was to initiate a shift in perspective among physicians and therapists, recognizing fascial distortions as a significant cause of pain and functional limitations.

This altered perspective on the etiology and treatment of various clinical presentations is the central element of the Fascial Distortion Model. At the same time, this change in approach is probably the most challenging aspect to convey.

In my experience as an FDM instructor, the key to understanding the concept of the FDM is its clinical and practical application using the Typaldos method. This makes it possible to experience the effects of fascial distortion correction directly and to assess the relevance of the model for the treatment of patients.

The aim of this textbook is to present this practice-oriented approach and to emphasize the close interconnection between Typaldos' concepts and their implementation in clinical practice.

The Typaldos method is a non-invasive approach for treating a wide range of conditions affecting the human body. The focus of the method is the correction of fascial distortions, which, according to the Fascial Distortion Model, are considered to be the underlying cause of pain and functional limitations. Specific manual techniques or mechanical therapeutic devices are used for this purpose.

Which techniques of the Typaldos method are used depends on which fascial distortions can be identified with the help of a specific form of clinical diagnostics. The perception of the problem by the patients themselves plays a particularly important role in this process. Their verbal and non-verbal descriptions significantly guide both the diagnosis and the treatment of fascial distortions.

The theoretical Fascial Distortion Model (FDM) and the practical-clinical Typaldos method are two interlinked concepts.

Fundamentals for understanding the Typaldos method, and thus for its adequate application in clinical practice, are therefore

- a detailed knowledge of the Fascial Distortion Model
- knowledge about the diagnosis of fascial distortions and
- understanding the role of patients as experts on their own symptoms

When therapists treat patients according to the FDM, this is usually done using manual techniques of the Typaldos method. It is divided into a

- typical course of treatment and
- treatment approaches for all known fascial distortions in order to correct them directly and through mechanotherapy

Background Information
The terms FDM and Typaldos method are often used synonymously in clinical practice and were also usually not strictly distinguished by Typaldos himself.

However, differentiating between model and method is important, as the Fascial Distortion Model is fundamentally a method-neutral theory and is therefore open to implementation with a wide variety of therapeutic approaches.

Typaldos was convinced that the FDM could be applied in various fields of medicine to solve clinical problems and to develop efficient treatment strategies. He considered pharmacological applications based on the Fascial Distortion Model to be just as possible as surgical interventions specifically tailored to the correction of fascial distortions. To date, such therapeutic procedures have not yet become established. The Typaldos method is the independent manual therapy form based on the Fascial Distortion Model and is the focus of this textbook.

Structure of the Textbook
The book is divided into two sections.

The **first part** examines the Fascial Distortion Model. The first chapter deals with the fundamental premises of the model. In the second chapter, the six fascial distortions are presented with their specific characteristics. FDM diagnosis, with the special role of patients in the diagnostic process, is the subject of the third chapter.

Building on this, the **second part** is dedicated to the Typaldos method, its manual techniques and treatment approaches. After a general description of the diagnostic and treatment process in the fourth chapter, the fifth chapter demonstrates the specific manual techniques for targeted direct correction of fascial distortions. The selection of techniques presented is based on the curriculum of the European Fascial Distortion Model Association (EFDMA).

The appendix contains flowcharts developed by Typaldos for the treatment of shoulder complaints, as well as a glossary of important terminology. An additional graphic shows the six fascial distortions in direct comparison.

Typaldos regarded the correction of fascial distortions as an opportunity to address the challenges of clinical practice and to push the boundaries of what is possible in medicine. This book is intended to support practitioners in demonstrating the significance of fascial distortion correction, implementing treatment approaches correctly or adapting them when necessary, without losing focus on fascial distortions.

Fundamentals of the Textbook

Stephen Typaldos published his findings in professional journals and presented his concepts to colleagues around the world. He authored a textbook on the FDM and its clinical-practical implementation with the Typaldos method, which was published in four editions. Since his passing, however, these works have only been available in their original form to a limited extent.

The publications of Stephen Typaldos from 1992–2002 remain the standard for conveying his concepts to this day, especially the latest edition of his textbook entitled "FDM – clinical and theoretical application of the fascial distortion model within the practice of medicine and surgery". For the present book, these publications [1–6] form the substantive basis. The texts are summarized and explained for this purpose. The aim is to provide readers with the most complete, original, and practice-oriented understanding possible of the Fascial Distortion Model and the Typaldos method.

References

1. Typaldos S (1992) The fascial continuum model. A new philosophical and practical approach for enhancement of athletic performance and treatment of musculoskeletal dysfunction and pain. https://www.fascialdistortion.com/the-fascial-continuum-model/
2. Typaldos S (1994) Introducing the Fascial Distortion Model. AAO J 4(2):14–18, 30–36. https://afdma.com/articles/introducing-fascial-distortion-model/
3. Typaldos S (1994) Triggerband technique. AAO J 4(4):15–18, 30–33. https://afdma.com/articles/triggerband-technique/
4. Typaldos S (1995) Continuum technique. AAO J 5(2):15–19. https://afdma.com/articles/continuum-technique/
5. Typaldos S, Meddeb G (1997) Orthopathic Medicine. The connection between orthopedics and osteopathy through the Fascial Distortion Model. Verlag für Ganzheitliche Medizin Wühr, Kötzing/Bavarian Forest
6. Typaldos S (2002) Clinical and theoretical application of the Fascial Distortion Model within the practice of medicine and surgery, 4th ed. Orthopathic Global Health Publications, Brewer

The Fascial Distortion Model describes six specific deformations of human fascia, called fascial distortions, which individually or in combination cause impairments of the musculoskeletal system and various other organ systems. The model places the consequences of changes in the shape of fascia on the functional capacity of the human body at the center and expands the conventional medical concept of pain and functional limitation.

The clinical application of the model offers the possibility of interpreting a wide variety of complaints as a result of fascial distortions. The goal is to use the model to develop effective and practically applicable treatment strategies that lead to clear, immediate, and measurable results.

The fundamental elements of the Fascial Distortion Model can be outlined as follows:

- *Fascia:* They serve as the explanatory basis for the relationships described by the FDM and are at the center of any therapeutic intervention. Their important role in the structure and functional capacity of the body makes it possible to establish connections between patients' complaints and fascial distortions.

- *Distortion:* Instead of assuming damage to bodily structures, the FDM focuses its therapeutic approach on the deformation of fascial structures due to physical trauma or overload. This makes it possible to successfully treat both acute and chronic complaints, regardless of the time of onset and the degree of tissue injury.

- *Model:* A model makes it possible to render complex issues understandable by reducing them to their essential influencing factors. With the model of fascial distortions, clinical information can be analyzed, interpreted, and practically applicable conclusions for treatment with the Typaldos method can be derived.

Example

A female patient sprains her ankle while playing sports. The joint subsequently swells significantly. The athlete feels pulling pain on the outside of her foot and can only move forward with a limp. The intensity of the symptoms prompts her to go to the hospital. There, the ankle is examined according to conventional medical criteria and an X-ray is taken to rule out a fracture. Since there is no bone fracture, the attending physician diagnoses a lateral ligament sprain. The patient is advised to wear a stabilizing bandage, rest, and apply ice to manage the pain. A

© The Author(s), under exclusive license to Springer-Verlag GmbH, DE, part of Springer Nature 2026
S. Anker, *Fascial Distortion Model in Clinical Practice*, https://doi.org/10.1007/978-3-662-72081-3_1

follow-up appointment is scheduled for three weeks later.

This example describes a typical situation following physical trauma. As a rule, such injuries are treated in the hospital according to a more or less standardized protocol. After ruling out serious pathologies that would require surgical intervention, standard treatment is provided, such as prescribing anti-inflammatory medication or immobilization. In this specific case, the approach is justified by the need to allow the pain-causing inflammation to subside. Immobilization is intended to support the healing of potentially sprained ligament structures, so that after a certain period of time, full weight-bearing of the ankle can again be expected.

Typaldos criticizes this approach. He considers it nonspecific and argues that it ignores the fascial anatomical causes of the patient's functional impairment. This can lead to treatment failure and prolonged rehabilitation times.

He analyzes such trauma using the Fascial Distortion Model based on four criteria:

- The *mechanism of injury* and the specific injury position provide an initial indication of the type and extent of fascial deformation.
- The patient's *subjective complaints* provide information about which distortions are present and how they can be treated.
- The *clinical examination* clarifies the indication and contraindication for treatment and collects objective findings, which in turn point to specific fascial distortions.
- The *interpretation of body language* makes it possible to use the patient's intuitive perception of the problem to identify and specifically correct fascial distortions.

The analysis of this clinical information explains the patient's complaints in a way that differs from the conventional medical perspective and consequently leads to different therapeutic consequences. While the physician in the example prescribes immobilization and treats the inflammation, the FDM addresses the fascial distortions caused by the injury. The goal is to correct the fascial anatomical causes of the complaints and thereby achieve immediate pain reduction as well as improvement in mobility and load-bearing capacity. Immobilization and anti-inflammatory treatment can thus become obsolete (despite the ligament sprain diagnosed by conventional medicine). ◄

1.1   Typaldos' View of Anatomy

When Typaldos began developing the Fascial Distortion Model in 1991, there was significantly less scientific knowledge about fascia than today. At that time, fascia was regarded in medicine primarily as a form of connective tissue, which, in contrast to bones, muscles, or ligaments, played a secondary role in the structure and function of the human body.

For Typaldos, however, fascial tissue proved to be a crucial bridge between his clinical observations in practice and the way patients perceived complaints, how injuries affected bodily functions, and how these could be influenced by targeted treatments.

As an osteopath, he was familiar with the fascial concept of A. T. Still, the founder of osteopathy. For Still, fascia represented a central element for human anatomy, physiology, and pathophysiology [1]. Typaldos based his theoretical considerations on osteopathic publications and his own anatomical studies, which were conducted during his time as Clinical Assistant Professor at the Texas College of Osteopathic Medicine.

Building on this, Typaldos developed his understanding of fascia, which he summarized in 1992 in the so-called "Fascial Continuum Model". This established an independent perspective on anatomy, in which fascia played a central role.

Typaldos considered his model as a way to explain the fundamental relationship between structure and function of the body in osteopathy. Subsequently, with the help of the appropriate basic scientific research, a new concept of anatomy, physiology, and pathophysiology was able to emerge.

The following three premises characterize the Fascial Continuum Model:

> *Fascia occurs in the form of fascial bands throughout the body.*

Their significance is underestimated by anatomy, as classical dissection divides the human body, contradicting the nature of continuous fascial connections. However, injuries to fascial bands are common and provide a suitable concept to explain a range of pain and functional limitations of the musculoskeletal system.

> *Fascia has functions in the human body that have not yet been described.*

Due to its close connection to the muscular system, fascia appears to play a decisive role in movement coordination. Through a kind of "fascial memory," repeated movements are stored and locally coordinated within the fascial system. This relieves the central nervous system. In addition, fascia transmits, distributes, and buffers a micro-electric tension. This explains why injured fascial bands negatively affect muscular strength, coordination, and performance.

> *Fascia is an interwoven continuum of various structures and enables their adaptation.*

This continuum is of a fluid nature. It includes bones as well as ligaments, tendons, or aponeuroses. These can change in their constitution according to the influence of intrinsic and extrinsic forces explaining physical adaptations due to fascial disorders, such as the calcification of tendons or the decalcification of the involved bone.

The following section describes Typaldos' fascia concept. In addition, an overview of the current state of knowledge on fascia is provided. The aim is to highlight points of connection between Typaldos' considerations and the current state of research. This textbook draws on publications by renowned authors from the *Fascia Research Society*, which was founded following the first Fascia Research Congress in 2007.

1.1.1 Typaldos' Definition of Fascia

In his 2002 textbook, Typaldos describes fascia as primary connective tissue, which is found throughout the body and manifests in a wide variety of anatomical structures, for example as part of tendons, ligaments, aponeuroses, adhesions, and various coverings of organs (e.g. the pericardium or the meninges) or of muscles (perimysium and epimysium). Fascia not only connects different structures, but also envelops them down to their smallest muscle fibers, it wraps and separates tissues from each other, and protects bones, nerves, muscles, and various other tissues from external forces.

Fascia plays a crucial role in force transmission within the body, its capacity for movement and load-bearing, and in pain perception. It is living tissue and represents a fluid transport network. Its metabolism functions less through blood supply and more through the exchange of interstitial fluid. This ensures the supply of nutrients and oxygen and the removal of metabolic waste products, a prerequisite for the resilience that characterizes healthy fascia.

1.1.1.1 Current State of Knowledge

Typaldos' view of fascia as an anatomical structure with functional significance was ahead of its time. The definition of fascia in medicine and science was inconsistent at that time and remains a subject of controversy today. Originally, a perspective had become established that described fascia based on anatomical and histological characteristics. For example, the Federative International Programme for Anatomical Terminology defines fascia as "sheath, sheet, or other dissectible connective tissue aggregations that forms beneath the skin to attach, enclose and separate muscles and other internal organs." [2]

With increasing knowledge about the function of fascia in the human body, it became increasingly clear that a narrow anatomical definition does not do justice to its real significance. For this reason, the Fascia Nomenclature Committee developed a proposal for a more comprehensive terminology from 2014 onwards, which also reflects the functional aspects of fascia [3]:

- Fascia includes connective tissue sheaths and sheets beneath the skin, which both connect and envelop other anatomical structures and organs, as well as separating them from each other (histological-anatomical definition).
- The fascial system is a three-dimensional continuum of soft, collagenous, loose and dense connective tissue that extends throughout the body. It includes, for example, adipose tissue, nerve and vascular sheaths, aponeuroses, joint capsules, ligaments, and inter- and intramuscular connective tissue. It surrounds and permeates all organs, muscles, bones, and nerves, and establishes a functional structure and environment which enables integrated function of the body (functional definition; fig. 1.1a and b).
- Fascia is therefore part of the fascial system, which in turn is part of the connective tissue. (The latter's definition includes tissues of mesenchymal origin such as bone, cartilage, and also blood).

Science increasingly provides insights into the important functions of fascia in the human body. Fascia influences the form and structure of all tissues, fulfills biomechanical and neurological

functions, and is integrated into a cellular signaling network [4].

The following points are of particular importance for understanding fascia-oriented treatment concepts:

- Fascia is involved in the transmission of forces within the body and thus influences biomechanics [5, 6 and 7].
- Fascia is densely innervated and plays a role in self-perception within the framework of proprioception, nociception, and interoception [8, 9 and 10].
- Fascia has an important function in regeneration and wound healing [11, 12].

1.1.1.2 Fascia and Connective Tissue

Fascia can be described as the soft tissue components of connective tissue. Connective tissue consists of *cells, fibers, and ground substance.* The latter two form the *extracellular matrix.* Connective tissue arises from mesenchymal cells and, depending on functional requirements, presents in different forms with varying proportions of its three basic components. In tendons and ligaments, the fibrous components predominate over the cells, resulting in a firm, organized connective tissue structure. In contrast, loose connective tissue has a reduced fiber content and is dominated by ground substance, giving the tissue a more gel-like consistency.

Connective tissue fulfills various functions in the body:

- It forms a structural framework and maintains the shape of the body, organs, and systems.
- It connects the various structures of the body.
- It protects and separates organs. It enables their smooth movement relative to other structures.
- It serves a metabolic function. It is involved in nutrition, the removal of waste products, and the distribution of various substances throughout the body.
- It is an energy store (in the form of adipose tissue).
- It plays a central role in wound healing.

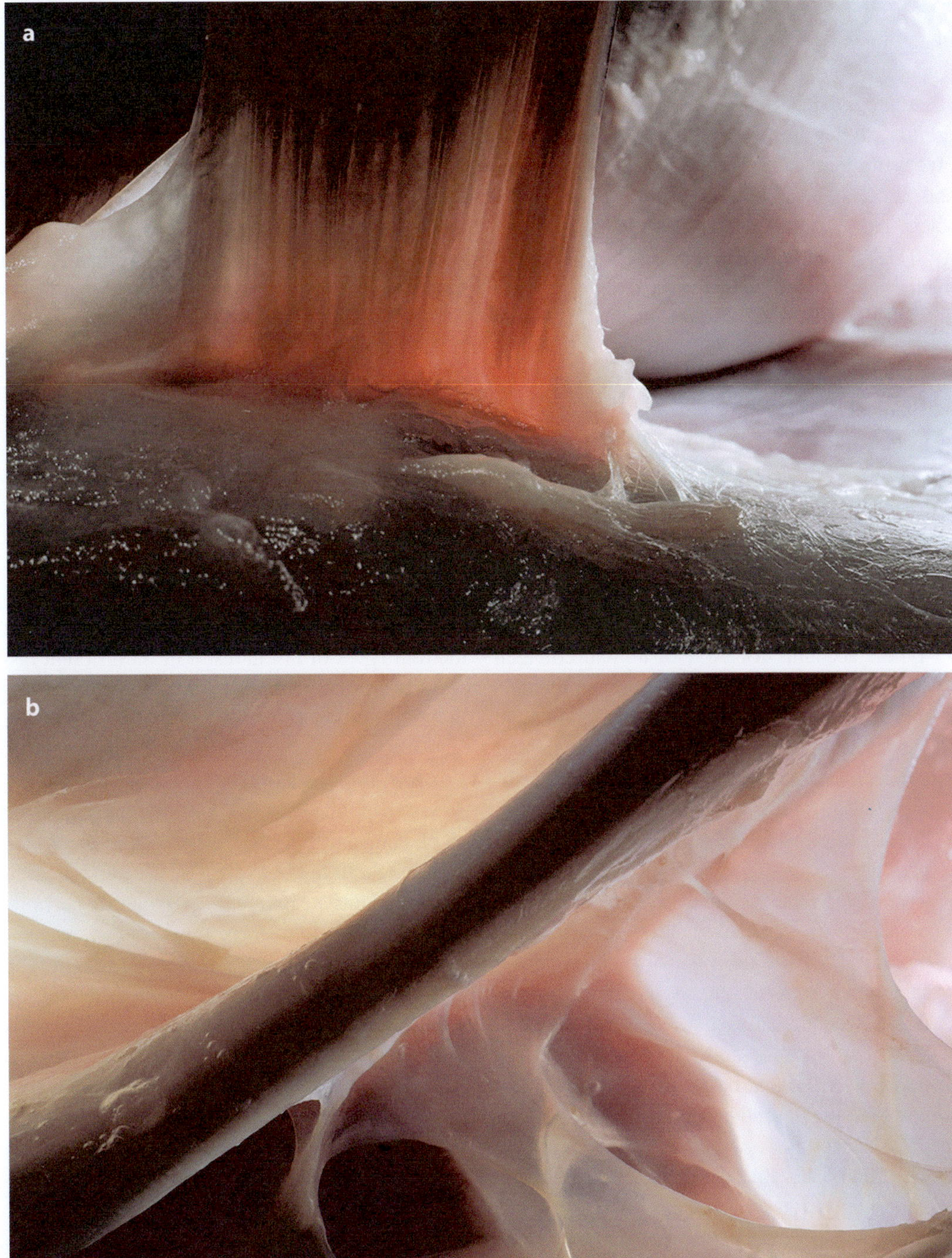

Fig. 1.1 **a** and **b** fascia. (© Fascialnet.com. Photographer: Thomas Stephan)

The *ground substance* is an amorphous, gel-like substance that surrounds the cells. It contains proteoglycans, to which various glycosaminoglycans (such as hyaluronan, chondroitin sulfates, or heparin) are attached. The glycosaminoglycans carry a negative charge and attract water. This gives the ground substance its gel-like volume and viscoelasticity. The ground substance serves as a transport medium for metabolism on the one hand, and on the other hand, it fulfills a mechanical function. It allows the smooth gliding of fibers, shock absorption, and shape retention after mechanical stress [13].

Connective tissue contains two types of *fibers:* collagen fibers and elastic fibers.

Collagen fibers are generally oriented according to their mechanical load. Depending on fiber thickness, four types of collagen fibers can be distinguished:

- Type I accounts for 90% of human collagen and is found, among other places, in the dermis of the skin, in bone, fascia, and organ capsules. It is characterized by bundles of connective tissue fibers, which give this type high tensile strength.
- Type II has finer fibers and is found mainly in cartilage.
- Type III has even finer fibers, which are organized in a reticular rather than bundled pattern. They are the type of connective tissue from which all other types develop (e.g. during wound healing).
- Type IV forms a kind of connective tissue network and is a basic component of the basal lamina of epithelia.

Elastic fibers are thinner than collagen fibers and are interwoven with them. They are responsible for the elastic behavior of connective tissue and protect it from mechanical damage [14].

The *cells* of connective tissue are fibroblasts, adipocytes, and undifferentiated mesenchymal cells. In addition, connective tissue also contains, among others, macrophages, mast cells, lymphocytes, and white blood cells.

Fibroblasts produce fibers for the extracellular matrix and are stimulated, for example, by mechanical stress. They also play a crucial role in wound closure by secreting type III connective tissue. A special subtype should be mentioned: myofibroblasts are found in tendons, fascia, and scars. They have contractile ability and draw the wound edges together.

Adipocytes store energy and are involved in hormone synthesis [15].

1.1.2   Four Types of Fascia

Based on his own research and empirical observations, Typaldos assumed that fascia can be distinguished in the body according to their structure and function. He developed a concept of four types of fascia, each with a typical structure and localization, as well as specific functions and risks of deformation. Deformations of the four types of fascia result in six different fascial distortions, which can cause pain and functional limitations:

- **Band-like fascia (also called banded fascia)** is dense, tensile tissue with a high proportion of connective tissue fibers, which are found throughout the body. Its structure and orientation adapts to its respective load. It plays an important role in force transmission, protects tissues such as bone, muscle, and vessels, and adapts to their movements without resistance. The flow of interstitial fluid in the tissue is oriented along band-like fascia. According to Typaldos, this is also the type of fascia whose state of tension significantly influences body perception. Deformations in this area are referred to as triggerbands or continuum distortions (fig. 1.2a).
- **Smooth fascia** appears as supple, adaptable fascial planes found in the area of joints and internal organs. It is less resistant than banded fascia, but its gliding ability allows for great mobility. If this type of fascia is deformed, we refer to herniated triggerpoints or tectonic fixations (fig. 1.2b).

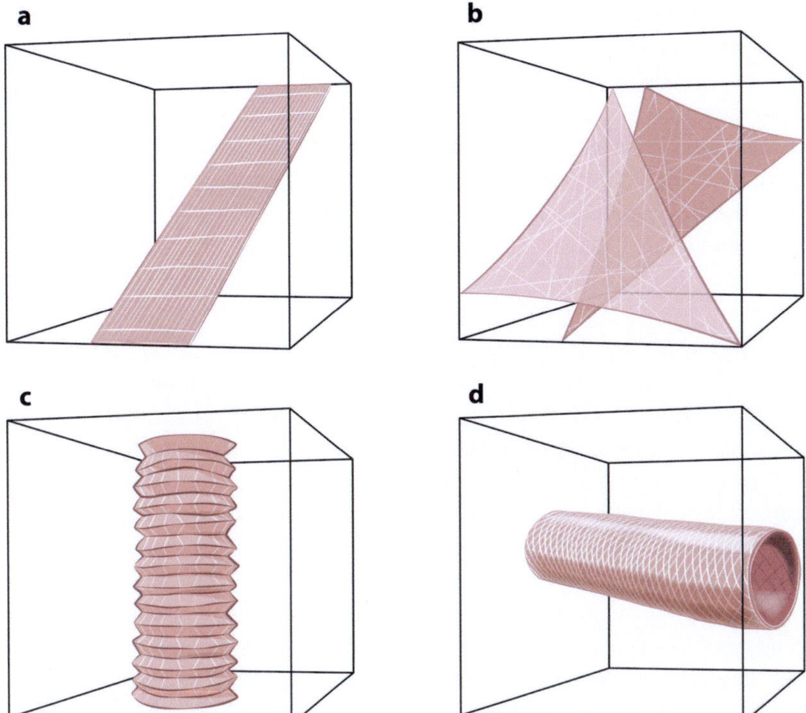

Fig. 1.2 The four types of fascia according to Typaldos. The FDM describes band-like (**a**) and smooth fascia (**b**), which differ particularly in the concentration and orientation of their fascial fibers and thus in their strength. In addition, two shock absorber systems are described: folding fascia (**c**) in the area of joints and cylinder fascia (**d**) for soft tissues and vessels.

- **Folding fascia** is found in the area of joints (in the form of joint capsules and other structures surrounding a joint). Muscle septa and the interosseous membranes are also considered folding fascia. Its folded structure allows the tissue to be unfolded or refolded without being damaged. It functions as a kind of shock absorber for jointed areas. This potential is limited when a folding distortion, a deformation of this type of fascia, occurs (fig. 1.2c).
- **Cylinder fascia** is a spirally constructed structure enveloping soft tissues such as muscles, vessels, nerves, and internal organs in several layers. Like the coils of a spiral, this type of fascia can be stretched apart or compressed together and, like folding fascia, serves as a shock absorber for non-articular areas. Deformations of this type of fascia are referred to as cylinder distortions (fig. 1.2d).

Basically, all four fascia types are present in every person. However, individual fascia types may be more or less developed in each person, which influences both the functional capacity of the body and its susceptibility to injury:

- People whose band-like tissue is particularly well developed have the advantage that these stable fascial structures provide a good foundation for the exertion of strength. However, the disadvantage is a tendency toward the formation of adhesions and, as a consequence, movement restrictions, especially if immobilization of a body region is necessary due to injury.
- Dominance of folding fascia allows for good mobility, but also results in a certain susceptibility to folding distortions with their typical symptoms of painful or unstable joints.

- People with pronounced jumping ability and elastic tissue have a high proportion of cylinder fascia, but are also prone to cramps or diffuse pain syndromes.
- Finally, a high proportion of smooth fascia tends to have a negative effect on the general resilience of the body, making injuries and overuse more likely.

> **Background Information**
> Knowing the four fascia types and their distribution in the body can help in diagnosing fascial distortions. Depending on the location of the problem, certain types of distortions may be more likely than others. For example, the tissue in the anterior neck region is required to have a great deal of adaptability and deformability in order to ensure simultaneous free movement of the head and shoulders. Smooth fascia plays a key role here. In clinical practice, we see that movement restrictions in this region often also involve this fascia type, and the corresponding deformation patterns (herniated triggerpoints or tectonic fixations) tend to occur.

1.1.2.1 Scientific Consideration of Fascia Types

Anatomically, loose connective tissue is distinguished from dense connective tissue [16]:

- *Loose connective tissue* is the most common connective tissue in the body. It is characterized by a high proportion of ground substance. Compared to dense connective tissue, it contains fewer cells and fibers and forms a net-like, multidirectional structure. Loose connective tissue serves transport and storage functions. It facilitates the gliding of various structures (e.g. muscles) against each other, fills spaces between organs thereby stabilizing their position, and acts as a shock absorber.
- *Dense connective tissue* can be subdivided into regular, irregular, and elastic connective tissue. Structures such as ligaments, tendons, or aponeuroses have a regular, parallel-oriented structure with a high proportion of collagen fibers. Muscle fasciae, on the other hand, are also regular but are organized in several overlapping layers.

Fascia, as part of the connective tissue, can be divided into four layers [17]:

- The *superficial fascia* (fascia superficialis; panniculus layer) is located in the subcutaneous tissue and separates superficial from deep fat tissue. It is in contact with the deep fascia [18].
- The *deep fascia* (fascia profunda; trunk or muscle fascia) is divided into aponeurotic fascia (e.g. the thoracolumbar fascia) and epimysial fascia (e.g. muscle fascia in the arms and legs). Both are organized fascial layers that mainly differ in their thickness and location. They connect various structures and are involved in force transmission [19].
- The *meningeal fascia* surrounds the nervous system and includes, for example, the dura mater.
- The *visceral fascia* lines the body cavities and is involved in the formation of conduit layers for neurovascular bundles (e.g. the mediastinum).

Typaldos' distinction of four fascia types is not based on this anatomical consideration—at least, there is no explicit reference to such in his publications. However, the characteristics he describes for each type can certainly be reconciled with this view. For example, dense connective tissue corresponds more to the band-like fascia, while loose connective tissue is more similar to the cylinder fascia.

Typaldos also draws a connection between the topography of fascia in the body and a specific (primarily mechanical) function. This idea arose partly from clinical observations of the relationship between certain symptom patterns and specific physical constitutions in patients. On the other hand, Typaldos identified structural differences in the course of anatomical studies on specimens. Current research is developing a similar perspective, according to which fasciae fulfill different functions depending on their location and architecture [20]. However, the explicit assignment of functions such as shock absorption or joint stability to individual fascia types remains a concept that is particularly helpful for the clinical practice of the Typaldos method.

1.1.3 Fascial Continuity Model

The Fascial Distortion Model promotes a perspective on the human body that centers on the continuity of tissues. Fascial fibers traverse the body in its entirety, thereby connecting different tissue types, and forming a framework for all structures of the organism (fig. 1.3).

This results in the following clinical phenomena:

- Fascial deformations are not limited to specific structures such as bone or muscle, but depending on the injury, may affect, for example, the fascia of the bone and simultaneously the fascia of the associated soft tissues.
- The continuous fascial fibers are under a baseline tension, which is integrated in the central nervous system as mechanical information. This relationship forms the basis for self-perception, within which changes in tension (for example due to fascial distortions) can be perceived. This mechanism is crucial for movement coordination and the adjustment of muscle tone.
- The model of continuity further explains why fascial distortions can have not only local effects but also distant effects. Due to the continuity of fascial fibers, deformations and the resulting changes in mechanical tension can be transmitted to more distant areas, causing symptoms or further deformations at those sites.

1.1.3.1 Anatomy and Architecture of Fascia

The fascial continuity model promoted by Typaldos is still not the standard perspective in anatomical literature. In accordance with the concept of anatomy, which involves dissecting the body into individual parts to make its structure comprehensible, most anatomists divide the fascia into individual sections. These are named after the structures with which they are associated (such as the fascia cruris or the fascia renalis). This segmentation is in contradiction to the embryological development of fascia from the mesoderm. Fascia differentiates according to the functional requirements in the body. It forms a continuous, fibrillar, and tensioned framework [21]. Along this framework, various bodily structures develop organically [22]. From this perspective, the continuity of fascial

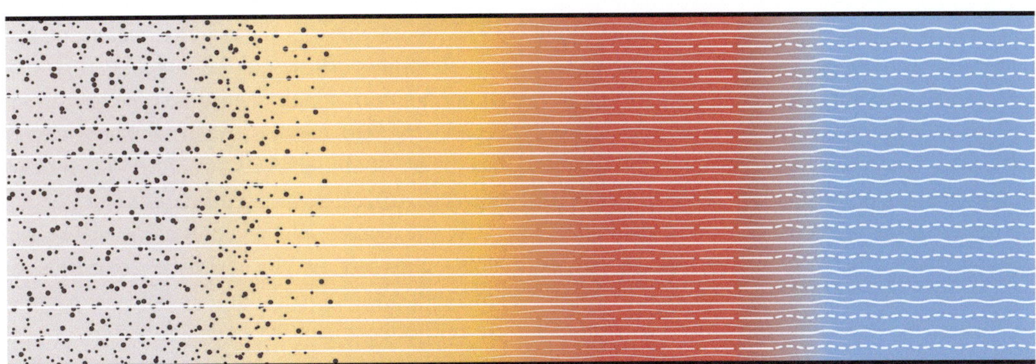

Fig. 1.3 Continuity of tissues from Typaldos' perspective. Continuous fascial bands run throughout the entire body. They connect different structures from bone (beige), through ligaments and muscles (yellow-red), to loose connective tissue (blue). (© Anker 2022)

fibers, as described by Typaldos, is clearly comprehensible.

In the scientific field, the term fascial architecture is increasingly being established. This reflects the fact that, in addition to anatomical localization, the manner in which fascia is arranged in the body also plays a role:

- When fascia is aligned parallel to other structures, it functions as a separating layer that, for example, enables gliding movements or separates pressure compartments. Typaldos attributes such a function to the so-called smooth fascia.
- In a serial arrangement, there are sometimes fluid transitions between muscles, ligaments, and fascial structures, as described by Typaldos within the framework of the continuum theory (see sect. 1.1.4). This concept is supported by the distribution of mechanoreceptors along these serial tissues. They are more likely to be localized along functional force lines in the body and concentrated on distinct anatomical structures [23].

The self-perception of changes in fascial tension explained by Typaldos on the basis of fascial continuity has not yet been proven. However, in light of current knowledge, it appears plausible.

Fascia possesses a baseline tension, which can be explained by its close connection with the muscles. In addition, it has inherent tension (due to elastic fibers) and fascia-specific contractile elements (myofibroblasts). The tonicity of fascia is further influenced by the pH value of the tissue, temperature, and humoral factors such as inflammatory mediators [24].

The architecture of the body aims to ensure maximum mobility and adaptability while simultaneously providing resistance to mechanical forces. If the organism is viewed as a tensegrity structure, these functions appear to be ensured and understandable.

Tensegrity—tensional integrity—is a model from architecture that can be applied to biological structures in the form of biotensegrity. According to this construction principle,

structures such as muscles, bones, tendons, or cell membranes are arranged in a specific manner, consisting on the one hand of pre-tensioned elements (e.g. fasciae) and on the other hand of compression-resistant elements (e.g. bones) without direct contact. As a result, these structures are under a baseline tension that stabilizes and buffers applied forces. The fascial system, characterized by continuity, plays a key role in this [25]. Consequently, Typaldos' consideration that fascia, depending on its arrangement and localization, assumes certain mechanical functions (such as stabilization, force transmission, or shock absorption) becomes more plausible (see sect. 1.1.2).

Typaldos describes the fascial system as a tension receptor, whose information is integrated in the nervous system. Fascia possesses the various mechanoreceptors necessary for this in large numbers. These receptors are not only concentrated in the periarticular area. They are found especially in the area between the superficial and deep fascial layers [26]. Through its connection to the nervous system, fascia can indeed be regarded as a sensory organ for our proprioception, nociception, and interoception [27].

1.1.4 Continuum Theory

With the continuum theory, Typaldos describes the plastic behavior of fascia, which he regards as a continuous anatomical structure. As described in his Fascial Continuum Model in 1992, he emphasizes the adaptive nature of fascial structures. These can be considered part of a continuum in which one tissue type transitions seamlessly into another. Each of these tissues has the ability to adapt its structure to that of an adjacent tissue type along this continuum.

At the center of the continuum theory are bones and soft tissues (such as ligaments or tendons), which, according to this perspective, are not independent structures. Band-like fibers traverse both tissue types, thereby ensuring their tensile stability. The bones are further reinforced by mineral components, which gives them the

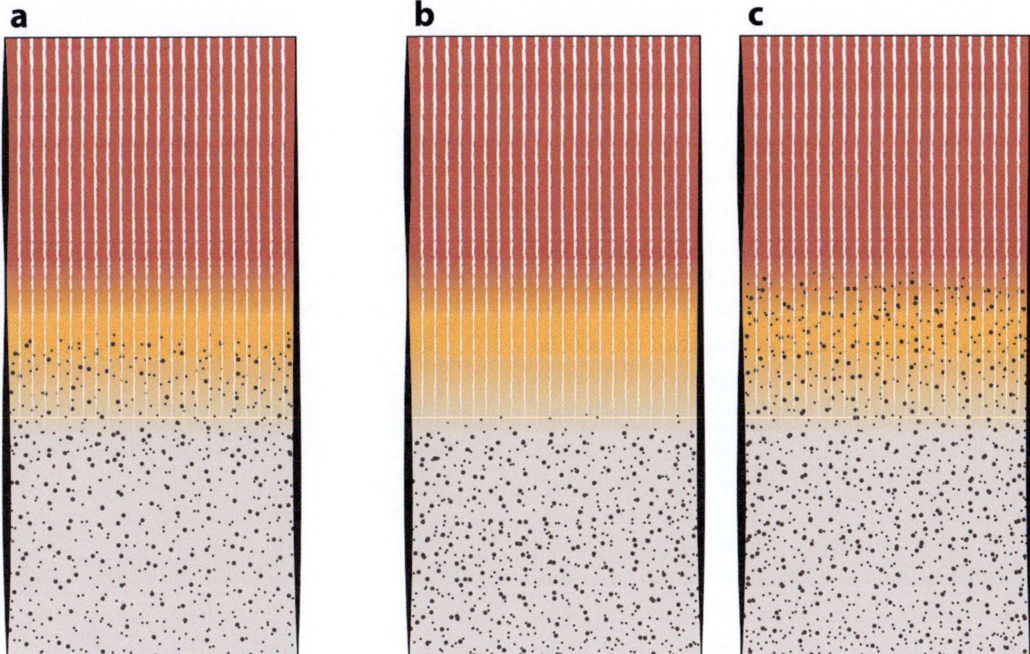

Fig. 1.4 Continuum theory. The transition zones between bone and soft tissue allow for complete adaptation from a neutral configuration (**a**) to a ligamentous (**b**) or bony (**c**) configuration. (© Anker 2022)

potential to maintain their shape against gravity. Complementarily, the ligaments provide flexibility for movement.

Typaldos locates a *transition zone* at the interface between bone and soft tissue, in which both tissue types are present simultaneously (fig. 1.4a). Depending on the type of force applied (Typaldos distinguishes between unidirectional and multidirectional forces in this context), a structural adaptation of the transition zone occurs in favor of either bone or soft tissue (fig. 1.4 b and c). This dynamic adaptation operates through the adjustment of mineral concentration in the transition zone. These minerals are transported via the interstitial fluid along the band-like fascia. Through this mechanism, transition zones can stabilize and provide an optimal basis for the transmission of forces. However, they can also reduce their stiffness to allow for elastic movement behavior.

According to Typaldos, these adaptation processes can occur abruptly, allowing the tissue continuum to respond immediately to the respective demand and ensuring optimal function. However, fascial distortions can impair the flow of interstitial fluid and thus this adaptive capacity. This can not only lead to local complaints (as is the case with the continuum distortion described in the second chapter), but also impair the metabolism of soft tissues and bone in the long term.

1.1.4.1 Fascial Plasticity

Two traditional explanatory models for fascial plasticity are mechanical in nature [28]:

- The thixotropic effect, the change in viscosity of the fascia due to pressure, is a temporary phenomenon. This partly explains the release, the yielding of (fascial) tension perceived by therapists and patients during manual treatment. However, it does not explain the lasting structural change that Typaldos describes in the development of a continuum distortion.

- Fibroblasts exhibit piezoelectric behavior and are stimulated by pressure to synthesize collagen fibers. However, this synthesis takes time. The formation of collagen fibers could explain the medium-term adaptations of a continuum disorder, but not the abrupt change in the sense of a (usually trauma-induced) continuum distortion.

Typaldos places the transport of fluid along the band-like fascia at the center of his argument. Its dynamics and the associated transport of calcium phosphate enable the adaptability of the fascia. This is fundamentally plausible, since especially the gel-like component of the fascia, the extracellular matrix, significantly influences the architecture and function of fascial tissues [29, 30].

As described by Typaldos, the architecture of the tissue also appears to play a role. Fluids move along interfaces such as fiber bundles or cell membranes [31]. It is conceivable that deformations (e.g. adhesions) impair this fluid movement and subsequently lead to a morphological adaptation of the fascia. This would explain medium-term effects of a continuum disorder (e.g. calcification of soft tissues). However, even the impairment of fluid transport does not provide a satisfactory explanation for the purely mechanical, abrupt onset of a continuum distortion.

Neurological mechanisms of action could play a role in this context. Typaldos did not comment on such a possible connection. From a scientific perspective, stimulation of the mechanoreceptors present in fascia leads to an immediate change in sympathetic tone, a change in local blood supply, and consequently an adjustment of the viscosity of the ground substance. Myofibroblasts also play an additional role in this context. They have the ability to contract and can also regulate fascial tone [32, 33]. It is therefore conceivable that a continuum distortion is not purely a mechanical phenomenon, but that neurological mechanisms are also involved in its development and functional effects.

FDM and Science
Typaldos cited as the greatest weakness of his model the lack of scientific evidence on the subject of fascia, fascial bands, and the anatomical transition areas between different tissue types. As the greatest strength, he described the associated opportunities to develop treatment approaches for previously difficult-to-treat diseases based on a fascial anatomical perspective, and to draw practice-oriented conclusions for the therapy of various complaints.

Typaldos was interested in scientific research on the subject of fascia, as this opened up possibilities for treating complaints even more specifically and effectively.

To what extent today's state of knowledge would have fundamentally influenced his considerations cannot be answered. Typaldos often does not provide scientifically substantiated explanations for the mechanisms of action he describes with the FDM. He justifies the phenomena observed by clinicians with pragmatic concepts of different types of fascia. These concepts are based partly on the knowledge of his time, and partly on hypotheses that have proven themselves in practice. However, the ongoing confirmation of hypotheses through practice is not scientific proof of their accuracy.

The current state of research on fascia is still incomplete and unsatisfactory. Partly, this state of research can be interpreted as supporting Typaldos's concepts. On the other hand, contradictions also emerge that still need to be clarified and have not yet led to a fundamental questioning, revision, or improvement of the Fascial Distortion Model. The sometimes insufficient evidence base makes it difficult to accept the Fascial Distortion Model in an evidence-based medical practice, which Typaldos himself has always aimed for. However, the lack of verifiability does not change the function and logic of the model and is therefore not a reason to prevent its application in clinical practice.

Scientific findings could enrich the FDM and its clinical application. For example, it is conceivable that new methods for detecting fascial deformations could influence and expand the existing concept of FDM diagnostics. New treatment modalities are possible if we better understand how mechanical forces during manual therapy affect the body.

complaints, independent of the conventional medical diagnosis. Typaldos was also convinced that this could open up possibilities for specific surgical and pharmacological treatment interventions.

1.2   Fascial Distortions

Fascial distortions lead to dysfunctions of the affected tissue and other related structures. They deform the fascial architecture in a characteristic manner and trigger changes in tension, resulting in symptoms such as movement restrictions or pain. Fascial distortions thus make it possible to interpret symptoms as the result of changes in the shape of the fascia and to expand the conventional medical understanding of functional impairments.

Background Information

To what extent these distortions also structurally alter fascia remains unclear, as to date fascial distortions cannot be detected using imaging techniques.

The concept of fascial distortions developed from the clinical observation that defined patterns of complaints can be specifically and predictably resolved through targeted, mechanically acting manual techniques and therapeutic approaches. Typaldos was unable to classify these phenomena using conventional pathophysiological medical models, and subsequently postulated that many symptoms described by patients can be attributed to a defined fascial deformation. This makes it possible to investigate the effects of various therapeutic interventions on the potentially altered fascial architecture. As a result, it can be deduced how certain therapeutic measures affect specific

1.2.1   Discovery of Fascial Distortions

From 1986, Typaldos worked as a Doctor of Osteopathic Medicine (DO) in the USA and practiced at various hospitals in several states. There, he treated a broad spectrum of patients, from injured athletes to individuals with chronic diseases or disorders of internal organs. He was familiar with osteopathic medicine according to Dr. Andrew Taylor Still and was willing to use manual therapeutic interventions in a hospital setting. Despite his commitment, however, the therapeutic concepts he had learned during his osteopathy studies and, previously, in chiropractic training, often yielded only insufficient treatment success. Even the use of standard therapies such as prescribing anti-inflammatory medications or immobilization was often ineffective. This led to personal dissatisfaction and motivated him to seek more effective therapeutic approaches, which ultimately resulted in the development of the Fascial Distortion Model.

Starting in 1991, Typaldos discovered and characterized six different fascial distortions in a process that spanned several years. In this, random events in his life as a physician played a decisive role:

One day, a patient consulted him with severe pain in her upper back. After the medical examination, however, it was unclear to Typaldos which treatment could help with her complaints. He discussed the situation with the patient, who urged him to treat her complaints according to her own ideas and perceptions. She asked Typaldos to apply strong manual pressure to specific areas of her back, expecting relief from this intervention. After some hesitation and without a clear idea of the exact treatment procedure, Typaldos finally agreed and began to carry out the obviously painful procedure. To his surprise, the patient was able to explain step by step what he should do next, until a marked and lasting alleviation of her symptoms was ultimately achieved.

Typaldos was astonished by the effect of the treatment. From a medical perspective, he could not explain why the patient knew exactly what would help her pain. Furthermore, he lacked a plausible explanation for the mechanism of action of the successful manual treatment.

Another key experience for Typaldos was the fracture of his own forearm, which led to a persistent limitation in rotational movement. Although there was no objective reason for this blockage, neither he nor his medical colleagues were able to resolve it. Ultimately, Typaldos decided to develop a treatment for the problem himself, as the application of the medical concepts known to him did not lead to any improvement. Based on his self-perception and considerations regarding the cause of the movement restriction, he forcefully manipulated his arm with considerable effort until mobility was restored, accompanied by a loud cracking sound.

From this peculiar experience, he drew the following conclusions:

- As a patient, he had a precise idea of what improvement was possible regarding his own problem, while his medical colleagues were unable to assess this.
- Based on his perception, he was able to devise a concept for how he could resolve his complaints himself.

He began to question his perspective on diagnosis and therapy and found that many patients had precise ideas about which type of treatment might be appropriate for them. This intuitive knowledge led to sometimes unusual treatment interventions that immediately resolved complaints. Typaldos could not explain the often surprising effectiveness of these interventions based on his previous medical knowledge.

He discovered correlations between the type of complaints and their mechanism of injury. He also recognized that patients, regardless of their conventional medical diagnosis, often described similar pain patterns or limitations. When he focused treatment on directly resolving these patterns instead of therapy according to the conventional medical diagnosis, many symptoms disappeared immediately and sustainably.

Of particular importance, especially for diagnostics, was ultimately the realization that patients indicated their complaints not only verbally but also non-verbally in the form of specific gestures on their own bodies. This form of body language seemed to occur in a typical and comparable manner among different patients and provided important clues as to where and how the complaints could best be treated. At first, he thought that the observable gestures pointed to specific anatomical structures such as nerves or vessels. However, such a connection was often not comprehensible.

The omnipresent fascial system therefore seemed to him to be the key to explaining the phenomena he observed. His theoretical considerations ultimately resulted in the characterization of six patterns of fascial deformation between 1991 and 1995. These fascial distortions form the core of the Fascial Distortion Model as it is known today.

1.2.2   Deformation versus Destruction

In order to understand the concept of fascial distortion, it is necessary to emphasize the plasticity of human anatomy, rather than perceiving it as a rigid arrangement of various structures. Typaldos describes that physical trauma or overloading of tissues leads to a change in shape in the area of the fasciae, but their integrity remains preserved. This view of injuries stands in contrast to the common understanding that mechanical forces damage tissue and create a wound, which is responsible for pain and loss of function. Conventional medicine focuses on the diagnosis and treatment of such damage. However, from Typaldos' perspective, this concept often hinders immediate functional rehabilitation, which he aims to achieve using the Fascial Distortion Model and the Typaldos method.

Background Information

The FDM does not question the possibility of tissue injury and does not offer an alternative explanatory model for conventionally defined medical diagnoses. Treatment according to the FDM does not aim to heal or repair structural-anatomical damage, but rather focuses on correcting fascial deformations. From the perspective of the model, restoration of the optimal fascial form is possible at any time after the occurrence of the distortion.

Fascial distortions are usually caused by external or internal mechanical forces and can likewise be corrected with mechanical force.

Each of the six distortions is characterized by a typical, visualizable type of deformation of individual fascial types (fig. 1.5a to f).:

- **Triggerband (TB):** distorted fascial band.
- **Herniated triggerpoint (HTP):** protrusion of tissue through an adjacent fascial layer.
- **Continuum distortion (CD):** alteration of the transition zone between different tissue types within the fascial continuum.
- **Folding distortion (FD):** three-dimensional deformation of folding fascia.
- **Cylinder distortion (CyD):** tangling of coils of the cylinder fascia.
- **Tectonic fixation (TF):** loss of gliding ability of smooth fascia.

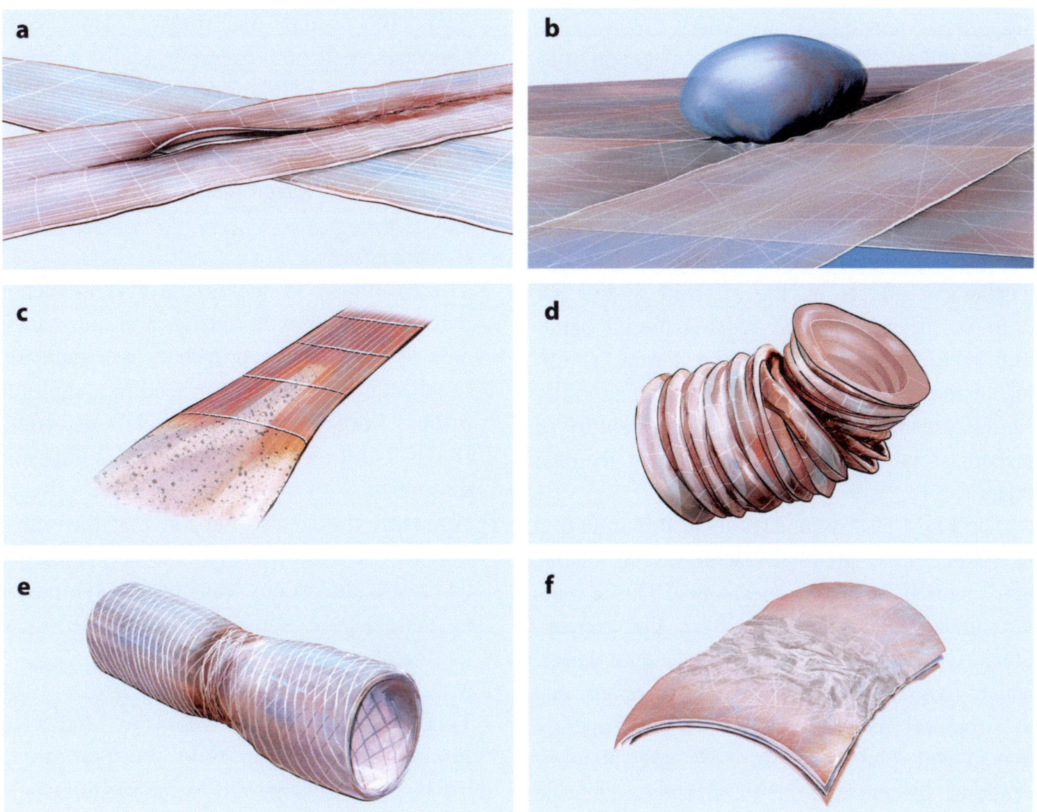

Fig. 1.5 Depiction of the six fascial distortions: triggerband (**a**), herniated triggerpoint (**b**), continuum distortion (**c**), folding distortion (**d**), cylinder distortion (**e**), tectonic fixation (**f**). (© Anker 2022)

1.2.3 Pain and Functional Impairment from the Perspective of the Fascial Distortion Model

Based on the six distortions and the associated changes in fascial architecture, the FDM explains a wide variety of symptoms such as pain, movement restriction, or loss of strength.

Typaldos regards fasciae as receptors of mechanical tension. Fascial bands, which run throughout the entire body, possess an individual baseline tension and are stimulated by movement. This leads to a kind of vibration, which is integrated into the nervous system as information and significantly influences proprioception. Fascial distortions can alter the tension of the fascial bands and thus the vibration (Typaldos calls this "pitch"). The nervous system interprets this as pain, whereupon muscular coordination or contraction adapts. Pulling, burning discomfort, tension, or weakness are possible consequences. The interaction between fasciae and the nervous system also explains the immediate effect in terms of pain relief or functional improvement when fascial distortions are resolved.

Regardless of the nervous system, certain symptoms can also be explained by the direct mechanical effects on the affected tissue. For example, triggerbands as twisted fascial bands can lead to shortening of the tissue, resulting in movement restriction. Reduced mobility can also result from a loss of gliding ability of planar fascial structures, as occurs in tectonic fixation.

The FDM also associates local inflammation or degenerative processes with fascial distortions, namely as their consequence. This reveals the fundamental difference from the conventional view of musculoskeletal complaints, which focuses on inflammatory processes due to structural damage. These are subsequently treated with pharmacological or surgical interventions. In contrast, the FDM emphasizes the connection of these processes with tissue deformations, thereby expanding the consideration of pain as a neurochemical process to include a fascial-anatomical dimension.

1.2.4 Effects of Fascial Distortions

Fascial distortions affect the tissues of the body in various ways, both directly and indirectly:

- *Local effect*
  The change in fascial architecture leads to symptoms at the site of the distortion. The FDM generally assumes that the location of the fascial distortion coincides with the location of the symptoms. If the fascial distortion is therefore corrected locally and the tension relationships are thereby normalized, the symptoms disappear. This explains why the intuitive perception of symptoms and their localization by the patients themselves is a significant element in the diagnosis of fascial distortions. (This view contrasts with other neurologically or muscularly based pain models, which describe a different localization of the pain generator and the perceived pain. The concept of projected or referred pain can be cited as an example.)
- *Remote effect*
  The continuity of the fascial system means that local changes in tension and the associated symptoms can propagate mechanically to adjacent areas. This can lead to symptoms distant from the original fascial distortion. If this is corrected, these remote symptoms disappear.
  However, it can also happen that the transmitted tensions lead to the formation of additional distortions, causing the symptoms to spread and subsequently require local treatment.
- *Roadblock effect*
  This phenomenon describes the effects of fascial distortions on fluid transport along the fascial bands as well as the medium- and long-term effects on fascial metabolism. The interstitial fluid ensures the supply of

nutrients, the removal of metabolic products, and the transfer of minerals between bone and adjacent soft tissues. This fluid can be considered a transport medium. All six fascial distortions can act as a mechanical obstacle to fluid dynamics and slow it down.

Possible consequences are

- impairment of metabolism and, as a result, reduced tissue resilience,
- subsequently, an increased risk for the development of additional fascial distortions,
- persistent, localized swelling,
- the redistribution of calcium phosphate from bone into soft tissues (as corresponds to the picture of osteoarthritis in conventional medicine),
- and the triggering of diffuse, regional symptoms.

1.2.5   Prevention of Fascial Distortions

Fascial distortions become apparent primarily through the symptoms they cause in patients and, consequently, can only be inadequately detected in the absence of complaints. This naturally limits the possibilities for preventing fascial distortions.

The best possible treatment of individual complaints is considered to have a preventive value, as incompletely corrected underlying fascial distortions can, based on experience, lead to the development of new distortions, even after a period of time.

Apart from this, Typaldos points out in his textbooks the importance of resilient, healthy fasciae and the role of a well-functioning fascial metabolism. However, he does not describe any specific measures for maintaining health in order to prevent fascial distortions.

Current research in this context emphasizes the positive effect of movement and loading, as compared to immobilization and rest, on the fasciae. This supports Typaldos' approach of enabling patients to return to their usual activities as soon as possible [34, 35].

1.3   A Model for Clinical Practice

When Typaldos described the first fascial distortion in 1991, it was unclear how many distortions were yet to be discovered, and where these insights would lead. Over the years, however, it became apparent that the relationships between symptoms and fascial distortions could be formulated in increasing detail. This created the need to formally summarize the large number of clinical observations and empirically verified relationships, making them comprehensible and teachable for his medical colleagues.

To this end, Typaldos chose the term Fascial Distortion Model (FDM) to describe the connection between fascial distortions and patients' symptoms. Over the years, he used other terms to name his concept. "Orthopathic Medicine," composed of the terms orthopedics and osteopathy, was for several years, from his perspective, the appropriate designation for his clinical approach. Ultimately, however, he abandoned this term and returned to "Fascial Distortion Model."

Background Information

For Typaldos, the FDM was a self-contained, independent concept. However, he did not rule out further development. Although the FDM with its six fascial distortions proved effective in clinical practice, Typaldos was repeatedly confronted with persistent symptom patterns and therefore remained open to possible further insights he could integrate into the FDM. For example, he considered the possibility of a seventh fascial distortion, even though he did not discover it before his death.

1.3.1   Model of Fascial Distortions

The general aim of a model is to reduce complex relationships to the essential influencing factors. A model is not a depiction of reality, but rather deals with the factors that are relevant to the real process and in the context of the model. The specific aim of the Fascial Distortion Model is to illustrate the relationships between clinical phenomena and fascial distortions. This creates a guiding structure for the analysis and interpretation of symptoms, from which practice-relevant conclusions for treatment can be derived.

In medical practice, models are used daily to clarify clinical questions. The biomedical model is a standard in the treatment of a wide variety of symptoms. It assumes that the cause of diseases and their symptoms arises from disturbances of bodily functions that can be demonstrated biochemically or physically. This, among other things, leads to laboratory findings or imaging procedures having great significance in medical diagnostics.

The biomedical model is also used for musculoskeletal complaints. The focus of diagnosis is on identifying structural damage or inflammation, which are then treated with anti-inflammatory medications, immobilization, or surgical interventions. The individual functional loss that patients experience in everyday life in this context often plays a subordinate role as a diagnostic parameter. This is often incomprehensible to patients, as these functional limitations are usually the reason they seek medical or therapeutic care. This lack of understanding is further exacerbated for patients because measures such as immobilization or the administration of pain-relieving medications are often used reflexively, even when this cannot be deduced from the diagnostics performed or when corresponding findings are not even obtained.

Typaldos contrasts the biomedical model with his anatomical model of fascial distortions. He postulates that deformation of the fasciae is primarily responsible for patients' functional impairment, and that inflammatory processes or degenerative changes should rather be regarded as consequences of these fascial distortions. Thus, he attributes decisive importance to the form of the fasciae and considers how changes in fascial architecture affect bodily function. As a result, he focuses his diagnostics and therapy on these distortions and, based on the Fascial Distortion Model, formulates an independent etiology of symptoms. His sometimes controversial approaches led to discussions and opposition among his medical colleagues, which Typaldos countered with his often astonishing treatment results.

The Fascial Distortion Model is characterized by the following theses:

- Pain and functional limitations are primarily the result of fascial distortions and are therefore caused by changes in the form of the fasciae.
- The prevailing concept of conventional medicine disregards this anatomical component of pain and dysfunction, leading to an underestimation in medical practice of the mechanical effect of various therapeutic methods on such complaints.
- Inflammation and degeneration can be regarded as consequences of fascial distortions, as can circulatory impairments and certain neurological disorders. Therefore, therapy aimed at the causes is linked to the correction of fascial distortions.
- Autonomously occurring regeneration processes, pharmacological therapies, surgical interventions, or conservative treatment approaches develop a mechanical effect in the tissue that can contribute to resolving fascial distortions. Chronification arises from adhesions in the area of the fasciae, which structurally impair their regenerative capacity.
- Because patients are able to perceive changes in fascial tension in their own bodies, they play a crucial role in diagnosis and therapy. They are the experts on their own symptoms. Their expertise cannot be replaced by conventional technical diagnostic procedures.

1.3.2 Areas of Application of the Fascial Distortion Model

The Fascial Distortion Model makes it possible, on the one hand, to examine existing medical concepts and treatment approaches for their effects on fascial distortions, and on the other hand, to develop mechanotherapeutic treatment strategies for a wide range of clinical issues.

Through his work as an osteopath in various hospitals and outpatient clinics, Typaldos was frequently confronted with acute injuries and chronic complaints of the musculoskeletal system. Based on these practical experiences, the clinical application of the model developed particularly in this area.

However, Typaldos assumed that the FDM could, in principle, be applied in a wide variety of medical fields, and he formulated concepts for its implementation in internal medicine, particularly in cardiology, as well as in neurology and rehabilitation. He envisioned surgical methods based on the model as well as pharmacological interventions to influence fascial distortions with medication.

Background Information
Typaldos wanted to improve the form of medicine familiar to him. The FDM seemed to be an effective means for this purpose. Therefore, from the outset, he published his findings in osteopathic journals and wrote four textbooks on the subject. He gave lectures and led training courses in the USA, Europe, and Japan. In doing so, he primarily aimed to reach his medical colleagues, so that in the future, the diagnosis and correction of fascial distortions would become standard practice in medicine.

Since Stephen Typaldos' death in 2006, the target audience for teaching the model has expanded, and more and more physiotherapists, chiropractors, and rehabilitation specialists are using the FDM to treat musculoskeletal complaints. As a result, the model is increasingly being established in conservative orthopedics and rehabilitation.

Example

The following clinical examples illustrate the possible uses of the Fascial Distortion Model:

- Conservative medical treatment of injuries such as strains, dislocations, or sprains generally consists of immobilizing or relieving the affected body part. This is intended to support the autonomously occurring healing process of potential tissue injuries. The Fascial Distortion Model shortens this process by correcting the fascial-anatomical causes of the complaints as soon as possible after their occurrence, thereby restoring mobility and load-bearing capacity. This creates the conditions for the fastest and most complete regeneration possible and also reduces the side effects of immobilization.

- Degenerative disc damage and joint wear are often associated in orthopedics with persistent, therapy-resistant complaints. Conventional medical diagnostics focus on identifying structural changes, even though these are hardly influenced by conservative methods. As a result, therapy is usually symptom-oriented. In contrast, the FDM analyzes which distortions need to be corrected in order to achieve functional improvement for the patient (despite the tissue degeneration, which in many cases is clearly visible, e.g. on X-rays). Correction of the distortions is possible at any time, making a range of chronic conditions potentially treatable.

- Circulatory disorders are often associated with the diagnosis of arteriosclerosis, which reduces vascular flow. Typaldos postulates that, in addition, constrictions of the affected vessels by surrounding fasciae are possible, thereby expanding the common explanatory model for such complaints. In his view, future therapeutic methods such as specific surgical interventions could be developed that focus on decompression of vessels by correcting these fascial distortions. ◄

References

1. Stark J, Pöttner M (2007) Stills Faszienkonzepte. Eine Studie. Jolandos, Pähl
2. Drake RL (2011) Federative international programme on anatomical terminologies FIPAT Terminologia Anatomica. International anatomical terminology, 2nd edn. Georg Thieme, Stuttgart, p 33
3. Adstrum S, Hedley G, Schleip R, Stecco C, Yucesoy C (2017) Defining the fascial system. J Bodyw Mov Ther 2:173–177
4. Adstrum S, Hedley G, Schleip R, Stecco C, Yucesoy C (2017) Defining the fascial system. J Bodyw Mov Ther 2:176
5. Huijing PA (2009) Epimuscular myofascial force transmission between antagonistic and synergistic muscles can explain movement limitation in spastic paresis. In: Huijing PA, Hollander P, Findley WT et al (eds) Fascia research II. Basic science and implications for conventional and complementary health care. Elsevier, Munich, pp 40–56
6. Huijing PA (2022) Epimuscular myofascial force transmission: an introduction. In: Schleip R, Stecco C, Driscoll M, Huijing PA (eds) Fascia. The tensional network of the human body, 2nd edn. Elsevier, London, pp 206–209
7. Levin SM, Scarr G (2022) Biotensegrity and the mechanics of fascia. In: Schleip R, Stecco C, Driscoll M, Huijing PA (eds) Fascia. The tensional network of the human body, 2nd edn. Elsevier, London, pp 232–238
8. van der Wal J (2022) Proprioception. In: Schleip R, Stecco C, Driscoll M, Huijing PA (eds) Fascia. The tensional network of the human body, 2nd edn. Elsevier, London, pp 160–168
9. Hoheisel U, Taguchi T, Mense S (2022) Nociception: the thoracolumbar and crural fascia as sensory organs. In: Schleip R, Stecco C, Driscoll M, Huijing PA (eds) Fascia. The tensional network of the human body, 2nd edn. Elsevier, London, pp 179–187
10. Schleip R, Calsius J, Jäger H (2022) Interoception: a new correlate for intricate connections between fascial receptors, emotion, and self-awareness. In: Schleip R, Stecco C, Driscoll M, Huijing PA (eds) Fascia. The tensional network of the human body, 2nd edn. Elsevier, London, pp 173–175
11. van den Berg F (2022) The physiology of fascia. An introduction. In: Schleip R, Stecco C, Driscoll M, Huijing PA (eds) Fascia. The tensional network of the human body, 2nd edn. Elsevier, London, pp 260–261
12. Hinz B (2022) Extracellular matrix. In: Schleip R, Stecco C, Driscoll M, Huijing PA (eds) Fascia. The tensional network of the human body, 2nd edn. Elsevier, London, pp 283–284
13. Stecco C (2015) Functional atlas of the human fascial system. Elsevier, Edinburgh, pp 1–4
14. Stecco C (2015) Functional atlas of the human fascial system. Elsevier, Edinburgh, pp 4–5
15. Stecco C (2015) Functional atlas of the human fascial system. Elsevier, Edinburgh, pp 5–8
16. Stecco C (2015) Functional atlas of the human fascial system. Elsevier, Edinburgh, pp 8–20
17. Willard, FH (2022) Somatic fascia. In: Schleip R, Stecco C, Driscoll M, Huijing PA (eds) Fascia. The tensional network of the human body, 2nd edn. Elsevier, London, pp 29–34
18. Stecco C (2015) Functional atlas of the human fascial system. Elsevier, Edinburgh, pp 21–24
19. Stecco C (2015) Functional atlas of the human fascial system. Elsevier, Edinburgh, pp 51
20. van der Wal J (2009) The architecture of the connective tissue in the musculoskeletal system. An often overlooked functional parameter as to proprioception in the locomotor apparatus. In: Huijing, PA., Hollander, P., Findley, WT et al (eds) Fascia research II. Basic science and implications for conventional and complementary health care. Elsevier, Munich, pp 21–35
21. Guimberteau JC (2022) Human living microanatomy. In: Schleip R, Stecco C, Driscoll M, Huijing PA (eds) Fascia. The tensional network of the human body, 2nd edn. Elsevier, London, pp 239–240
22. van der Wal J (2009) The architecture of the connective tissue in the musculoskeletal system. An often overlooked functional parameter as to proprioception in the locomotor apparatus. In: Huijing, PA., Hollander, P., Findley, WT et al (eds) Fascia research II. Basic science and implications for conventional and complementary health care. Elsevier, Munich, pp 22–24
23. van der Wal J (2009) The architecture of the connective tissue in the musculoskeletal system. An often overlooked functional parameter as to proprioception in the locomotor apparatus. In: Huijing, PA., Hollander, P., Findley, WT et al (eds) Fascia research II. Basic science and implications for conventional and complementary health care. Elsevier, Munich, pp 34–35
24. Schleip R, Jäger H, Klingler W (2022) Fascia is alive. How cells modulate the tonicity and architecture of fascial tissues. In: Schleip R, Stecco C, Driscoll M, Huijing PA (eds) Fascia. The tensional network of the human body, 2nd edn. Elsevier, London, pp 267–270
25. Levin SM (2002) The tensegrity-truss as a model for spine mechanics: biotensegrity. J Mech Med Biol 02(03–04):375–388. https://doi.org/10.1142/S0219519402000472
26. van der Wal J (2009) The architecture of the connective tissue in the musculoskeletal system. An often overlooked functional parameter as to proprioception in the locomotor apparatus. In: Huijing, PA., Hollander, P., Findley, WT et al (eds) Fascia research II. Basic science and implications for conventional and complementary health care. Elsevier, Munich, pp 294–334

27. Schleip R (2022) Fascia as an organ of communication. In: Schleip R, Stecco C, Driscoll M, Huijing PA (eds) Fascia. The tensional network of the human body, 2nd edn. Elsevier, London, pp 156–159

28. Schleip R (2003) Fascial plasticity. A new neurobiological explanation: part 1. J Bodyw Mov Ther 7(1):11

29. Hinz B (2022) Extracellular matrix. In: Schleip R, Stecco C, Driscoll M, Huijing PA (eds) Fascia. The tensional network of the human body, 2nd edn. Elsevier, London, p 276

30. Rutkokwski JM, Swartz MA (2012) A driving force for change: interstitial flow as a morphoregulator. In: Chaitow L, Findley TW, Schleip R (eds) Fascia research III. Basic science and implications for conventional and complementary health care. Kiener, Munich, pp 21–24

31. Meert GF (2022) Fluid dynamics in fascial tissues. In: Schleip R, Stecco C, Driscoll M, Huijing PA (eds) Fascia. The tensional network of the human body, 2nd edn. Elsevier, London, pp 295

32. Schleip R (2003) Fascial plasticity. A new neurobiological explanation: part 2. J Bodyw Mov Ther 7(2):105–109

33. Schleip R, Jäger H, Klingler W (2022) Fascia is alive. How cells modulate the tonicity and architecture of fascial tissues.. In: Schleip R, Stecco C, Driscoll M, Huijing PA (eds) Fascia. The tensional network of the human body, 2nd edn. Elsevier, London, pp 269–273

34. Zügel M, Maganaris CN, Wilke J, Jurkat-Rott K, Klingler W, Wearing SC, Findley T, Barbe MF, Steinacker JM, Vleeming A, Bloch W, Scheip R, Hodges PW (2018) Fascial tissue research in sports medicine: from molecules to tissue adaptation, injury and diagnostics. 6–7. Br J Sports Med 52:1497. https://doi.org/10.1136/bjsports-2018-099308

35. van den Berg F (2022) The physiology of fascia. An introduction. In: Schleip R, Stecco C, Driscoll M, Huijing PA (eds) Fascia. The tensional network of the human body, 2nd edn. Elsevier, London, pp 259–261

Six Fascial Distortions

2

The Fascial Distortion Model recognizes six types of fascial distortions:

1. Triggerbands (TB—Trigger Band)
2. Herniated triggerpoints (HTP—Herniated Triggerpoint)
3. Continuum distortions (CD—Continuum Distortion)
4. Folding distortions (FD—Folding Distortion)
5. Cylinder distortions (CyD—Cylinder Distortion)
6. Tectonic fixations (TF—Tectonic Fixation)

These six fascial distortions (as well as additional subtypes) can be recognized and differentiated by therapists based on

- their mechanism of injury
- the subjective complaints described by the patients
- the objective findings, as well as
- the body language of the patients

As part of the FDM diagnosis, information is collected which allows conclusions to be drawn about one or more of the six fascial distortions, thereby making the problem explainable on the basis of the Fascial Distortion Model.

2.1 Triggerbands (TB—Trigger Band)

A triggerband is defined as a twist in the area of the band-like fascia and is the first distortion described by Typaldos in 1991 (fig. 2.1). The discovery of this fascial distortion is considered the starting point for the development of the Fascial Distortion Model.

2.1.1 Formation of Triggerbands

Triggerbands arise in the area of band-like fascia and can, in principle, occur anywhere in the human body. In clinical practice, they frequently—but not exclusively—occur *in connection with physical trauma or overuse syndromes*. In addition, Typaldos assumes that triggerbands are also possible in the area of the heart, lungs, and other organ systems, and can thus be the cause of complaints in these areas.

The band-like fascial type is characterized by a high proportion of fascial fibers that are oriented according to the respective functional requirement. They are compactly connected by stabilizing **crosslinks** (fig. 2.2a). This form of fascia is tensile and thus predestined to transmit and adequately distribute forces within the tissue. It fulfills a connecting and protective

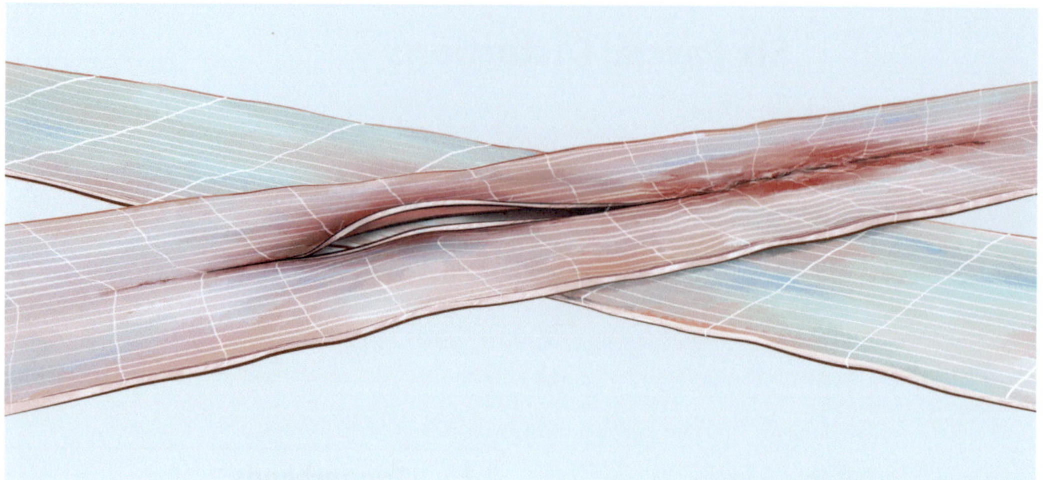

Fig. 2.1 Triggerband. (© Anker 2022)

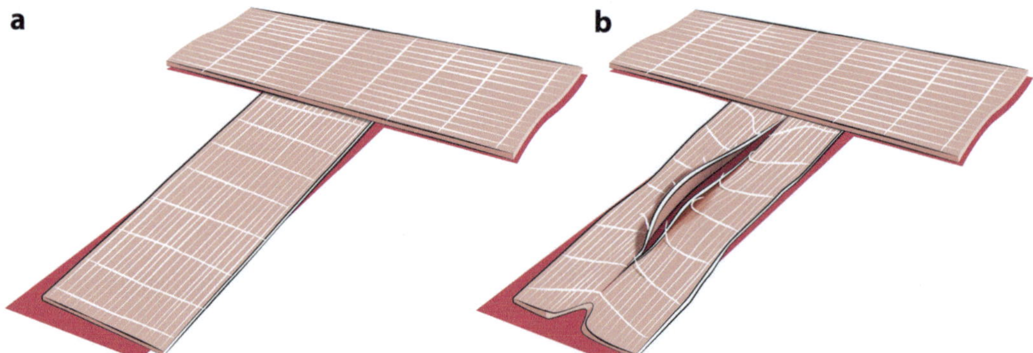

Fig. 2.2 Mechanism of injury of a triggerband. Intact band-like fascia (**a**). Twist in the fascial band (**b**). (© Anker 2022)

function, while at the same time dynamically adapting to body movements. It also serves as an important guiding structure for fluid transport and thus for the metabolism of the fascia. Possible symptoms such as weakness, restricted movement, or swelling in the event of a distortion of this fascia type are derived from these functions.

Typically, triggerbands are caused by shear forces. In a first step, this leads to damage in the area of the crosslinks, causing the compact connection of the fascial fibers to partially dissolve and the fibers to drift apart. As a result, the structure deforms three-dimensionally. It loses its functional orientation and thus—partially or completely—its function.

The decisive element of the triggerband is a more or less pronounced distortion of the band-like tissue, which Typaldos refers to as a "twist". This **twist** in the fascial band is responsible for the symptoms perceived by patients in connection with triggerbands. In order to reduce these complaints, this twisting of the banded fascia must therefore be corrected (fig. 2.2b).

The extent of the twist and the corresponding symptoms depend on various factors such as the mechanism of injury and the individual properties of the patient's tissue. In addition, anatomical conditions also influence the extent of the twisting. Typaldos refers to structures arranged at a right angle to the course of a fascial band as **crossbands**. These can be retinacula or aponeuroses, which are located in the area of joints or at prominent bony points (for example, the mastoid process). Crossbands have a stabilizing effect and slow down or stop the drifting apart and twisting of the fibers during the formation of a triggerband. For this reason, triggerbands often start or end in these areas.

Typaldos assumes that in triggerbands, the affected fibers of the band-like fascia primarily deform but do not tear. Their continuity is preserved. This concept is also derived from the observation that after successful correction of a newly formed triggerband, mobility and load-bearing capacity can be immediately and sustainably improved, even if, from a conventional medical perspective, the injured region has not yet healed or healing is no longer expected.

However, if the deformation persists, the potential for force transmission and fluid transport subsequently suffers. As a result, the still functionally intact portions of the banded fascia are additionally stressed and less well supplied with nutrients. This increases the risk of progressive deformation, which, in individual cases, can result in tears transverse to the course of the longitudinal fibers (as we associate with a (partial) rupture from an orthopedic perspective).

ZIPLOC ® Analogy
Typaldos often used everyday objects to illustrate the mechanisms of formation of fascial distortions or their corrections. A resealable plastic bag equipped with two plastic lips serves as a visual aid for the triggerband:

By pulling the plastic lips apart at a right angle, the bag opens, causing the ends of the closure to be drawn together (fig. 2.3a and b). The opening can be closed again by pressing the plastic lips together precisely. The closure thus regains its original shape and length.

The same occurs with the triggerband. Due to shear forces, the fibers of the band-like fascia separate from each other and deform in the process, without being damaged. However, the length of the fascial band decreases. By realigning the fibers, e.g. using the triggerband technique (see sect. 5.1), the distortion of the fascia is corrected. As a result, the fibers regain their length and the tissue is immediately stabilized.

Possible Progressions of a Triggerband after its Formation

The prerequisite for the formation of triggerbands is the partial rupture of stabilizing crosslinks, which allows the twisting of the band-like fibers. This causes an injury to the band-like tissue and initiates autonomous wound healing. In addition to the well-known

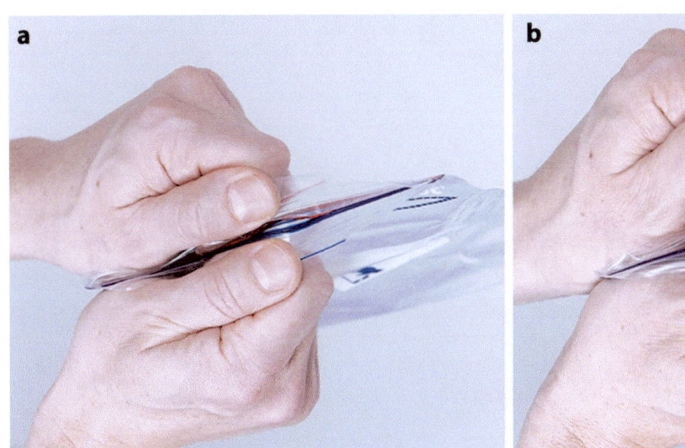
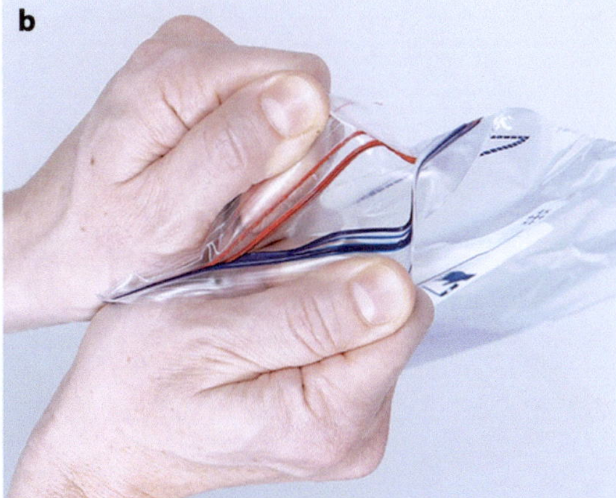

Fig. 2.3 **a** and **b** ZIPLOC ® analogy. (© Anker 2022)

physiological processes, Typaldos considers the healing of a wound as a mechanism aimed at reducing the twist in the fascial band. The manifestation of a triggerband is therefore not a completed sequence, as this healing process leads to various possible further developments of a triggerband:

- It is possible that the deformation of the fascial band is reduced by the rejoining of the stabilizing crosslinks. As a result, the symptoms of the fascial distortion, such as restricted movement or reduced load-bearing capacity, gradually disappear. Typaldos describes this process as **healing of the triggerband**. When we think of minor injuries we sustain in everyday life or during sports, which often disappear on their own, this seems plausible.

- However, this process can also be incomplete, and the twist in the fascial band remains as a whole or in part, even though wound healing can largely restore the integrity of the stabilizing crosslinks. Typaldos describes this as an **acute triggerband,** which, in contrast to a chronic triggerband, does not develop excessive adhesions in the tissue. However, the twist persists, and subsequently its acute symptoms only partially resolve. In that case, therapeutic intervention to correct the underlying twist in the fascial band is necessary (fig. 2.4a).

- If, during the healing process, excessive adhesions form or the restoration of the ruptured crosslinks does not correspond to the original fascial architecture, the twist in the fascial band can become structurally fixed. In this context, we refer to a **chronic triggerband.**

A hallmark of chronification is the permanent loss of function of the affected fascia due to the formation of adhesions. A progressive process begins, which generates shear forces on the surroundings of the triggerband and involves previously undeformed tissue in the distortion. This leads to an increasing, locally spreading symptomatology characterized by persistent pain and movement restrictions. As a result, the metabolism of the affected structures also suffers, and additional distortions may occur, even after a period of time (fig. 2.4b).

Chronification from Typaldos' Perspective
By definition, chronification requires the presence of triggerbands with adhesions. The triggerband is the only one of the six fascial distortions that can be considered a tissue wound and has the potential to develop adhesions. From Typaldos' perspective, chronification is therefore a structural process that is reversible by resolving the adhesions. In this way, he

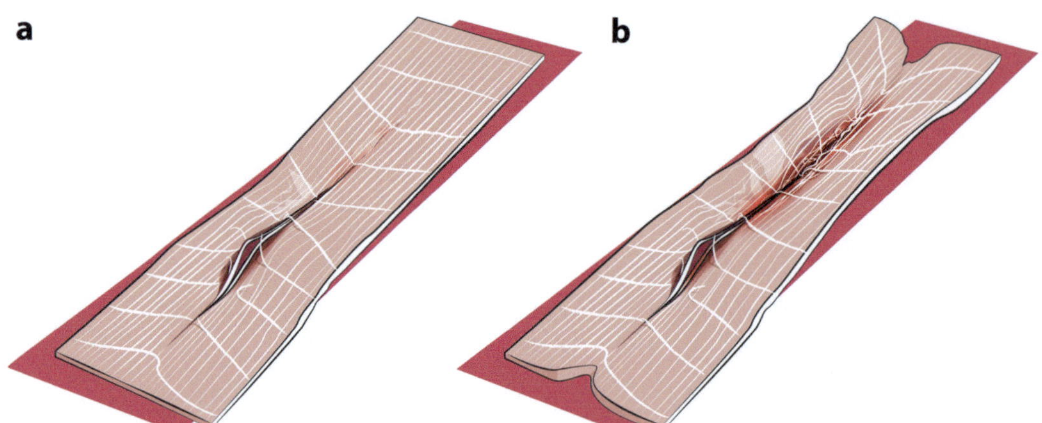

Fig. 2.4 Possible progressions of a triggerband. Acute triggerband (**a**). Chronification of a triggerband (**b**). (© Anker 2022)

expands the definition of conventional medicine, which focuses on the persistence of therapy-resistant symptoms.

Whether and when triggerbands become chronic varies individually. The process can begin more or less directly after an injury, develop very slowly over weeks and months, or not occur at all. Therefore, the FDM does not define a specific point in time from which a problem should be considered chronic.

However, immobilization of the affected tissue could be a risk factor. Clinical observation shows that active movement reduces the formation of adhesions or can be used to resolve adhesions. As a result, we assume that shorter immobilization periods or complete avoidance of immobilization are associated with a reduced risk of chronification.

To correct the twist as the cause of triggerband symptomatology independently of wound healing, Typaldos used the so-called *triggerband technique*. This technique anticipates the mechanical effect of wound healing by manually resolving the twist in the fascial band. This offers the possibility of immediate improvement in mobility and load-bearing capacity, regardless of the time elapsed since the formation of the triggerband. Furthermore, the risk of chronification due to pain-induced immobilization of the tissue is reduced.

2.1.2 Subjective Complaints with Triggerbands

Triggerbands cause *pulling, burning pain* of varying intensity. These symptoms can occur with or without loading and generally become more pronounced the more the triggerband is under tension. *Nocturnal symptoms* can occur as well as *start-up pain* at the beginning of movement after a period of rest. The symptoms may appear during certain movements or only in specific loading situations, as triggerbands *reduce the load-bearing capacity of the tissue*. The intensity of the pain can also change over time, as the deformation can autonomously progress as described.

The twist in the fascial band leads to a *shortening of the affected tissue*. This explains the perception of pulling pain, but above all the movement restriction in several planes of motion that is typical for triggerbands. This is usually associated with pain and is often dependent on the position and tension of the affected region.

Loss of strength and weakness can also be associated with triggerbands. The deformation of the fascial fibers reduces their capacity to transmit force. Furthermore, the twist in the fascial band may be localized in the area of a muscle, thereby impairing its full contractile ability. In both cases, symptoms can range from a subjective feeling of weakness to an objectively measurable loss of strength. Additionally, the deformation can also affect inter- and intramuscular coordination. Possible consequences range from balance difficulties in single-leg stance to reduced movement speed to cogwheel-like movement execution.

Triggerbands can lead to *local swelling*. Basically, the band-like fascia functions as a fluid transport system, which transports nutrients into the fascia and metabolic products out of the fascia via the interstitial fluid. The twist impedes or blocks fluid transport along the fibers. Local, sometimes persistent tissue swelling can result. If the deformation persists for a longer period, the metabolism of the affected fascia suffers. As a result, further weakening of the tissue may occur, with an increased risk of new fascial distortions (as described with the roadblock effect in the first chapter).

2.1.3 Objective Findings in Triggerbands

Triggerbands are *typically tender to manual pressure* along their entire course. The patient recognizes the triggerband when the therapist applies pressure to the distortion and thereby elicits the familiar pain. For this reason, the patient can provide feedback on the exact location of the distortion.

Typaldos describes that triggerbands are *palpable as tissue changes for the therapist*. He mentions various qualities such as linear twists, nodules of different sizes, or grainy roughness similar to a grain of salt (fig. 2.5a to e). This can be helpful in the treatment of the triggerband, as the corrective force applied can be adapted to the type of deformation. However, therapists should not be tempted to diagnose triggerbands solely by palpating the tissue. Like all other fascial distortions, triggerbands are characterized by their specific pattern of symptoms, which allows for diagnosis. The singular finding of tissue changes is of little significance without this clinical context.

The mobility of patients with triggerbands can be visibly altered both quantitatively and qualitatively. As previously mentioned, *movement restrictions* can occur to varying degrees and often in several planes of movement. Measuring mobility is well suited for assessing the effect of treatment, as both the patient and the therapist can easily perceive changes.

Obviously, *changes in movement quality* can also be triggered by triggerbands. Symptoms such as reduced movement speed, cautious movement behavior, and jerky force development are notable here. Finally, a local, visible tissue swelling associated with triggerbands can also be a measurable criterion. After correction of the distortions and the resulting improved fluid transport, the swelling often reduces immediately.

2.1.4 Body Language with Triggerbands

With the discovery of the connection between fascial distortions and a body language typical for each of the six distortions, Typaldos elevated

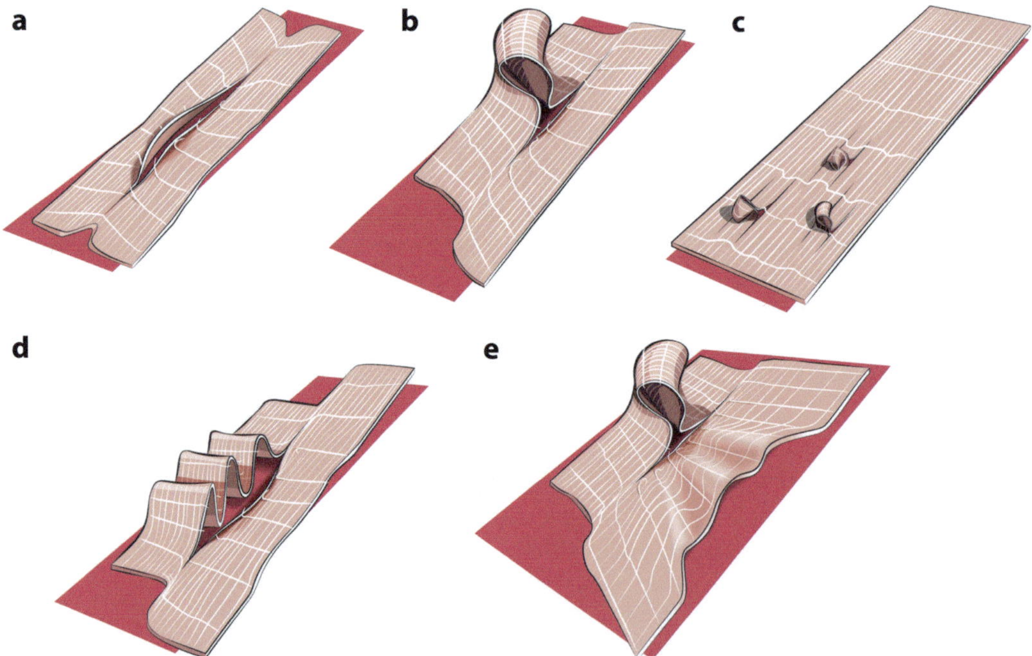

Fig. 2.5 Subtypes of triggerbands. Different forms of triggerbands can be distinguished based on palpation, symptomatology, and response to specific treatment approaches: the twist (**a**), the nodule or pea (distinguishable by size and consistency, **b**), the grain of salt (**c**), and the crumple (**d**). Triggerbands can also cause waves in the adjacent tissue (**e**). (© Anker 2022)

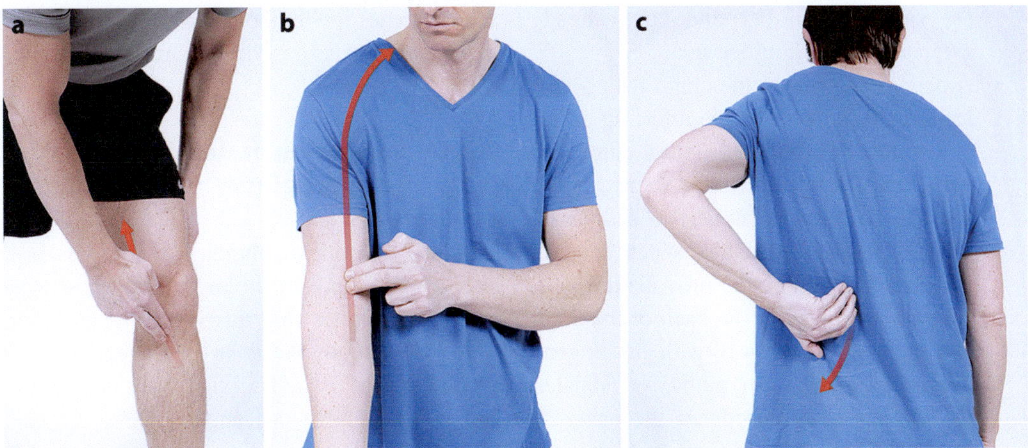

Fig. 2.6   a to **b** Typical body language in triggerbands. Usually, patients indicate the course of the trigger band with several fingertips using a dynamic gesture. It is less typical when the triggerband gesture is indicated with only one finger. (© Anker 2022)

the observation of patients to a decisive criterion in diagnosis. Typaldos describes the typical gesture with which patients indicate a triggerband as a *dynamic stroking with the fingers (usually with the fingertips) along a pathway* (fig. 2.6a to c).

The gesture can provide further information about the location, the extent of the twist, and the effective direction of treatment:

- The more pressure is applied with the fingers during the body language to indicate the pathway, the more likely the triggerband is located in deeper tissue layers.
- The longer the indicated pathway, the greater the extent of the twist.
- If the dynamic stroking occurs in a specific direction, we see more success in practice when we perform the treatment in accordance with this direction.
- If the correction is performed in the posture and position in which the patient reports the pain, the effectiveness also increases, as in this provocation position the triggerband appears to be pre-tensioned and can therefore be treated more specifically.

2.1.5   Summary and Examples

Cardinal symptoms of triggerbands are pulling, burning pain and movement restrictions.

In addition, the typical body language confirms the diagnosis and provides further information on the exact location of the triggerband and clues for optimal adaptation of the treatment. However, the striking gesture alone should not be used as the sole diagnostic criterion for this fascial distortion. A triggerband diagnosis is substantiated when the mechanism of injury, subjective complaints, and objective testing are also consistent. This is of particular importance in triggerbands, as their treatment is usually painful for patients and can cause side effects.

Clinical Patterns from Practice

- A patient sprains his ankle while playing sports. Twisting the foot causes pain and swelling in the area of the lateral ankle, which extends to the area of the outer metatarsal bones. The patient is able to bear weight on the foot but complains of pulling pain along a line he indicates in the injured area.
- A female patient describes persistent burning neck pain for three weeks, which increasingly restricts neck rotation. She also reports particularly severe pain in the morning after getting up, which improves after a few minutes of movement but does not disappear completely. She also has the impression that the symptoms

are spreading further and have already extended to the shoulder area.

- A patient presents to the clinic with severe leg pain. According to the referring orthopedist, this is associated with a diagnosed herniated disc in the back. A corresponding result from a magnetic resonance imaging scan is available. When bending forward, the patient can provoke the typical pain localized on the back of the thigh and indicate it precisely with his fingers. Pressure on the pain pathway indicated in this way also reproduces the pain. By interpreting these symptoms as those of a triggerband and following local treatment, the symptoms decrease significantly. ◄

2.2 Herniated Triggerpoints (HTP—Herniated Triggerpoint)

The second distortion described by Typaldos is the so-called "herniated triggerpoint," or HTP for short.

The herniated triggerpoint is defined as a tissue protrusion through an adjacent fascial layer (fig. 2.7). The concept of the herniated triggerpoint is based on the mechanism of injury of a hernia, as known from conventional medicine, and combines it with the symptom characteristics of triggerpoints as described in manual therapy.

2.2.1 Formation of Herniated Triggerpoints

Typaldos describes common locations of herniated triggerpoints in the area of the torso and pelvis and argues that this is due to the dominance of smooth fascia in these regions. This type of fascial tissue is designed for adaptability and gliding ability, which, compared to band-like fascia, contains fewer fibers and therefore offers less stability. In contrast, herniated triggerpoints appear to be less likely outside the torso, as the tissue configuration in these area is much more strongly dominated by band-like fascia. As a result, the risk of tissue protrusion is lower but cannot be completely ruled out in individual cases with clear diagnostic evidence.

A herniated triggerpoint arises (like a hernia from a conventional medical perspective) not from tissue wounding, but as the result of *entrapment of tissue* within a physiological existing anatomical corridor. For this reason, this distortion cannot be considered a wound that can heal on its own, but rather remains a permanent deformation in the tissue until it is corrected.

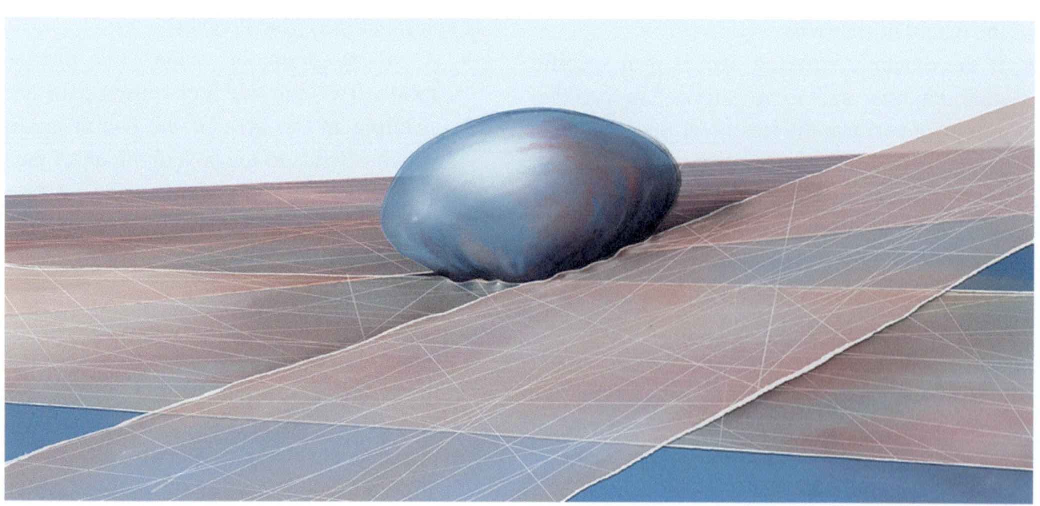

Fig. 2.7 Herniated triggerpoint. (© Anker 2022)

Background Information

Although Typaldos does not explain the mechanism of formation in detail, both pressure differences or abrupt increases in pressure in the body and also the structure and quality of the fascial tissue appear to be the main factors in their formation. This can be inferred from the clinical examples he describes in connection with a herniated triggerpoint. Acceleration trauma, falls, or severe coughing are cited in his books as possible causes. This is consistent with clinical observations that herniated triggerpoints can develop from heavy lifting or straining in daily life as well as during childbirth. Obesity or significant fluctuations in body weight also appear to promote the development of herniated triggerpoints.

In detail, the mechanism of formation of a herniated triggerpoint can be described as follows:

The body is divided into compartments with different pressure conditions. However, these compartments are not completely separated from each other, but must allow the passage of various structures such as vessels, nerves, or entire organs. Such connections exist in the body between many different tissue spaces. A clear example is the passage of the esophagus, accompanied by vessels and nerves, through a physiological gap in the diaphragm, while at the same time maintaining a lower pressure in the thoracic cavity compared to the upper abdomen.

These contradictory functional requirements are managed by a kind of sluice system at the transition points from one compartment to another. Here, tissue layers are arranged in such a way that a kind of adaptive closure is formed, which both separates and connects (fig. 2.8a). However, if there is an increase in pressure combined with a widening of this passage (e.g. due to severe coughing during an expansive movement), there is a risk of tissue displacement along the pressure gradient (fig. 2.8b and c). As a result, this protrusion can become entrapped when the sluice closes again, which explains the typical symptoms of a herniated triggerpoint. This entrapment is considered permanent, as it cannot resolve on its own due to the different pressures (fig. 2.8d).

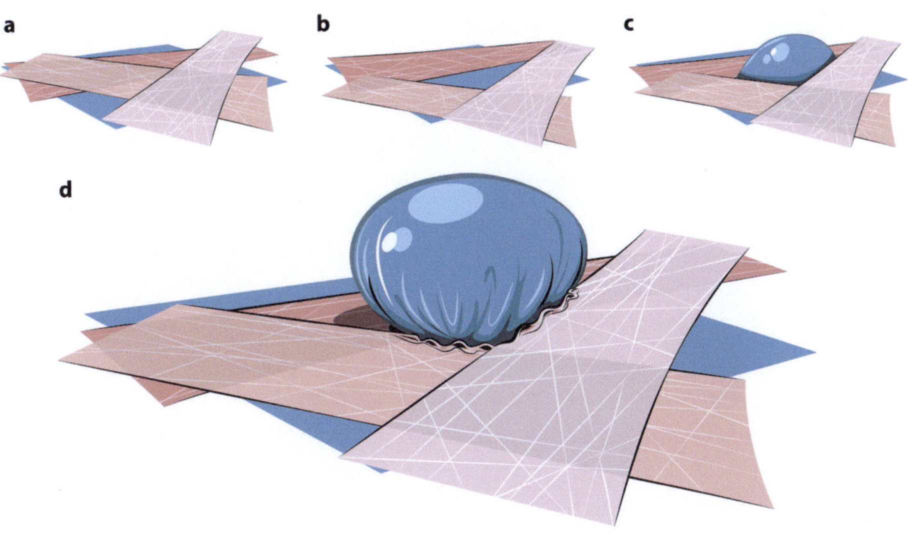

Fig. 2.8 Mechanism of formation of a herniated triggerpoint. Adaptive closure in the area of the smooth fascia (**a**). Opening of the closure along the pressure gradient (**b**). Formation (**c**) and entrapment of the protrusion (**d**). (© Anker 2022)

2.2.1.1 Types of Herniated Triggerpoints

Typaldos differentiates between various types of herniated triggerpoints, which differ in their development and symptomatology and respond to different treatment methods:

- The *classic* **herniated triggerpoint** is a tissue protrusion **through a smooth fascial plane** (non-banded HTP). The typical symptom of this deformation is a painful restriction of movement, which can be corrected by repositioning the protrusion.
- Distinct from this is the special form of the **herniated triggerpoint in the area of banded fascia** (banded HTP). In this distortion, there is a protrusion through banded tissue, which is additionally twisted by a triggerband. This results in a stronger strangulation of the entrapment and an increased risk of chronicity of the involved triggerband, which can lead to particularly persistent symptoms (fig. 2.9a).
- **Pseudo-herniated triggerpoints** are overlapping triggerbands that appear as nodular changes in the tissue and can therefore be mistaken for herniated triggerpoints on palpation. This subtype is not a protrusion and does not respond to the herniated triggerpoint technique (see sect. 5.2). This form is typical in patients with fibromyalgia (fig. 2.9b).

2.2.2 Subjective Complaints with Herniated Triggerpoints

The herniated triggerpoint can cause a *restriction of movement*, which primarily affects the joints in the immediate vicinity of the distortion. Smooth fascia ensure the frictionless gliding and adaptability of adjacent tissues, which should ideally be able to move against each other with minimal resistance. The entrapment of the protrusion leads to a restriction of movement, which patients often describe as a (more or less painful) blockage in the area of the soft tissues.

The following patterns are typical:

- The supraclavicular herniated triggerpoint (SCHTP) in the shoulder girdle area causes a restriction of neck rotation and abduction or internal rotation of the shoulder on the affected side.
- The herniated triggerpoint in the gluteal region (bullseye HTP) can restrict forward flexion of the trunk, while a protrusion in the lower back area tends to impair trunk extension.
- There is often an association between restricted hip flexion and external rotation and a herniated triggerpoint in the groin area.

If the herniated triggerpoint causes *pain*, it is usually localized in the area of the protrusion

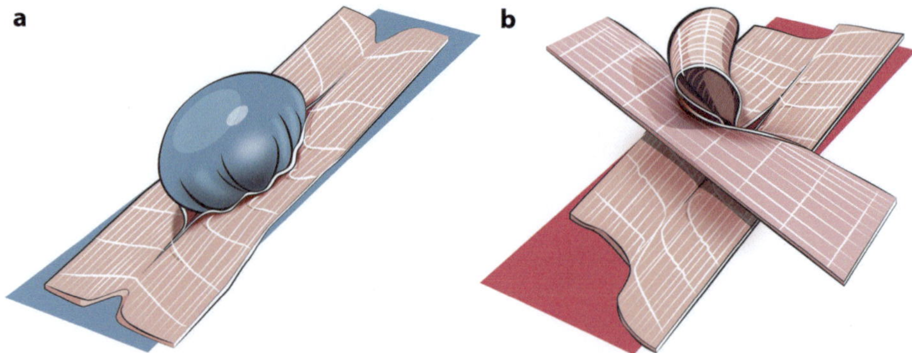

Fig. 2.9 Subtypes of herniated triggerpoints. Herniated triggerpoint in the area of banded fascia (**a**). Pseudo-herniated triggerpoint (**b**). (© Anker 2022)

and in its immediate vicinity. However, similar to triggerpoints, it can also have a certain referred effect. For example, the SCHTP can cause diffuse symptoms in the arm and upper back. The same applies to herniated triggerpoints in the pelvic or lower back area, which can lead to pain in the legs.

Muscle tension and tension-related pain patterns such as headaches or back pain can also be associated with herniated triggerpoints. The blocked mobility of the tissues leads to regional symptoms, with the protrusion often located at the center of the complaints.

The herniated triggerpoint is considered a *permanent distortion,* which permanently deforms the fascial architecture. However, this does not necessarily mean that the corresponding symptoms, especially pain and muscle tension, are permanently present. Rather, the permanence creates tissue vulnerability, and symptoms can easily flare up again when additional factors such as stress or mechanical strain occur.

Sometimes it is helpful in diagnostics to know which symptoms are not typically associated with a specific fascial distortion. In the case of the herniated triggerpoint, night pain, weakness, and swelling are uncharacteristic.

2.2.3 Objective Findings in Herniated Triggerpoints

The herniated triggerpoint can be identified by its functional effects. Imaging diagnostics, which are used to detect hernias in conventional medicine, do not play a decisive role here.

As mentioned, a herniated triggerpoint can significantly restrict active mobility. Therefore, active movement tests are an important parameter to confirm a corresponding suspicion. Especially in the shoulder girdle area, Typaldos describes this association and interprets a restricted active abduction of the arm as a direct indication of the existence of a supraclavicular herniated triggerpoint (SCHTP).

Herniated triggerpoints are *tender to pressure* and thus are clearly *perceptible and localizable* for patients *during palpation.* Typaldos also assigns typical palpatory findings to the herniated triggerpoint and compares its size and consistency to a small, soft marble or a firm-elastic, lens-shaped induration. In practice, palpation and the pain provoked by it can confirm and precisely localize the protrusion.

However, it should be noted here that the singular palpation of a focal tissue change without associated symptoms of a herniated triggerpoint has little diagnostic relevance. Conversely, if corresponding symptoms are present and patients can clearly localize the distortion even though the therapist cannot perceive it by palpation, treatment can still be appropriate.

2.2.4 Body Language with Herniated Triggerpoints

Typaldos describes the typical body language of a herniated triggerpoint as *pressing with several fingers, the knuckles, or the thumb into a soft tissue area* (fig. 2.10a to c). In contrast to the body language of the triggerband, where patients trace a linear path into the tissue, the herniated triggerpoint is characterized by local deep pressing without movement along the skin.

2.2.5 Summary and Examples

Herniated triggerpoints are associated with painful movement restrictions and are often the key to their mobilization. They are permanent distortions. This means they can permanently impair the fascial architecture, therefore patients often report recurrent symptoms.

- A female patient has been suffering from unilateral tension headaches for months. Neck mobility is restricted in rotation toward the painful side, and the patient presses several fingers into the shoulder girdle when localizing her muscle tension.

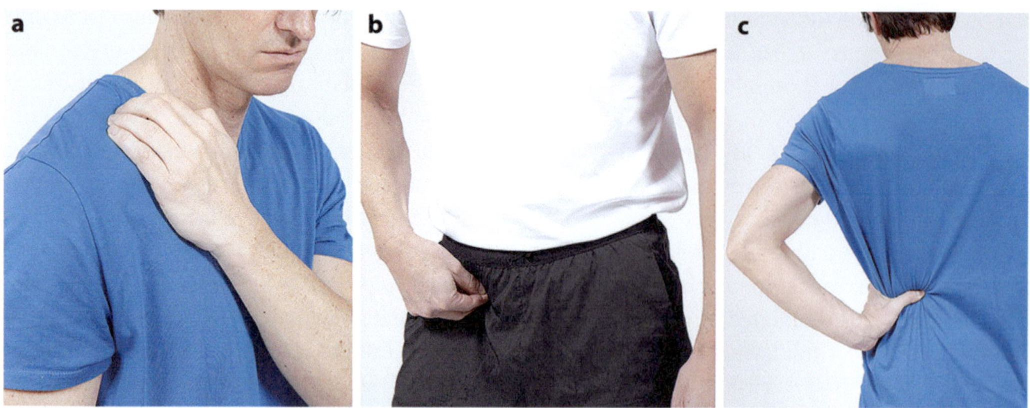

Fig. 2.10 Typical body language with herniated triggerpoints. Gestures for a herniated triggerpoint at the shoulder, the so-called SCHTP (**a**), at the groin (**b**), and at the back (**c**). (© Anker 2022)

- A patient develops a movement restriction in the shoulder after a fall. Abduction of the arm is particularly impaired and only possible up to about 30°. When he attempts the movement, he describes a sensation of movement blockage and pain in the shoulder area.
- A female patient presents to the emergency department with acute back pain. She reports having felt severe pain after lifting a heavy box. Since then, she has been unable to fully straighten up. While explaining the situation to the doctor, she supports her back with one hand and presses her fingers into the soft tissues at specific points. ◄

2.3 Continuum Distortions (CD—Continuum Distortion)

Continuum distortions are fundamentally possible between all structures of the tissue continuum. As a rule, we find them in the transition zone between bone and various soft tissues such as tendons, ligaments, or muscles (fig. 2.11).

The basis for understanding continuum distortion is the **continuum theory** explained in the first chapter. This theory states that the different tissues of the body can be considered as part of a continuum. Adjacent tissue types transition smoothly into one another and can structurally adapt within the area of transition zones (fig. 2.12a). Unidirectional loading (by compression or tension) provokes a "bony configuration" of the entire transition zone by increasing the concentration of stabilizing minerals (such as calcium phosphate) in this area (fig. 2.12b). This improves the capacity for force transmission. In contrast, when multidirectional forces occur, the transition zone shifts into its "ligamentous configuration" by transporting the same minerals out of the zone. This allows it to respond more elastically and protects the adjacent structures from injury (fig. 2.12c).

A prerequisite for these configuration changes is adequate fluid transport along the banded fascia. This continuous flow of fluid ensures the transport of minerals into and out of the transition zone. This enables a smooth and rapid switch from a neutral to a bony or ligamentous configuration and back again at any time. Loss of this physiological adaptive capacity is a sign of a continuum distortion.

2.3.1 Formation of Continuum Distortions

A continuum distortion arises when this transition zone is simultaneously subjected to uni- and multidirectional forces, thereby demanding both configurations at the same time. The cause is often a *physical trauma or overload* in the area of the band-like fascia.

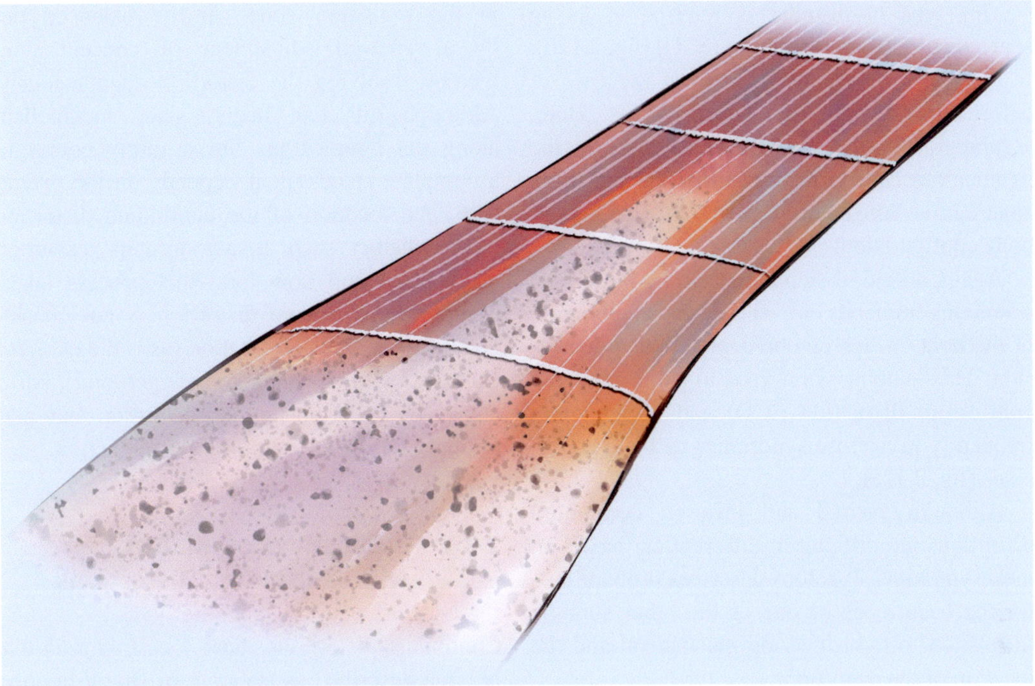

Fig. 2.11 Continuum Distortion. (© Anker 2022)

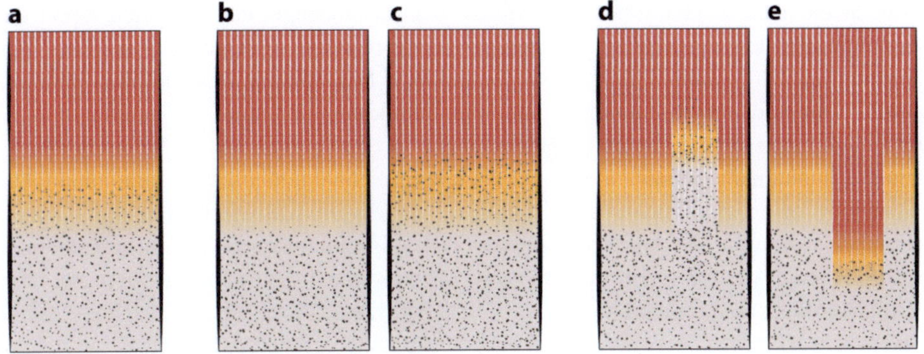

Fig. 2.12 Formation of continuum distortions. Neutral transition zone (**a**). Transition zone in ligamentous (**b**) or bony configuration (**c**). Everted continuum distortion (eCD) (**d**). Inverted continuum distortion (iCD) (**e**). (© Anker 2022)

If, in the context of the mechanism of injury, unidirectional forces predominate (e.g. due to strong traction in a joint or bone trauma) and these forces exceed the adaptive capacity of the affected transition zone, an "overshift" occurs. In this process, a subregion of the transition zone is deformed, and becomes stuck in the bony configuration, and thereby loses the ability to fully return to the neutral or ligamentous configuration.

This "hardening" can be illustrated as a step-like deformation, as if a bony protrusion were projecting into the transition zone. This results in tension both in the affected soft tissues and on the bone side, which the nervous system typically interprets as localized pain.

This type of disorder is referred to as an **everted continuum distortion** (eCD) (fig. 2.12d).

A reverse mechanism occurs in the case of deformation by multidirectional forces. Here, a subregion of the zone becomes stuck in the ligamentous configuration, so that the transition zone can no longer fully switch to a neutral or bony configuration.

Again, a kind of step is formed, in which the stabilizing minerals are absent in a subregion of the bone, which can be depicted as a depression. This subtype is referred to as an **inverted continuum distortion** (iCD) and occurs more frequently in overuse syndromes or bone contusions (fig. 2.12e).

Although everted and inverted continuum distortions are difficult to differentiate based on their symptoms, Typaldos describes probabilities for the occurrence of one or the other subtype in relation to the triggering mechanism and the location of the distortion:

- Physical traumas (with the exception of bone contusions), such as ligament sprains or injuries at the muscle-tendon-bone junction, more frequently lead to everted continuum distortions.
- Repeated overload without trauma, e.g. in the case of tennis elbow, tends to produce inverted continuum distortions.
- A clustering of inverted continuum distortions is also seen in the back and pelvis, whereas in the ankle and wrist, everted continuum distortions predominate.

Like triggerbands, continuum distortions impair fluid transport along the fascia. As a result, the metabolic potential in the affected area is reduced, leading to a medium-term decrease in tissue resilience. On the other hand, continuum distortions themselves can be the result of this roadblock phenomenon, when calcium phosphate becomes trapped in atypical areas of the tissue continuum and forms calcifications (e.g. in the context of soft tissue calcification or calcifying tendinitis).

The impairment of fluid transport also reduces the possibility that the step formation in the transition zone can be balanced out by a renewed adjustment of concentration, thereby resolving the distortion spontaneously. Although this can occur, since metabolism along the ligamentous fascia rarely comes to a complete standstill, it depends on the extent, type, and location of the continuum distortion as to whether such an autonomous resolution takes place and how long this process takes. Therefore, continuum distortion is not considered a permanent deformation (as is the case, for example, with the herniated triggerpoint), but it cannot be ruled out that the distortion may persistently impair the corresponding function.

2.3.2 Subjective Complaints with Continuum Distortions

Continuum distortions cause *localized pain* that is often described as stabbing or sharp/shooting and can be precisely localized by patients.

These complaints are often associated with *specific movement restrictions* and present as a painful blockage. Patients often report an exact body position in which the restriction occurs. When this position is abandoned, the pain also disappears.

Background Information
This demonstrates the difference from a movement restriction caused by a triggerband: In the case of a triggerband, the pain increases the more tension is applied to the area of fascial twisting, resulting in a painful movement trajectory. In contrast, with continuum distortions, we see a specific position in which the pain abruptly stops the movement. In addition, these symptoms occur less frequently during rest or at night than is the case with triggerbands.

Like triggerbands, continuum distortions can also lead to *local swelling* due to inhibition of fluid transport along the banded fascia.

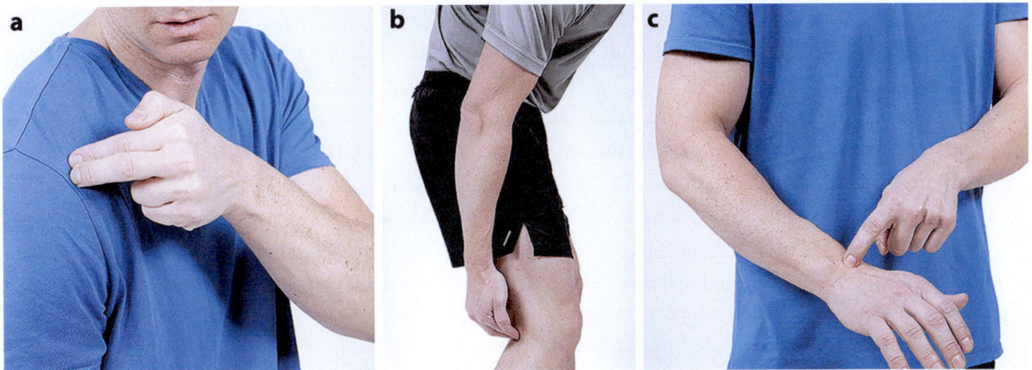

Fig. 2.13 Typical body language in continuum distortions. Pointing gesture at the shoulder (**a**), in the area of the popliteal fossa (**b**), and at the wrist, the so-called Posterior Wrist Continuum Distortion PWCD (**c**). (© Anker 2022)

Weakness and coordination disorders are also typical, although in continuum distortions, these symptoms are primarily pain-related.

2.3.3 Objective Findings in Continuum Distortions

The most striking objective sign of a continuum distortion is its *tenderness to manual pressure.* With millimeter precision, the patient can be guided to localize the continuum distortion and provoke pain. The pain does not radiate or shift under the provoking pressure. (This only occurs if palpation compresses structures such as nerves or vessels in the vicinity of the distortion, or if a triggerband is also present.)

If a continuum distortion leads to *swelling,* it is usually localized in the area of the distortion. Weakness due to a continuum distortion is also usually not generalized, but highly dependent on a specific position in which the continuum distortion is bothersome.

Typaldos describes that continuum distortions can also be *perceived by the therapist through targeted palpation.* The everted continuum distortion can be felt as a raised area on the bone, at most one to two millimeters in size, while the inverted continuum distortion is described as a tiny, difficult-to-palpate depression. Frequently, several continuum distortions may be present in a small area.

2.3.4 Body Language with Continuum Distortions

The body language for both the everted and the inverted continuum distortion is clearly defined as "pointing with the fingertip to a spot" (fig. 2.13a–c). Although Typaldos notes in his books that the index or middle finger is usually used for this, in practice, depending on the accessibility of the relevant body region, certain variations are seen: several fingers may be used simultaneously to indicate the spot, and sometimes patients dynamically search in the soft tissues until they can precisely locate the continuum distortion and then pause.

2.3.5 Summary and Examples

Continuum distortions cause localized pain and precisely localizable movement restrictions. They frequently occur in connection with injuries and overuse in the musculoskeletal system and play a key role in mobilizing the ankle, knee, and wrist in trauma-related movement restrictions.

Clinical Patterns from Practice

- A patient sprains her wrist during gymnastics. The area is swollen and she can only actively extend it to a limited degree. If she tries to move it anyway, she describes a single, clearly localized pain point at the joint.

- A patient comes for treatment after knee surgery. He can walk and extend the knee, but flexion beyond 90° causes him severe pain in the popliteal fossa, which he indicates precisely with his fingertip.
- A patient fell from a ladder three weeks ago and bruised her shoulder. Although the symptoms have significantly improved, a stabbing pain in the anterior shoulder area persists stubbornly. The movement is particularly painful when she tries to reach for the seatbelt in the car. Apart from that, mobility is neither restricted nor painful. ◄

2.4 Folding Distortions (FD— Folding Distortion)

Typaldos defines folding distortions as *three-dimensional deformations of folding fascia* and distinguishes between an *unfolding distortion* (uFD - un Folding Distortion) and a *refolding distortion* (rFD - re Folding Distortion; fig. 2.14). This differentiation is based on different mechanisms of injury, different symptoms, and different treatment concepts for the two subtypes.

Folding fascia is located in the area of joints, between parallel bones (for example, in the forearm), and between different muscle groups in the arms and legs. Accordingly, unfolding and refolding distortions can occur in the area of joints, the *interosseous membrane* (IOM— Inter Osseous Membrane), and the *muscle septa* (IMS—Inter Muscular Septum).

2.4.1 Formation of Folding Distortions

Folding fascia acts as a shock absorber in jointed regions and ensures stability while maintaining good mobility. To fulfill this function, the tissue must be able to repetitively compress under load and return to its original state when unloaded, similar to a coil spring. However, if the folding fascia is deformed, this shock-absorbing function is impaired and the typical symptoms of a folding distortion arise.

In principle, folding distortions are caused by externally applied forces. These are often associated with *physical trauma*. Less commonly, folding distortions (especially in the area of

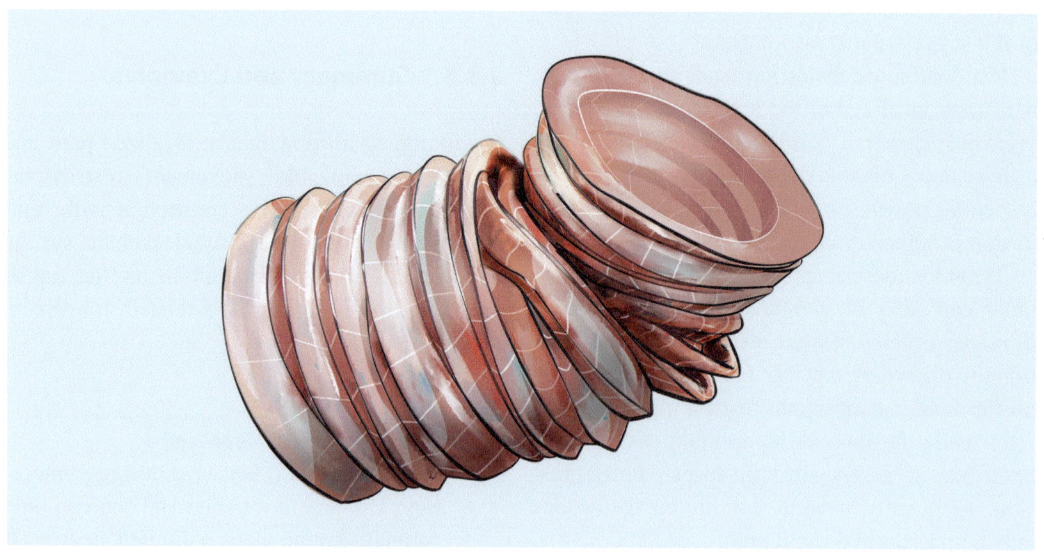

Fig. 2.14 Folding distortion. (© Anker 2022)

muscle septa) result from repetitive movements in the sense of overuse.

The cause of the development of an **unfolding distortion** (uFD) is a traction-torsion, a combination of traction and additional rotational and shearing forces. In this process, the folds of the fascia are pulled apart and simultaneously twisted. As a result, they lose the ability to return completely to their resting position and to be compressed without resistance (fig. 2.15a to c).

In contrast, the formation of a **refolding distortion** (rFD) is caused by a compressive force that occurs in combination with a shearing and rotational movement. As a result, the folds of the fascia are compressed and, due to an additional dislocation, are blocked in this compressed position. Consequently, the folding fascia can no longer fully relax (fig. 2.16a to c).

Background Information

To understand these mechanisms of formation, it is important to know that pure traction or compression, without the occurrence of additional shearing and/or rotational movements, does not cause folding distortions. Hanging from the arm or jumping on one leg are movements that, with good shock-absorbing function, are unproblematic and do not endanger the shape of the folding fascia. However, if it is already deformed, such activities can trigger symptoms.

By analyzing the respective mechanism of injury, it is possible to assess how the folding fascia is likely deformed. An unfolding distortion is more likely to occur in connection with a dislocation (for example in a shoulder dislocation). A refolding distortion, on the other hand, is more likely to be caused by a sprain (such as a fall onto the wrist). In cases where the mechanism of injury cannot be precisely determined, the therapist must analyze the patient's symptoms to assess which type of folding distortion is likely present.

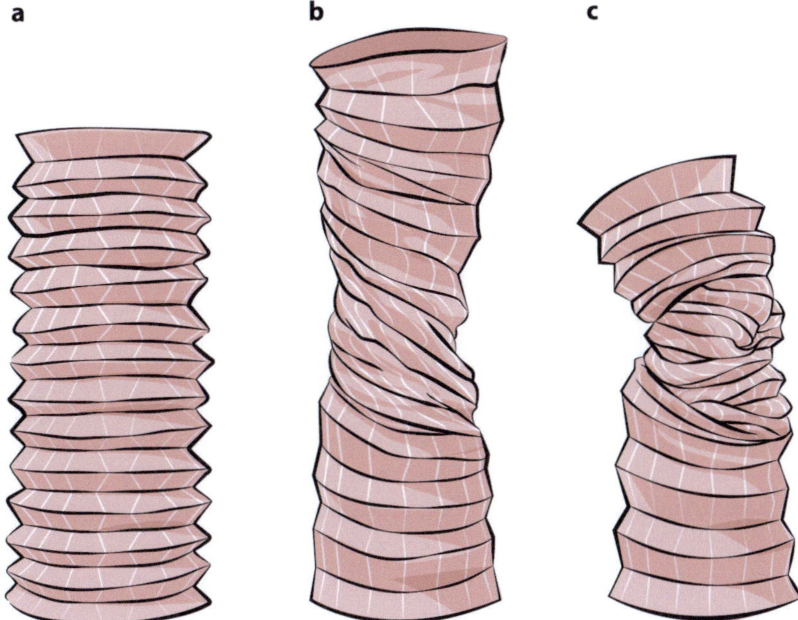

Fig. 2.15 Mechanism of injury of an unfolding distortion. Intact folding fascia (**a**). Causative traction-torsion (**b**). Unfolding distortion (**c**). (© Anker 2022)

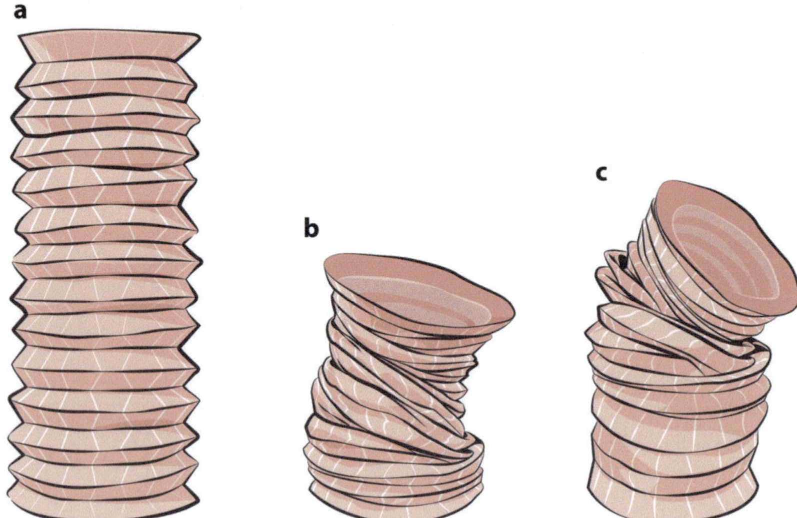

Fig. 2.16 Mechanism of injury of a refolding distortion. Intact folding fascia (**a**). Causative compression and dislocation (**b**). Refolding distortion (**c**). (© Anker 2022)

Folding distortions (like herniated trigger-points and continuum distortions) are not tissue wounds and therefore cannot heal.

Folding distortions are deformations that remain permanently in the tissue until they are corrected and can trigger symptoms even after a period of time. A certain exception in this context are refolding distortions in the area of the legs and back, which may sometimes resolve spontaneously in everyday life due to the effect of gravity.

Due to the *permanence of the deformation*, symptoms may not (or not only) be associated with a current trauma, but also with previous injuries (and possibly with uncorrected folding distortions related to them). In addition, the roadblock effect can also be caused by folding distortions, thereby triggering symptoms at a time interval after the deformation.

2.4.2   Subjective Complaints with Folding Distortions

Cardinal symptoms of folding distortions in the area of joints are pain on movement and loading, instability, and joint swelling. This also applies to folding distortions of the interosseous membranes and muscle septa, which can additionally be responsible for significant movement restrictions.

A typical indication of folding distortions is *pain on loading in the joint*. The symptomatology differs depending on the origin of the deformation:

- As described, a combination of traction and shear forces leads to the development of an unfolding distortion. Due to this dislocation, the folding fascia can no longer be fully compressed, which reduces its shock-absorbing capacity. Clinically, this results in pain that increases with loading and compression, while relief reduces the symptoms. Consequently, activities such as standing, jumping, or supporting oneself often exacerbate the pain, whereas lying down is reducing the pain. This relationship is also evident in the fact that symptoms tend to increase over the course of the day, as the effect of gravity places stress on the area of the unfolding distortion.

- The opposite is true for refolding distortion. Through a combination of compression and shear forces, the fascia is excessively compressed and becomes stuck. As a result, the folding fascia can no longer fully relax, but renewed compression is possible. This explains the typical symptoms of a refolding distortion. Loading and activity tend to relieve the symptoms more than unloading and immobilization. Over the course of the day, pain is more pronounced in the morning than in the evening and is often accompanied by a sensation of morning stiffness.

Folding distortions can cause *pain on movement despite good mobility*, which often increases with repeated movement. Mobility itself is usually less impaired than with triggerbands or herniated triggerpoints. Typical for a folding distortion is pain at the end of the range of motion; significant movement blockades are rather rare.

In this context, two exceptions should be mentioned:

- Joint swelling due to a folding distortion (for example when caused in the context of an acute joint trauma) can impair mobility, at least temporarily.
- Folding distortions of the interosseous membranes and muscle septa, in contrast to folding distortions of joints, can lead to persistent restrictions. For example, folding distortions in the area of the interosseous membrane of the forearm are considered the main cause of limited pronation and supination after a fracture in this region.

Instability is considered a typical indication in unfolding and refolding distortions. This ranges from a subjective feeling of lack of control over a joint to clinically demonstrable instability. As a result, many patients consciously or unconsciously adapt their daily activities. They move cautiously to avoid situations in which stability and joint control (such as jumping on one leg) are put to the test. Typaldos explains instability primarily not by lack of strength and coordination, but by reduced proprioception triggered by folding distortions. Consequently, treatment to improve stability focuses on correcting the folding distortion rather than on muscle training or proprioceptive exercises.

Another symptom of folding distortion is *joint swelling*. In contrast to triggerbands and continuum distortions, which are more likely to cause local swelling in the area of the soft tissues, folding distortions affect the intra-articular space. Due to the persistence of the deformation, there is a tendency for ongoing, mostly load-dependent swelling, which can vary in extent. In otherwise minimally symptomatic folding distortions, even a (mild) swelling of the joint can be a subtle but nonetheless typical clinical sign.

2.4.3 Objective Findings in Folding Distortions

Folding distortions cannot be provoked by palpatory pressure nor palpated by the therapist (in contrast to triggerbands, herniated triggerpoints, and continuum distortions). This matches the subjective description of the complaints as deep, located within the joint, and thus inaccessible to palpation.

Possible objective signs of a folding distortion are therefore potentially visible impairment of stability, corresponding movement restriction, and/or joint swelling. These can be compared before and after treatment.

2.4.4 Body Language with Folding Distortions

In folding distortions, *patients unconsciously place their hand on the affected region or grasp the area*. This behavior is visible in both unfolding and refolding distortions. The gesture remains static, meaning the hand does not move across the skin (fig. 2.17a to c).

Apart from this, there are further body language indicators:

- Intuitively, many patients relieve or compress the area of the folding distortion.

Supporting the arm in a refolding distortion of the shoulder or generally avoiding weight-bearing on the ankle in an unfolding distortion are examples from clinical practice.

- In a refolding distortion, *a dynamic horizontal stroking with the fingers across the joint* may be observed, which, according to Typaldos, is presented by about half of patients with refolding distortions (fig. 2.18a to c).
- In a folding distortion of the interosseous membrane, *patients often press several fingers between parallel-aligned bones or grasp them with the whole hand* (fig. 2.19a).

Sometimes, a kind of deep rubbing with the fingers (similar to the triggerband gesture) between the bones can also be seen (fig. 2.19b).

- The body language as an indicator of a folding distortion in the area of the muscle septa resembles the gestures in the area of the interosseous membrane, but is indicated in the area of the soft tissues. *Several fingers are pressed between muscles* or patients *pull at the muscles,* as if trying to create space in the affected area (fig. 2.19c). Deep rubbing with the fingertips is also frequently observed.

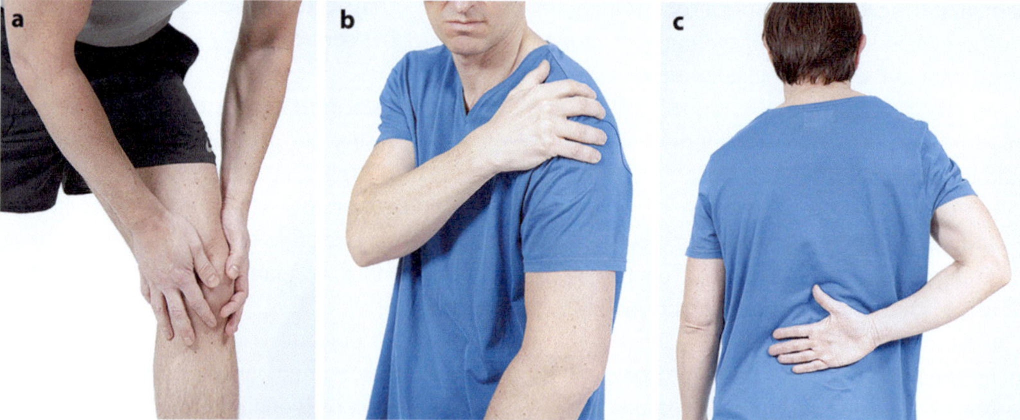

Fig. 2.17 Typical body language in folding distortions (in both unfolding and refolding distortions). Grasping the knee with both hands (**a**). Grasping the shoulder with one hand (**b**). Placing a hand on the back in a folding distortion of the lumbar region (**c**). (© Anker 2022)

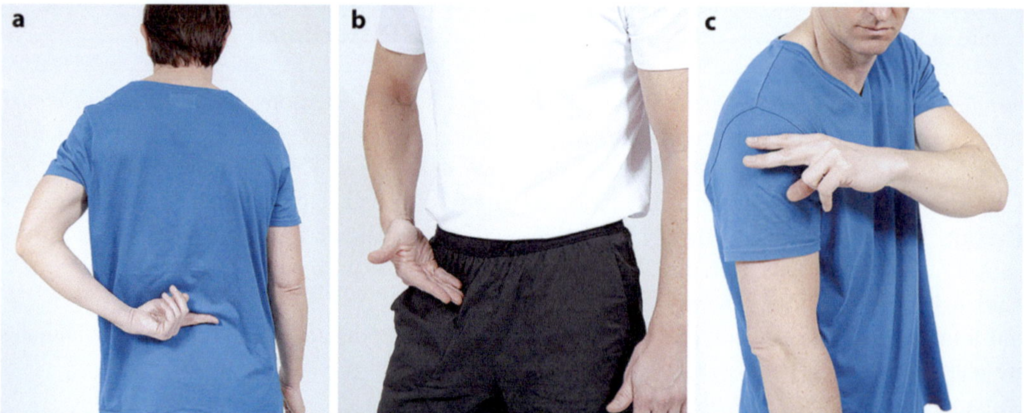

Fig. 2.18 Typical body language in refolding distortions. Horizontal stroking across the spine (**a**). Stroking with the edge of the hand along the groin (**b**). Horizontal stroking across the outer shoulder (**c**). (© Anker 2022)

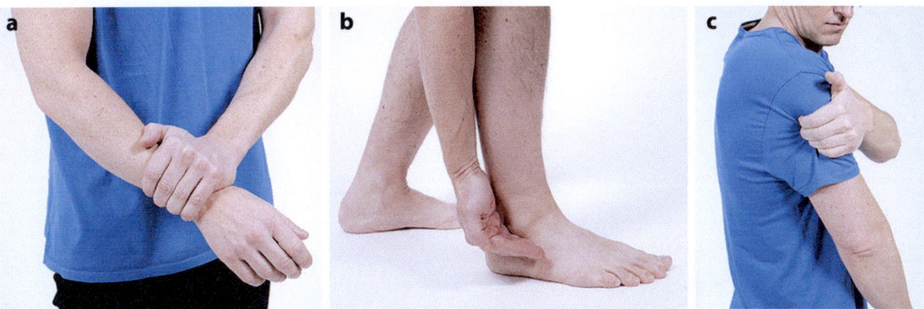

Fig. 2.19 Typical body language in folding distortions of the interosseous membrane or muscle septa. Grasping the forearm as a sign of a folding distortion of the interosseous membrane (**a**). Horizontal stroking with the edge of the hand below the lateral malleolus as a sign of a folding distortion of the interosseous membrane of the lower leg (**b**). Pushing several fingers between the muscles as typical body language in folding distortion of the muscle septa at the shoulder (**c**). (© Anker 2022)

2.4.5 Summary and Examples

Patients with folding distortions often describe the affected joint as "sprained" or "dislocated." Typically, this results in symptoms within the joint such as pain or a loss of stability. The initially pronounced symptoms may decrease over time. Nevertheless, without correction, the folding distortion usually remains permanent and can, even after a period of time, trigger symptoms again or be the cause of additional fascial distortions.

Clinical Patterns from Practice

- A female patient injures her anterior cruciate ligament during sports and subsequently undergoes surgery. Despite intensive exercise therapy, she continues to experience knee pain while running. In addition, the joint swells after prolonged activity. After correction of the unfolding distortion caused by the trauma, the symptoms disappear completely.
- A male patient presents to the clinic with acute lower back pain. He describes symptoms deep in the back that worsen throughout the day. When he lies flat on his back in the evening, the symptoms subside.
- A female patient dislocates her shoulder. After reduction in the hospital, she must wear a stabilizing bandage for several weeks. After completion of treatment, the joint still feels subjectively unstable and she avoids wide-ranging or rapid movements. ◀

2.5 Cylinder Distortions (CyD—Cylinder Distortion)

Cylinder fasciae envelop various structures in the body such as muscles, organs, or blood vessels. They act as shock absorbers for non-articular areas (in contrast to folding fasciae, which act as shock absorbers in the area of joints), and they can dynamically adapt to changes in volume and position of the enclosed structures.

When cylinder distortions develop, this microstructure of the cylinder fascia becomes deformed, impairing its adaptability and causing the enclosed tissue to become trapped (fig. 2.20).

2.5.1 Formation of Cylinder Distortions

Typaldos describes cylinder fascia as coils that wrap around tissue in various directions, forming a lattice-like structure. Each individual loop of this envelope system is freely movable relative to the other loops and to the enclosed structure. This allows the cylinder fascia to

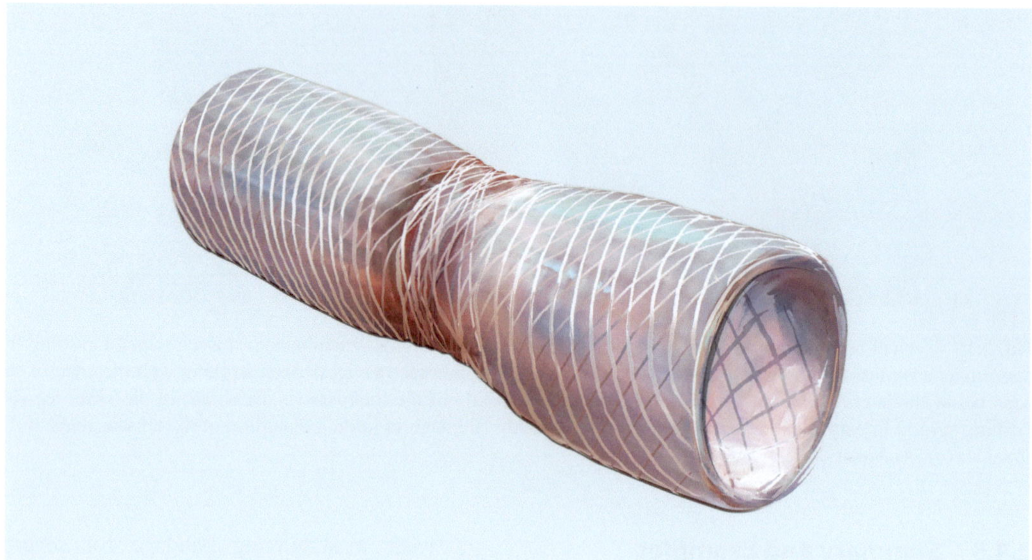

Fig. 2.20   Cylinder distortion. (© Anker 2022)

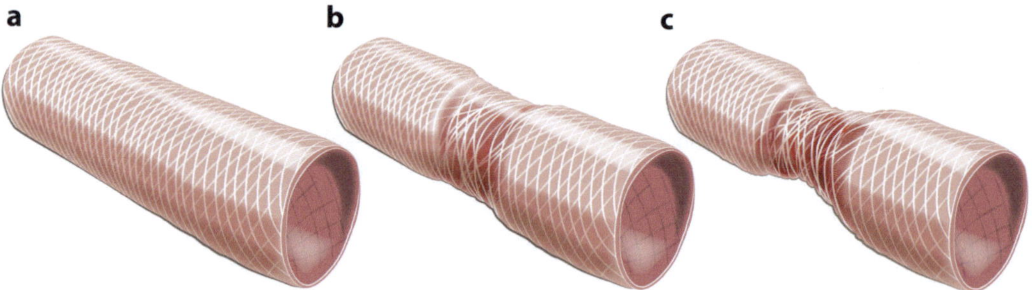

Fig. 2.21   Formation of a cylinder distortion. Intact cylinder fascia (**a**). Entanglement of the cylinder coils (**b**). Increasing constriction in a cylinder distortion (**c**). (© Anker 2022)

dynamically adapt to changes in volume and position by the individual coils being pushed apart and then elastically returning to their original position (fig. 2.21a).

However, twisting/traction forces or twisting/compression forces can lead to entanglements and overlaps of these coils, impairing their dynamic interplay. As a result, the cylinder fascia constricts the tissue they enclose (to varying degrees), thereby mechanically triggering a wide range of symptoms (fig. 2.21b and c).

The distortion can arise through various mechanisms. Physical trauma such as *soft tissue contusions, severe jolts, abrasions, or strains* as well as surgical interventions involving manipulation of the soft tissues can trigger a cylinder distortion. Typaldos also describes the possibility that *tight bandages or constricting clothing* can cause cylinder distortions. Also fitting into this group of seemingly harmless triggers are patient reports that their symptoms arose from *minor injuries* or from drafts. Often, there is a noticeable mismatch between the respective trigger and the severity of the symptoms.

Background Information
Apart from development due to external mechanical forces, there also appears to be a connection between viral or bacterial infections and cylinder distortions. Typaldos cites diffuse soft tissue pain during influenza as an example. He explains the connection by stating that

the inflammation and swelling of the soft tissues that occur during such infections lead to an increase in volume. This causes the cylinder coils to be pushed apart and become more susceptible to entanglement, so that even ordinary muscle contractions can trigger distortions.

This mechanism could also play a role in the association between injections and cylinder distortions, as patients may develop typical symptoms of a cylinder distortion in the area of the needle puncture. This also fits with reports from patients with cylinder distortions who develop even more symptoms after an injection treatment for pain management.

According to the mechanism of formation, we distinguish between the cylinder distortion, which arises from the coils being pushed apart and entangled, and its **compression variant** (Compression Cylinder Variant—CCV), which develops through compression and hooking of the coils. This differentiation is useful because the two subtypes respond to different therapeutic measures. However, based on the symptoms, they are usually difficult to distinguish.

Cylinder distortions are not wounds in the tissue. However, they are also not permanent deformations like herniated triggerpoints or folding distortions, which lead to a lasting change in the fascial architecture. On the contrary: cylinder distortions appear to be able to move.

This means that the position of the entangled coils, and thus the location and intensity of the symptoms, can change without any particular cause. This dynamic, characteristic of cylinder distortions, is referred to by Typaldos as the "phenomenon of jumping pain." The resulting great variability and unpredictability of symptoms often lead to confusion among patients and therapists, as the shifting location makes it seem impossible to identify the pain-triggering structure.

But the opposite can also be the case: pain caused by cylinder distortions can appear very persistent and stuck. Some therapists mistakenly interpret this as a sign of chronification. This is incorrect, because cylinder distortions do not cause adhesions and therefore always remain acute distortions.

Slinky Toy Analogy
According to Typaldos, this children's toy has a structure similar to that of the cylinder fascia. The coils of the spiral can be easily pulled apart and compressed (fig. 2.22a). However, if the coils become entangled, the elasticity of the spiral is reduced. As with a folding distortion, this impairs the shock-absorbing capacity (fig. 2.22b).

2.5.2   Subjective Complaints with Cylinder Distortions

The range of symptoms in cylinder distortions is broad. They are best summarized as diffuse, intense, and often unpredictable.

Cylinder distortions can cause *active movement restrictions*, while passive mobility is

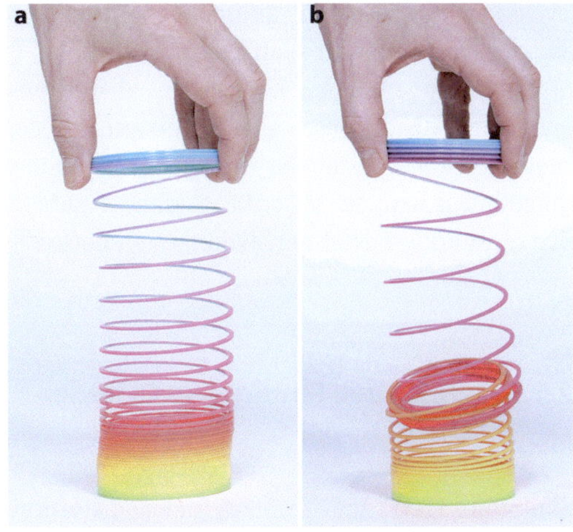

Fig. 2.22 Slinky toy analogy. (© Anker 2022)

generally not impaired. In some cases, these restrictions are so dramatic that, especially when associated with physical trauma, bone fractures or herniated discs are initially suspected. Sometimes, however, mobility may be almost normal, but the execution of movement appears uncoordinated or characterized by large compensatory movements.

Pain caused by cylinder distortions also presents very differently. It ranges from diffuse, superficial discomfort in a clearly defined area to severe, deep-seated pain syndromes affecting entire body regions, which can barely be alleviated by medication. Both the musculoskeletal system and internal organs (such as in painful abdominal cramps) can be affected.

Symptoms may also occur specifically at night. Thus, cylinder distortions, along with triggerbands, are among the most common causes of nocturnal pain.

For symptoms such as *cramps, muscle weakness, sensory disturbances, tremors, or autonomic symptoms such as sweating or a sensation of cold*, conventional medicine often suspects a connection with pathologies of the nervous or vascular system and initiates the corresponding diagnostics. However, examination results are often inconclusive, and the clinical effectiveness of the resulting therapeutic concepts is inadequate.

With the concept of cylinder distortion, Typaldos provides an alternative mechanical explanatory model for such symptoms.

Like triggerbands, continuum distortions, or folding distortions, cylinder distortions can cause *swelling* localized in the soft tissues. Sometimes, patients describe a kind of subjective sensation of swelling, even though no swelling is visible.

2.5.3   Objective Findings in Cylinder Distortions

Symptoms resulting from cylinder distortions are often localized deep within the soft tissues. It is therefore not surprising that cylinder distortions cannot be provoked by palpatory pressure.

There are two exceptions to this. One occurs in patients who report *marked sensitivity to touch*, making it impossible to manually examine the symptomatic region. The other can be observed through applying *traction on the skin* in the area of the cylinder distortion, which can trigger the characteristic pain. This skin traction test is helpful when, in cases of diffuse cylinder distortions, the question arises as to where an initial treatment intervention should be performed. This provocation test allows for a more precise localization of the affected area.

When testing active range of motion, pain-related limitations or disturbances in movement coordination may become apparent. Range of motion tests are therefore also a suitable means to objectify the effect of a treatment.

2.5.4   Body Language with Cylinder Distortions

Dynamic wiping, kneading, and pinching of the soft tissues with the fingers or the whole hand are the typical gestures performed by patients with cylinder distortions (fig. 2.23a to c). In addition, it is possible to derive further information about the qualities of the symptoms from body language. Diffuse complaints are often indicated by equally diffuse searching gestures. Constricting pain, on the other hand, is presented with pinching or kneading gestures. It can be important to perceive these differences, as they may provide clues for optimal treatment. Accordingly, widespread complaints often require a similarly broad treatment technique, whereas in cases of pronounced constriction symptoms, therapeutic approaches that lift the fascia from the underlying tissue may be advantageous.

2.5.5   Summary and Examples

Cylinder distortions explain many, sometimes dramatic symptoms that cannot be clearly assigned to specific pathologies by conventional medicine. Severe pain without inflammation,

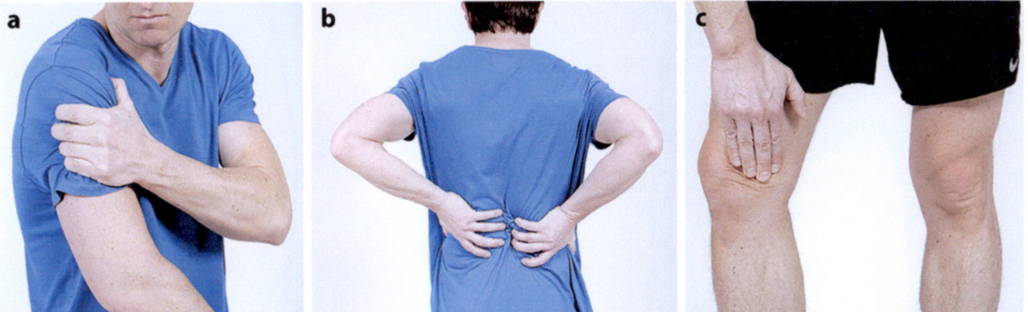

Fig. 2.23 Typical body language in cylinder distortions. Kneading gestures at the shoulder (**a**) and with both hands on the back (**b**). Dynamic rubbing with the fingers at the knee (**c**). (© Anker 2022)

symptoms that change location, or obvious neurological complaints without any evidence of a neurological disorder may be associated with cylinder distortions. These complaints become comprehensible through the concept of cylinder distortion and can subsequently be resolved by mechanotherapy.

Clinical Patterns from Practice

- A patient fractures his shoulder in a fall. After surgical treatment, he is plagued by severe nocturnal pain that cannot be controlled with medication. The patient describes the symptoms as deep, constricting, and sometimes cramp-like.
- After a contusion of the thigh, a female patient develops diffuse paresthesias in the leg. Since the neurological examination does not reveal a specific cause, the patient is unsettled. Further diagnostic workup also fails to explain the symptoms, so a psychosomatic cause is suspected.
- After a herniated disc twelve months ago resulting in weakness in the right calf, a patient still has reduced strength when standing on tiptoe. After initial improvement, recovery seems to have plateaued for the past two months. The neurologist interprets the residual symptoms as a cylinder distortion and treats them with specific manual techniques. After two therapy sessions, muscular activity is nearly identical when comparing both sides. ◄

2.6 Tectonic Fixations (TF—Tectonic Fixation)

Smooth fascia form gliding surfaces and thus have a decisive influence on the mobility and adaptability of various adjacent structures. When this gliding function is restricted, we speak of a tectonic fixation (fig. 2.24). Typaldos describes this as a physiological change that impairs the gliding ability of fascial tissue. As a result, freedom of movement, especially in joints and in the area of the internal organs, is reduced.

2.6.1 Formation of Tectonic Fixations

The development of tectonic fixation is explained by the reduction of synovial fluid between joint partners (fig. 2.25a). This can occur *in the context of physical trauma*, in which the affected structures are abruptly and forcefully compressed, squeezing the synovial fluid out of the (joint) space and subsequently making gliding movements more difficult. An example of this would be a vertebral blockage after a misstep, where the symptoms of tectonic fixation appear abruptly, similar to the mechanism of injury.

However, tectonic fixations can also *develop progressively due to other fascial distortions* that trigger increasing compression of the joint partners. As a result, even lubrication is restricted, resistance to movement increases,

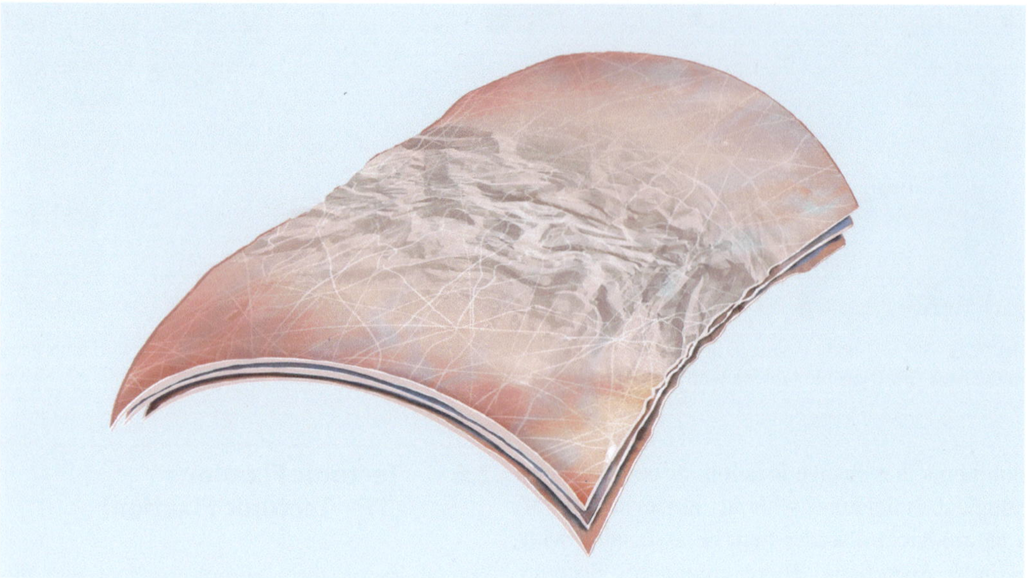

Fig. 2.24 Tectonic fixation. (© Anker 2022)

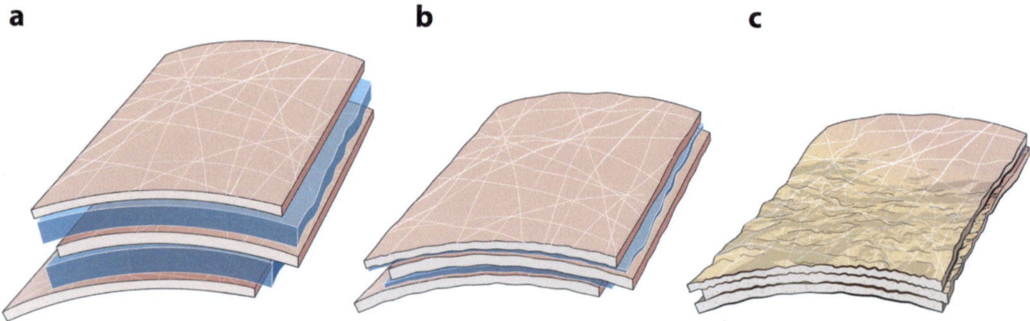

Fig. 2.25 Progressive formation of a tectonic fixation. Intact gliding ability of the smooth fascia (**a**). Reduced lubrication (**b**). Full manifestation of a tectonic fixation (**c**). (© Anker 2022)

and the smooth fascia is subsequently mobilized less. This in turn leads to a decrease in the quality of the joint fluid (it loses viscosity) and its new production is stimulated less, further reducing the gliding ability of the smooth fascia (fFig. 2.25b).

A classic example of this is a stiff shoulder ("frozen shoulder"): it develops in connection with chronic triggerbands, which lead to shortening of the band-like fasciae. This results in a restriction of movement, which initiates the cascade described above. The joint is moved less, which reduces the quantity and quality of synovial fluid, and ultimately a tectonic fixation develops, in which parts of the joint capsule virtually adhere to the bone and trigger the typical movement blockade (fig. 2.25c and 2.26c).

Typaldos describes the full manifestation of a tectonic fixation not only as a reduction in gliding ability, but as a state in which the joint partners adhere to each other like magnets. He compares this to tectonic plates around the globe, which are pressed together under high pressure. As long as this compression is maintained, there is hardly any possibility for movement. This explains the observation that tectonic fixation can also lead to a persistent reduction in mobility, and only resolves when increased play between the joint partners allows fluid to flow in, and gliding becomes possible again.

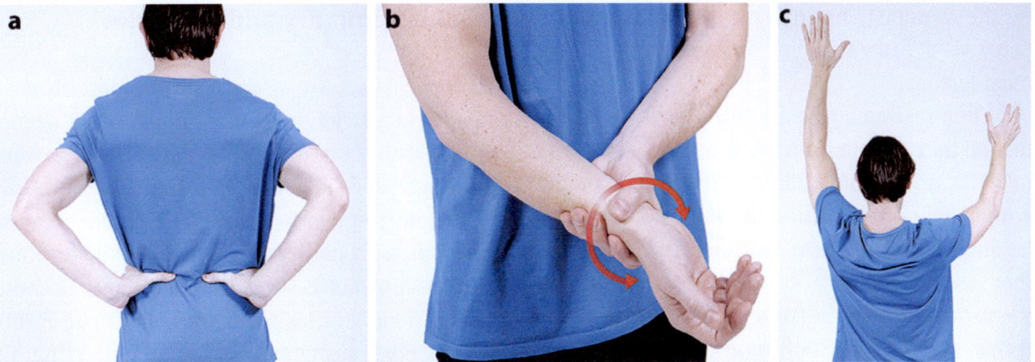

Fig. 2.26 Body language in tectonic fixation. Supporting both hands on the iliac crest as a sign of tectonic fixation of the lower back or hips (**a**). Grasping and actively mobilizing the forearm in tectonic fixation of the interosseous membrane (**b**). Typical restriction of shoulder elevation with compensatory movements (**c**). (© Anker 2022)

2.6.2   Subjective Complaints with Tectonic Fixations

The cardinal symptoms of tectonic fixation are *restriction of movement and stiffness.* Pain is not the main feature, but if present, it tends to occur at the end range of motion or during passive testing at the end of movement. (Typaldos describes only one exception to this, namely tectonic fixation of the lower back, which can cause pain in the midline of the spine.)

If pain occurs in connection with a tectonic fixation, we therefore assume in FDM diagnostics that additional distortions (apart from the tectonic fixation) are present.

Patients describe either a *blockage of a specific movement or a progressive loss of mobility in several directions,* which can also result in considerable limitations in daily activities.

In the progressive development of tectonic fixation—for example after a painful injury and associated pain-inducing fascial distortions—a correlation can often be observed between increasing restriction of movement and decreasing symptoms. The stiffer the joint becomes (that is, the more the tectonic fixation progresses), the less the fascial distortions associated with its development cause pain. This does not mean that these fascial deformations are resolved by the increasing stiffness, but only that they are less likely to be provoked. This mechanism can be interpreted as a natural reaction of the body to calm persistent symptoms. Although for different reasons, this principle is reflected in conventional medicine, where immobilization is used as therapy for painful conditions.

Symptoms such as weakness, swelling, or instability are not caused by tectonic fixation. However, tectonic fixations can prepare the ground for the development of corresponding fascial distortions, since reduced gliding and adaptability lead to less mobilization of tissue fluids and a subsequent reduction in metabolism (as described with the roadblock effect in the first chapter).

2.6.3   Objective Findings in Tectonic Fixations

Typaldos distinguishes between a subjective tectonic fixation and an objective tectonic fixation. In the first case, patients describe a feeling of blockage, which can be resolved by manual treatment or self-mobilization, but is hardly objectively measurable in terms of movement restriction. In the second case, reduced mobility, usually in several directions, can be quantified by the therapist. In addition, the therapist may perceive a firm end feel during passive movement testing.

When testing active mobility, *evasive* movements and compensatory movement patterns may be noticeable. For example, if a patient with a tectonic fixation in the shoulder area cannot abduct the arm sufficiently to the side, they will typically compensate by raising the arm more to the front or by extending the trunk backward. Such compensatory movements can also be observed in other regions of the body.

2.6.4   Body Language with Tectonic Fixations

While clearly defined gestures are described for the other five distortions, such gestures occur only in certain cases for tectonic fixation. For example, patients with a tectonic fixation of the lower back often support themselves with both hands in the posterior hip region (fig. 2.26a).

In general, the body language of tectonic fixation can rather be described as an *attempt at self-mobilization*. Either through active or passive movement, patients struggle against the restricted mobility (fig. 2.26b and c).

In clinical practice, however, it is more often the case history and examination of the patient which are the decisive factor when diagnosing a tectonic fixation, while body language is rarely an essential component of a diagnosis.

2.6.5   Summary and Examples

Tectonic fixation can generally be described as a painless restriction of mobility. When it occurs in isolation, it is usually in the form of a joint blockage that patients can specifically localize. More frequently, however, tectonic fixation develops as a consequence of other distortions. This circumstance should be taken into account during treatment, as tectonic fixation can rarely be resolved sustainably without correcting its underlying cause.

Clinical Examples from Practice

- A female patient fractures her metacarpal and is treated with a plaster splint. After six weeks of immobilization, the area is pain-free but severely restricted in movement.
- A male patient sprains his ankle when jumping from a wall and consequently develops bone marrow edema. Although the weight-bearing pain remains limited, increasing stiffness develops, which significantly impairs the rolling mechanism during walking.
- Due to a comminuted fracture in the knee joint area 15 years ago, a female patient has developed severe pain in the affected area, which could only be moderately alleviated by various therapies. It was only with increasing stiffness of the knee over the years that the symptoms became more tolerable for the patient. ◄

The diagnosis of fascial distortions (in short, the FDM diagnosis) is based on clinical criteria. On the basis of detailed knowledge of the six fascial distortions and the Fascial Distortion Model, a working diagnosis can be developed, which in turn forms the basis for the application of the Typaldos method to a wide variety of symptom patterns.

The diagnosis of fascial distortions differs from diagnosis in conventional medicine, where objectively verifiable findings such as imaging procedures or laboratory tests are often the focus. In contrast, the diagnosis of fascial distortions is strongly oriented towards the patient's self-perception and relies, among other things, on the verbal and non-verbal description of symptoms.

While conventional medical diagnostics focus on the identification of medically defined diseases, FDM diagnostics examine the relationship between the patient's individual symptomatology and fascial distortions. It consists of anamnesis, examination, and observation of the patient. The information thus obtained is correlated with the respective characteristics of the six fascial distortions or interpreted according to the Fascial Distortion Model. In this way, the question is answered as to which fascial distortion or combination of fascial distortions can explain the patient's symptoms.

Background Information

The diagnosis of fascial distortions is not intended to challenge conventional medical diagnoses, but rather to develop, in parallel, an independent, coherent, and practically applicable explanatory model for the patient's problem.

It is carried out by trained physicians and therapists as part of a medical treatment, so that the patient's health status is also assessed from a conventional medical perspective, and questions regarding indications and contraindications for treatment with the Typaldos method can be answered. This does not mean that the conventional medical diagnosis determines whether the Typaldos method can be used. The goal of treatment, according to the FDM, is to choose the most effective treatment approach for the patient at all times. Consequently, the therapist must weigh whether the FDM-based explanatory model for the patient's symptoms appears more plausible and likely to be more effective in practice than the conventional medical approach.

© The Author(s), under exclusive license to Springer-Verlag GmbH, DE, part of Springer Nature 2026
S. Anker, *Fascial Distortion Model in Clinical Practice*, https://doi.org/10.1007/978-3-662-72081-3_3

As already described in chap. 2, Typaldos describes four different sources of information that are used during examination and treatment to diagnose fascial distortions:

- The formation of symptoms
- The subjective symptoms of the patients
- The objectively verifiable findings in connection with the problem
- The interpretation of the patients' body language

In principle, the higher the number of individual pieces of information support the same diagnostic hypothesis, the more robust the diagnosis. This also applies to the FDM, so that, ideally, diagnostic details from the four sources of information mentioned above enable a coherent explanation of the patient's symptoms. It should be noted that information can and must be weighted depending on the situation. For example, Typaldos reports that in cases of acute trauma, the mechanism of injury and the interpretation of body language are particularly important for a diagnosis. In contrast, in chronic problems, the objectively verifiable findings and the detailed analysis of subjective symptoms can have a decisive influence on the working hypothesis for treatment.

The diagnostic process in the FDM can be divided into three phases (fig. 3.1):

Anamnesis as the entry point to diagnostics

At the beginning, the patient explains the origin of the symptoms and describes their subjective complaints. In practice, it is helpful to trace the chronological development of the individual symptoms in order to assess their dynamics.

The examination of the patient

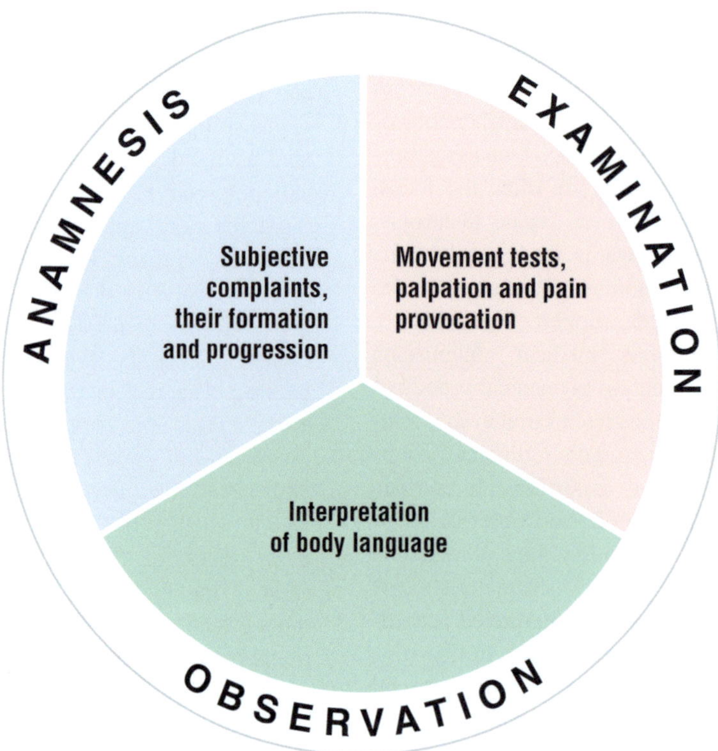

Fig. 3.1 FDM diagnosis model (© Anker 2022)

This is followed by an examination by the therapist using active movement and load tests as well as palpation of the affected area. Based on these objectively verifiable findings, conclusions can also be drawn regarding possible contraindications for treatment or the need for further conventional medical clarification.

Ongoing observation of the patient

In parallel with medical history and examination, the therapist continuously observes the patient's body language and behavior and interprets both in the context of the information obtained so far.

3.1   Formation of Fascial Distortions

A wide variety of symptoms are interpreted in the FDM as a consequence of deformation of the fascia. The analysis of how these deformations develop establishes a connection between possible symptom triggers, such as physical trauma or overuse, and the individual symptoms of the patient.

Questions about the formation of any fascial distortion are a good starting point for a medical history, as they provide an initial insight into potential   tissue deformation.   Symptom origin analysis allows conclusions to be drawn about individual types of distortion, their location, and their severity. Furthermore, questions regarding the indication or contraindication for treatment with the Typaldos method can sometimes be answered (fig. 3.2).

3.1.1   Causes of Fascial Distortions

Physical trauma and overuse are the main causes of the development of fascial distortions. In addition to these externally acting forces on the body, forces and tensions that arise within the body can also play a role, for example in fascial distortions associated with dysfunction of internal organs.

The extent to which the body's tissues can withstand such forces depends on their resilience. Typaldos describes risk factors that can lead to weakening of the fascia and thus

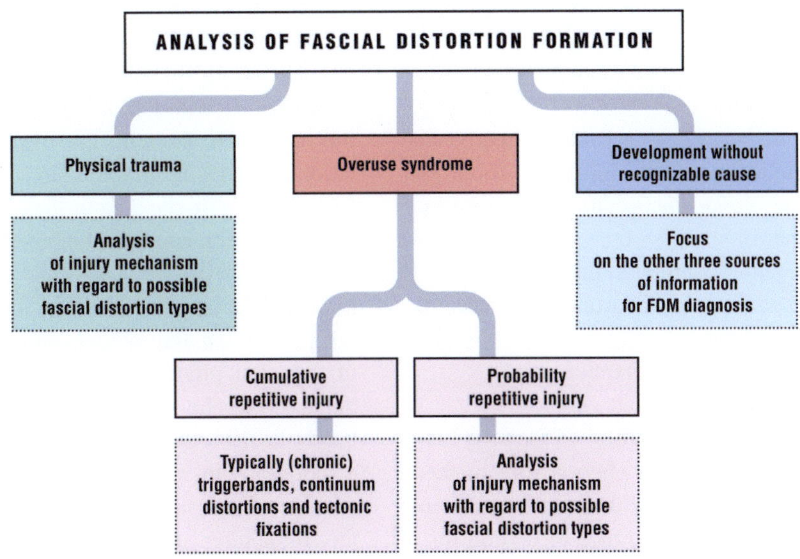

Fig. 3.2 Analysis of the fascial distortion formation (© Anker 2022)

promote the development of distortions. In this context, he mentions:

- Vitamin and nutrient deficiencies
- Bacterial or viral infections
- The roadblock effect, caused by pre-existing fascial distortions
- Genetic defects that lead to changes in the ground substance

3.1.2 Types of Fascial Distortion Development

Fascial distortions and therefore their symptoms can occur abruptly and without warning or develop slowly and progressively.

As a result of an injury, fascial distortions can, for example, occur abruptly. All six types of distortions can arise in this way and are potential causes of acute symptoms. The analysis of their formation and the specific injury position can help narrow down the involved distortion type(s) and their potential location. In clinical practice, typical correlations between mechanisms of injury and specific distortion patterns are often observed:

- *Soft tissue strain/overuse syndrome:* triggerband, continuum distortion, cylinder distortion
- *Sprain of a joint:* continuum distortion, refolding distortion
- *Strain or dislocation of a joint:* triggerband, continuum distortion, unfolding distortion
- *Soft tissue contusion:* cylinder distortion, triggerband
- *Bone contusion:* continuum distortion
- *Fracture:* continuum distortion, triggerband, folding distortion
- *Joint blockage:* tectonic fixation

Apart from this, the distribution of the four fascia types in the body also plays a role in this context. According to Typaldos, this results in different risks for the occurrence of certain distortions depending on the location of the problem. For example, herniated triggerpoints are considered unlikely in the extremities, as band-like tissue predominates in this region of the body.

In his textbooks, Typaldos also presents concepts on how conventional medical diagnoses and therapeutic approaches can be justified according to FDM criteria. These concepts do not replace the individual FDM diagnosis. Rather, they illustrate the independent etiology, which centers on fascial distortions and their functional consequences:

- *Fractures* can be considered to be extensions of fascial distortions in the osseous matrix. For example, spiral fractures correspond to the course of a triggerband in the bone. Avulsion fractures are more likely to be assigned to a continuum distortion, which arises when the transition zone cannot adapt quickly enough during physical trauma, resulting in a bone fracture.

  According to Typaldos, the fascial deformations of a fracture also cause the pain and functional limitations experienced by patients. Correction of the underlying fascial distortions, which can be identified through FDM diagnosis, can therefore restore the functionality of the affected region. Typaldos recommends performing these corrections before applying a cast or during surgical intervention. In his view, this optimizes the physiological conditions for fracture consolidation. In addition, it has been shown that this approach shortens the overall rehabilitation period after trauma. In certain stable fractures (e.g. in the area of the ankle or ribs), immobilization can even be omitted with this approach.

- *Ligament or tendon ruptures* are, from the perspective of the model, often the result of repeated physical overuse. The problem begins with the formation of local triggerbands in the affected structure. As a result, a portion can no longer fulfill its function of force transmission. Consequently, the remaining unaffected portion is overloaded, leading to further deformations, which increasingly spread across the entire cross-section of the tendon or ligament. The metabolism impaired by these deformations further reduces the resistance of the ligament or tendon, so that ultimately a complete rupture of the affected structure may occur. From this perspective, the treatment of partial ruptures is of great importance in order to stop the increasing deformation or to correct the deformation that is already present.

- *Muscle strains* are associated with triggerbands. They lead to a shortening of the fascial structures in the muscle and represent a mechanical obstacle to its full contractile capacity. This explains the typical symptoms of pulling pain and weakness. The conventional medical approach usually focuses on immobilizing the affected muscle to allow the injury to heal. The disadvantage of immobilization is a longer rehabilitation period and the risk of increased muscle atrophy. If, on the other hand, the twisted fascial band is corrected promptly, the load-bearing capacity and strength of the muscle improve immediately. In addition, it can be observed that the risk of recurrent injury is reduced.

- When patients complain of *sudden onset pain*, it is possible that similar pain episodes have occurred in the past. In this case, conclusions can be drawn about certain distortions, which, according to their characteristics, are considered permanent deformations of the tissue and can therefore repeatedly trigger new symptoms. The causes of permanent tissue deformation can be (chronic) triggerbands, herniated triggerpoints, and folding distortions.

- The analysis of the mechanism of injury is particularly important in situations where the onset and resulting symptoms do not appear to be related. We know that in such situations, cylinder distortions can be the cause. They can—sometimes without any apparent cause—trigger bizarre and dramatic symptoms. In general, the absence of any mechanical cause of symptoms should be understood as a prompt to analyze the clinical picture not only using the Fascial Distortion Model, but also from a conventional medical perspective.

For example, if a supposed triggerband suddenly appears in the calf after a long-haul flight, deep vein thrombosis should also be considered and further conventional medical evaluation initiated.

In addition to abrupt onset, fascial distortions can also develop progressively and cause increasing symptoms. Distortion types with dynamic development potential include, for example, triggerbands. They can become adherent, thereby causing complaints that become increasingly complex and spread regionally.

Furthermore, they can impair the metabolism of the tissue and thus create the basis for the development of additional distortions with further symptoms.

In practice, the term overuse syndrome is often applied to describe such progressively worsening clinical pictures. According to their mechanism of formation, Typaldos distinguishes two groups of overuse syndromes. This classification is of clinical importance, as different therapeutic strategies are generally effective for each group:

- *Cumulative repetitive injury* (CRI) develop over a longer period of time due to the repetition of a specific movement or load beyond the tissue's capacity. The repetitive overload leads to increasingly complex distortion patterns and, as a result, a reduced resilience of the tissue. Triggerbands and continuum distortions are frequently diagnosable in these cases. There is also a risk of chronification and the development of additional tectonic fixations.

  Accordingly, a dynamic increase in symptoms is observed. For example, at the onset of a cumulative repetitive injury, pain may only occur after a specific activity. With increasing chronification, this can develop into persistent pain that can significantly impair load tolerance.

  In treatment, the distortions must be corrected step by step over several therapy sessions. Due to the weakening of the tissue, new distortions may develop if the triggering activities are continued, which is why it is recommended to pause or at least reduce the intensity of loading during the initial phase of therapy until a stable reduction in symptoms is achieved. The treatment of cumulative repetitive injuries is continued until the tissue regains its original resilience. Subsequently, the focus is primarily on prevention of renewed overload (e.g. by adapting the (causative) physical training or by ergonomic modification of the workplace).

- *Probability repetitive injury* (PRI), on the other hand, occur without warning, even though the triggering movement has ultimately been repeated a thousand times. For example, an athlete may throw a ball hundreds of times without any problems until pain suddenly develops in the shoulder. In this case, all six fascial distortions may be considered as possible causes.

In contrast to cumulative overuse, discontinuing the causative movement is neither necessary nor advisable. The patient should be treated as quickly as possible to enable a return to usual activity. This approach is justified by the fact that, depending on the patient's activity level, the tissue is accustomed to a certain dose of loading, and both overload and underload can negatively affect its resilience. Immobilization or rest carries the risk of further fascial deformations. After successful correction, the likelihood of symptom recurrence is no higher than before the initial onset of symptoms. From the perspective of the FDM, additional preventive measures are therefore not necessary in these cases.

3.1.3 Further Development of Fascial Distortions and Progression of Symptoms

In addition to the mechanism of injury, the course and dynamics of symptoms after their onset are also important for diagnosis. The development of symptoms can provide clues to specific fascial distortions. In this context, it should be noted that each fascial distortion can potentially cause further distortions (fig. 3.3).

- Triggerbands can be considered as wounds that are capable of healing on their own, with their symptoms more or less completely disappearing. However, part of the fascial twisting may persist, so that specific symptoms (e.g. under load) continue. If triggerbands become chronic, it leads to an intensification of pain and movement restrictions, as the

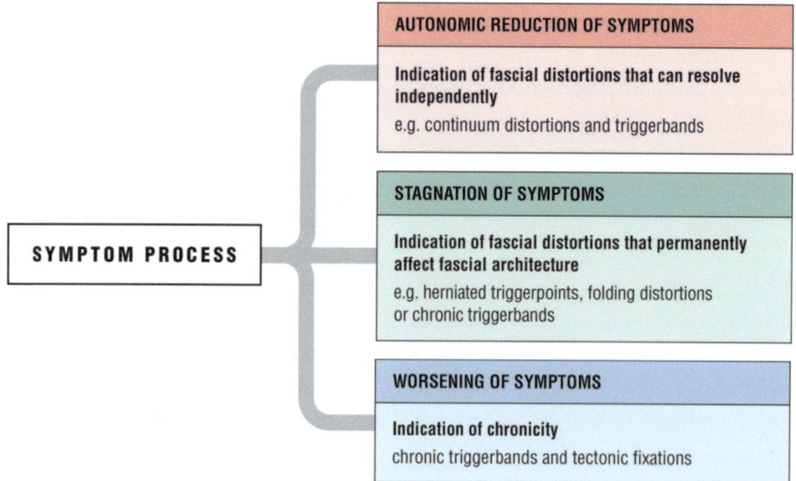

Fig. 3.3 Overview of symptom progression analysis. (© Anker 2022)

formation of adhesions causes the affected area to become deformed in an increasingly complex manner, and adjacent tissues become involved in the distortion process. As a result, continuum distortions may develop, since the twisted band-like fascia can exert excessive tension on the transition zone. Tectonic fixations also frequently occur, because triggerbands restrict mobility and thus impair fluid circulation in the tissue.

- Continuum distortions can resolve autonomously, as the flow of minerals along the band-like fascia can compensate for the step formation in the transition zone, thereby reducing symptoms. The pace of this development varies and ranges from days to months. In individual cases, this resolution process may also come to a halt along the way, so that continuum distortions, especially at the anterior ankle, in the popliteal fossa, and at the wrist, may persist. This carries the risk of triggerbands developing, as the continuum distortion also alters the tension in the adjacent area of the band-like fascia and causes shear forces.
- Folding distortions and herniated triggerpoints are considered permanent distortions and can cause persistent or recurrent symptoms. When these deformations occur for the first time, the corresponding painful symptoms are usually experienced more intensely and their effect is more apparent than they are further down the road. However, this phenomenon generally cannot be equated with an autonomous correction of the distortion.

An exception should be mentioned here: if these distortions cause a movement restriction, the symptoms usually remain constant both in subjective perception and in objective movement testing.

- Cylinder distortions can change unpredictably. The phenomenon of jumping pain, with an inexplicable change in the quality, quantity, and location of symptoms, is typical. However, cylinder distortions can also become persistent and cause ongoing, often very distressing local symptoms.
- Tectonic fixations, especially when they occur suddenly, can persist as a local distortion. If they develop progressively, increasing movement restriction and stiffness result. This is often associated with the chronification of triggerbands.

3.1.4   Significance of the Mechanism of Injury for Treatment

The mechanism of injury, especially the injury position, plays an important role in treatment. It can be advantageous to correct the existing distortions in a position similar to that same injury position (fig. 3.4a and b). This approach leads to better results, especially in the treatment of continuum distortions and folding distortions.

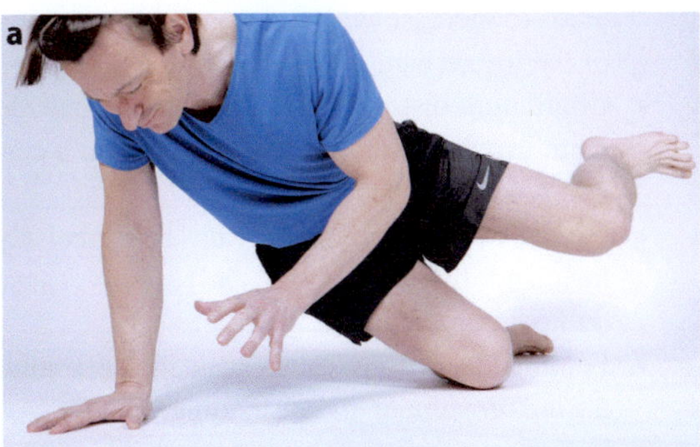
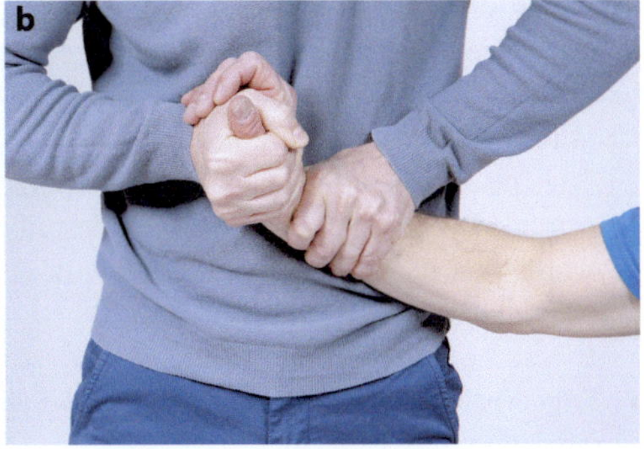

Fig. 3.4 Treatment of a folding distortion in the injury position. Fall onto the wrist as the cause of a refolding distortion (**a**). Refolding technique at the wrist (**b**). (© Anker 2022)

Knowledge of the dynamics of force application during injury can also influence treatment. High-velocity trauma often requires similarly dynamic treatment techniques, whereas chronic complaints that have developed over time require a more persistent approach in treatment.

3.2   Subjective Complaints of Patients

Each fascial distortion is characterized by typical symptoms that are triggered by it and described by the patient. The better the therapist knows the scope of complaint of the respective fascial distortion, the more precisely individual symptoms can be assigned and interpreted.

3.2.1   Fascial Distortions and Their Symptoms

The assignment of specific symptoms to individual fascial distortions is based on the mechanical effect each deformation has on the function of the body. In addition, over the course of development of the Fascial Distortion Model and the Typaldos method, empirical knowledge has been gained on which symptoms responded to which form of therapy. This, in turn, allows conclusions to be drawn on distortion type.

The patient's subjective complaints can be analyzed in a multifaceted way. A distinction of the respective fascial distortions can be made by observing the quality of the symptoms, their dynamics, or factors that lead to symptom relief or aggravation Every detail of a problem should be considered as an individual piece of the puzzle in forming a working hypothesis.

Each fascial distortion can be characterized by cardinal symptoms. Typaldos also describes keywords that patients frequently use with certain fascial distortions:

- Triggerbands: pulling, burning pain and restriction of movement
- Herniated triggerpoints: restriction of movement and dull, localized complaints or tension

- Continuum distortions: localized pain and local movement restriction, usually in the area of bony structures
- Folding distortions: pain in the joint during movement or loading as well as subjectively or objectively measurable joint region instability
- Cylinder distortions: diffuse, sometimes jumping or disproportionate pain as well as complaints similar to a neurological disorder
- Tectonic fixations: restriction of movement, stiffness, and a feeling of blockage; pain is not the main feature

If we look in detail at the relationship between the six fascial distortions and individual complaints, we find that certain symptoms can be triggered by different fascial deformations. Premature diagnostic conclusions can be avoided by first detecting all the symptoms and then considering them together. This comprehensive approach makes it possible to identify the causal relationships and to combine all details into a coherent explanatory model (fig. 3.5).

3.2.2   Fascial Distortions and Pain

Pain can in principle be triggered by all six distortions; least of all by tectonic fixation, which only leads to pain in exceptional cases.

Type of pain:

- Triggerbands cause pulling, burning pain that tends to increase with the degree of stretching of the triggerband.
- Continuum distortions cause clearly localized pain, usually in the area of the bone in a certain position or movement.
- Herniated triggerpoints can be precisely localized by the patient and usually cause dull pain or tension in the soft tissues.
- Folding distortions cause pain inside a joint during movement and/or loading.
- Cylinder distortions are responsible for a range of painful symptoms, from diffuse complaints to the perception of intense pain.

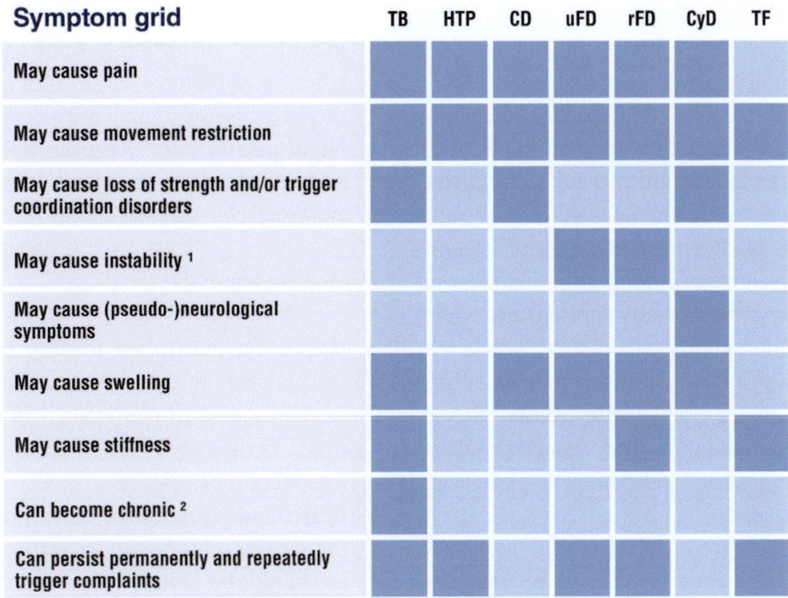

1) either as a subjective perception or as an objectifiable finding
2) in the sense of the Fascial Distortion Model (intensification and spreading of symptoms, increasing stiffness)

Fig. 3.5 Symptom grid. (© Anker 2022)

- With tectonic fixation, pain is rarely the main issue for the patient; rather, it is usually the feeling of blockage or a movement restriction with very little pain. A typical feature is the feeling of stiffness, which also occurs in the context of chronification (in connection with chronic triggerbands).

Location of pain:

- For complaints in the area of the soft tissues, triggerbands, herniated triggerpoints, or cylinder distortions are possible causes.
- In the area of the bone, continuum distortions or folding distortions are often the cause.
- Pain in the joint is a typical indication of a folding distortion.

Dynamics of pain:

- If pain occurs at the beginning of a movement and decreases with repeated movement, this is considered an indication of triggerbands. If complaints decrease with loading of a joint, a refolding distortion may also be the cause.
- Pain that increases with the duration or intensity of loading is explained by unfolding distortions. Triggerbands can also cause load-dependent symptoms, but in that case the pain is not localized in the joint.
- Jumping pain, changing in location, is a typical feature of a cylinder distortion.

3.2.3 Fascial Distortions as a Cause of Functional Impairment

Movement restrictions:

- Triggerbands often lead to restriction in more than one direction of movement.
- Herniated triggerpoints cause restrictions of adjacent joints.

- Continuum distortions can restrict a single specific movement—often, but not necessarily, in a painful way.
- Folding distortions can cause restrictions at the end of the range of motion. With the exception of folding distortions in the area of the interosseous membranes or muscle septa, they rarely lead to major mobility restrictions, apart from movement inhibition due to swelling or pain (which usually subsides over time).
- Cylinder distortions can cause various patterns of restriction. These range from restrictions of active mobility with full mobility on passive examination to pain-related protective postures, in which the patient tries to avoid any movement.
- Tectonic fixations cause local movement blockages or lead to increasing restriction of movement in several directions.

Disturbances of motor control:

- Loss of strength and disturbances of muscular coordination can be caused by triggerbands, continuum distortions, or cylinder distortions.
- A feeling of instability is a typical indication of folding distortions.
- Symptoms similar to a neurological disorder, such as impaired movement coordination, tremor, or cramps, are an indication of cylinder distortions.

Swelling:

- Local tissue swelling can be caused by triggerbands, continuum distortions, or cylinder distortions.
- Joint swelling should be considered an indication of a folding distortion.

3.2.4   Development and Response of Symptoms

Time-of-day dependence of symptoms:

- Morning movement pain and stiffness can be interpreted as an indication of triggerbands or refolding distortions.

- Over the course of the day, symptoms of unfolding distortions tend to increase, whereas symptoms of refolding distortions do not worsen and may even decrease.
- Night pain is usually caused by triggerbands and cylinder distortions; refolding distortions are less frequently the cause.

Response to activity:

- Active movement and loading are perceived by patients as (at least partially) relieving in the case of triggerbands, refolding distortions, certain cylinder distortions, and tectonic fixations.
- Relief and immobilization can reduce symptoms caused by fascial distortions. However, it should be noted that fascial distortions may trigger few symptoms due to immobilization, e.g. by a plaster cast,, but this does not necessarily lead to their autonomous resolution.
- Symptoms of cylinder distortions are often described as unpredictable and independent of specific activities. In contrast, symptoms caused by triggerbands, continuum distortions, or folding distortions can usually be more easily controlled by patients through the avoidance of certain activities.

Response to medications and physical measures:

- Steroid-containing medications can have a positive effect on continuum distortions and triggerbands. Non-steroidal anti-inflammatory drugs (NSAIDs) primarily act on folding distortions and, to a lesser extent, on triggerbands and continuum distortions. Cylinder distortions usually respond inadequately to various analgesics, even at high doses.
- Heat can, at least temporarily, relieve the symptoms of a tectonic fixation or a chronic triggerband. In contrast, especially in the case of cylinder distortions and triggerbands—particularly following their treatment—heat applications can intensify pain.
- Muscle stimulation through electrotherapy can, at least temporarily, reduce the symptoms of cylinder distortions.

In conclusion, it should be noted that symptoms may change during the course of therapy. Therefore, it is important to continuously analyze the patient's symptoms and, if necessary, adjust the treatment to the altered symptomatology.

3.3 Objective Findings

The examination focuses on

- the assessment of active range of motion,
- visual and palpatory findings of the symptomatic area, and
- manual pain provocation (fig. 3.6).

3.3.1 Active Range of Motion Testing

Testing mobility is not only important for diagnosis, all six fascial distortions can impair mobility in different ways, as described. Improved active mobility is also an important indicator of successful treatment and is readily apparent to both the patient and the therapist (in contrast to pain, which is subjectively perceived by the patient and can only be objectified or measured to a limited extent).

For range of motion testing, tests are used in which the patient independently moves the affected body region into the problematic range of motion. Typaldos used simple movements that could be performed spontaneously

and without aids. The aim is to identify typical patterns of restriction in patients with fascial distortions.

As a rule, these active tests are sufficient for FDM diagnosis. Additional passive examination of mobility, in which the therapist performs the movements on the patient, is not necessary, as it does not provide further clues to individual fascial distortions. Only a tectonic fixation can, in certain cases, be identified by passively restricted mobility with a firm end stop. Passive range of motion testing can also be helpful for clarifying symptoms from a conventional medical perspective.

3.3.1.1 Key Test Movements

In practice, the following active movement tests with and without loading have proven effective, and instructions for the patient are generally straightforward. In addition to these standard tests, further test movements—such as those specific to a particular sport—may be used in individual cases to determine the patient's functional limitation as precisely as possible.

Neck:

- Flexion ("Bring your chin to your chest")
- Extension ("Stretch the tip of your nose toward the ceiling")
- Rotation to the right/left ("Look over your right/left shoulder")
- Lateral flexion to the right/left ("Bring your ear to your shoulder")
- Additionally: shoulder range of motion testing

Test grid	TB	HTP	CD	uFD	rFD	CyD	TF
Typical pain can be triggered during palpation	●	●	●				
Objectifiable movement restriction possible	●	●	●	1)	● 1)	●	●
Palpable tissue changes	●	●	●				●

1) as a rule, predominantly end-range restriction of movement with the exception of folding distortions in the area of the interosseous membranes and the muscle septa

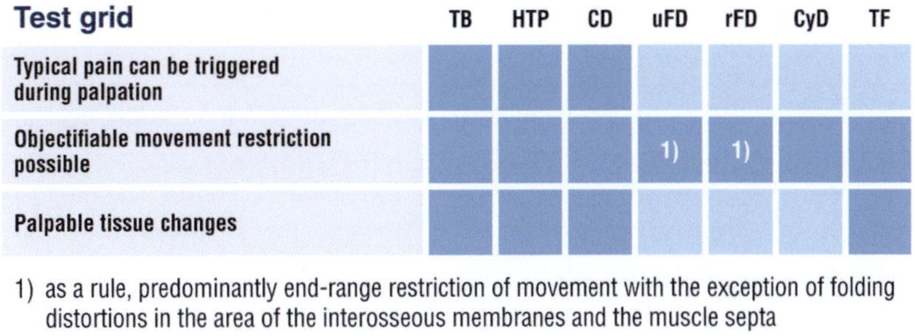

Fig. 3.6   Test grid. (© Anker 2022)

Shoulder:

- Abduction in the frontal plane ("With both arms straight, lift them sideways at the same time until your upper arms touch your ears")
- External rotation ("Clasp both hands behind your neck and push both elbows backward")
- Internal rotation ("Place the fingertips of one hand as high as possible on your back, then compare to the other hand")
- Adduction ("Touch your opposite shoulder with your hand")
- Flexion ("Stretch your arms forward as far as possible and lift them upward")
- Support ("Push off or support yourself with your hand from a seated position ")
- Lifting a weight
- Additionally: neck range of motion testing

Elbow:

- Flexion ("Touch your same-side shoulder with your fingertips")
- Extension ("Fully straighten your elbow")
- Pronation and supination of the forearm ("Bend your elbow to 90 degrees and keep it close to your torso, then rotate your forearm inward and outward as far as possible")
- Support ("Push off from a seated position with your hand and straightened elbow")
- Additionally: range of motion testing of the shoulder, neck, and hand

Hand:

- Flexion ("Touch forearm with fingertips")
- Extension ("Extend the hand as far as possible")
- Ulnar and radial abduction ("Move the little finger or thumb as far as possible toward the forearm without flexing or extending the hand")
- Support ("Push off from a seated position with a bent hand and extended elbow")
- Wringing out a towel
- Additionally: assessment of shoulder and elbow movement

Fingers:

- Flexion ("Make a fist")
- Extension ("Extend and straighten the fingers as much as possible")
- Abduction and adduction of the fingers ("Spread the fingers as far apart as possible or press them together as much as possible")
- Opposition and reposition of the thumb ("Touch the base of the little finger with the tip of the thumb or abduct and extend the thumb as much as possible")
- Support ("Push off from a seated position with extended fingers and a bent hand")
- Additionally: assessment of hand and elbow movement

Lower back:

- Flexion ("Touch the floor with your fingertips/palm")
- Extension ("Lean back as far as possible and look at the ceiling")
- Lateral flexion to the right/left ("Slide the middle finger along the side seam of the pants toward the toes")
- Rotation while sitting ("Rotate the upper body as far as possible to the right or left")
- Lifting a (heavy) object
- Additionally: assessment of hip movement

Mid-back and chest:

- Deep inhalation and exhalation
- Additionally: assessment of lower back movement (preferably in a seated position), neck, and shoulder

Hip:

- Flexion ("While standing, pull the knee toward the chest")
- Extension ("While standing, pull the heel toward the buttocks with the hand while extending the groin")
- Deep squat with legs more or less abducted
- Half-kneeling, single-leg stance, hopping on one leg or on both legs

- Additionally: assessment of lower back and knee movement, assessment of gait pattern

Knee:

- Flexion ("While standing, pull the heel toward the buttocks with the hand while extending the groin")
- Extension ("While standing, fully extend the knee")
- Additionally: assessment of ankle, foot, and hip movement

Ankle and foot:

- Extension ("Pull the dorsum of the foot toward the shin")
- Flexion ("Flex the toes and extend the dorsum of the foot")
- Inversion and eversion ("Rotate the soles of the feet toward each other or away from each other")
- Deep squat, single-leg stance, hopping on one leg or on both legs
- Assessment of gait pattern (is weight-bearing possible? Stepping length and heel-to-toe roll compared side to side? Compensatory movements?)
- Walking on tiptoes, on heels, on the outer and inner edges of the foot
- Additionally: assessment of knee movement

Toes:

- Flexion ("Curl the toes as much as possible")
- Extension ("Extend the toes as much as possible")
- Additionally: assessment of ankle and foot movement

Jaw:

- Abduction ("Open the mouth as wide as possible")
- Adduction ("Close the mouth and press teeth together")
- Protrusion/retrusion ("Move the lower jaw forward/backward")

- Laterotrusion: ("Relax the lower jaw and move it to the right/left")

3.3.1.2 Assessment Criteria for Movement Examination

- *Range of motion*
  The patient is asked to perform the respective movement to the maximum, possibly repeatedly. The range of motion can be determined by measuring the distance to reference points on the patient's body or in the room, with a measuring tape. Alternatively, the use of a goniometer is recommended.
- *Movement quality and compensatory movements*
  Good movement quality is characterized by smooth, rapid, and purposeful motion. Fascial distortions can impair this. However, it is difficult to attribute specific distortions to individual abnormalities such as jerky movements or movement slowing.
  In contrast, certain compensatory movements, such as lifting the arm forward in the case of restricted shoulder abduction, can indeed be assigned (in this case to a tectonic fixation of the shoulder).
- *Load tolerance*
  When movements are performed repeatedly, at full speed, or under load, distortions may become apparent that would otherwise remain hidden. Depending on the situation, the patient may, for example, be asked to move a weight in order to deliberately provoke symptoms and make the functional problem more clearly identifiable.

3.3.2 Visual Findings in the Area of Complaint

Visual diagnosis, aside from the interpretation of body language and movement assessment, plays a subordinate role in FDM diagnosis. Fascial distortions generally do not lead to externally visible changes such as skin discoloration or deformities. Even if such deviations are visible after an injury, for example, they usually cannot be directly attributed to specific fascial distortions.

However, interpreting the presence of swelling can be helpful. For example, subtle joint swelling may indicate a folding distortion. In contrast, large swellings, such as a joint effusion, cannot be clearly assigned to a specific type of distortion. Localized tissue swelling is more likely to be associated with triggerbands, continuum distortions, or cylinder distortions.

Hematomas can lead to adhesions in the tissue, which in turn are related to triggerbands. However, whether treatment using the triggerband technique is indicated should be decided based on the patient's symptoms, as hematomas often have no impact on bodily functions.

3.3.3　Palpatory Findings in the Area of Complaint

The significance of palpatory findings in FDM diagnosis also differs from that in conventional medical diagnostics. For example, a marked increase in tissue temperature or the detection of muscular guarding can provide clues for conventional medical diagnoses, whereas this information cannot be interpreted as direct evidence of specific fascial distortions.

Even though FDM diagnosis is fundamentally based on the patient's subjective perception, palpatory findings can be helpful. On the one hand, they allow for more precise differentiation of individual fascial distortions and their subtypes. On the other hand, palpatory findings play an important role in selecting the treatment technique according to the Typaldos method. The therapeutic forces applied must be adjusted according to the palpatory quality of the distortion, as certain deformations only respond to specifically tailored maneuvers (fig. 3.6).

In his textbooks, Typaldos describes various palpable tissue qualities in connection with the six fascial distortions. This information can be integrated into the diagnosis. However, it should not lead to relativizing the patient's subjective perception, as this is not in line with the FDM perspective. It is therefore important that the location of the palpable tissue change matches the patient's description.

- A triggerband may feel like
  - a twisted band, one to five millimeters wide,
  - small crumbs between muscle layers,
  - a firm nodule similar to a knotted rubber band,
  - soft peas,
  - grains of salt in the tissue (especially in the area of the hands, feet, and skull), or
  - wavy folds in the area of joints (see sect. 2.1.3, fig. 2.5).
- Herniated triggerpoints range in size from a raisin to a small almond. The consistency varies from jelly-like to firm/elastic.
- Typaldos describes continuum distortions as at most one to two millimeters in size. Everted continuum distortions may be perceived as small, firm roughness, while inverted continuum distortions may be felt as small depressions in the transition zone.
- Typaldos does not assign a specific palpatory finding to folding distortions, but he does describe increased tension in the surrounding tissue. The same applies to cylinder distortions.
- Tectonic fixations may be perceived as tissue densification and stiffness during passive movement testing.

3.3.4　Pain Provocation

Individual fascial distortions respond to manual pressure with pain (fig. 3.6). It is crucial that the symptoms familiar to the patient can be elicited by this provocation and that they fit the pattern of the respective FDM working hypothesis.

This must be distinguished from general pressure sensitivity. This should be interpreted with caution, as not every painful spot on the body corresponds to the location of a fascial distortion.

In principle, pressing along the course of a triggerband, on a herniated triggerpoint, or on a continuum distortion elicits characteristic pain that the patient recognizes. In contrast, with folding distortions and tectonic fixations, pain cannot be provoked by manual pressure. The same applies to cylinder distortions, in which, in rare cases, a form of touch sensitivity may be present, but this should not be misinterpreted as pressure sensitivity.

3.3.5 Imaging Techniques and Laboratory Findings

To date, fascial distortions cannot be visualized using standard imaging diagnostic techniques such as X-ray, magnetic resonance imaging, or ultrasound, even though Typaldos did not rule out such a possibility. The same applies to laboratory tests. Analysis of blood, urine, and other body fluids currently does not allow any conclusions to be drawn about fascial deformations.

The significance of these technical procedures lies primarily in their value for differential diagnostic clarification and for assessing whether there are contraindications to treatment according to the Typaldos method or whether treatment with other medical procedures appears more promising. It is therefore sensible to review existing findings or, in individual cases, to initiate further investigations in order to choose the best possible therapy for the patient.

3.4 Interpretation of Body Language

FDM captures body language particularly in the form of typical conscious and unconscious movements or postures that indicate specific fascial distortions. In general, this includes gesturing with hands and fingers, adopting protective postures, or forms of intuitive self-treatment. Specifically, it mainly refers to pointing gestures with which patients localize complaints on their own bodies and indicate information regarding the type of fascial deformation (fig. 3.7a to f).

Background Information
In communication research, the term body language also includes facial expressions and various, sometimes culture-dependent, behaviors. The interpretation of the patient's facial expressions plays little role in FDM diagnosis, apart from the typical distortion of facial features in pain. For monitoring the success of treatment, relaxation of the facial features is a useful sign.

3.4.1 Body Language and Proprioception

The interpretation of body language and its integration into diagnosis and therapy has shaped the Fascial Distortion Model from its development to its current application in clinical practice. Typaldos recognized the significance of body language through the observation that patients, while verbally describing their complaints, used supportive gestures. He found that this form of non-verbal communication occurred regularly and followed similar patterns: some patients pressed their fingers on their bodies, others indicated linear pathways, or massaged or mobilized themselves. He also recognized that different categories of gestures could be distinguished. On the one hand, patients used this body language to indicate the location of their individual complaints, and on the other hand, as a form of unconscious self-treatment.

He investigated the causes of this phenomenon. However, there appeared to be no connection between the observable gestures and specific anatomical structures such as nerves, muscles, or bones, which, from the perspective of conventional medicine, would be considered the source of the complaints. Hand signs did not provide any information that could be utilized in conventional medical terms. However, Typaldos discovered correlations between typical gestures, specific complaint patterns, and effective treatment approaches, independent of common diagnoses in conventional medicine. As a result, he developed a system of independent complaint patterns based

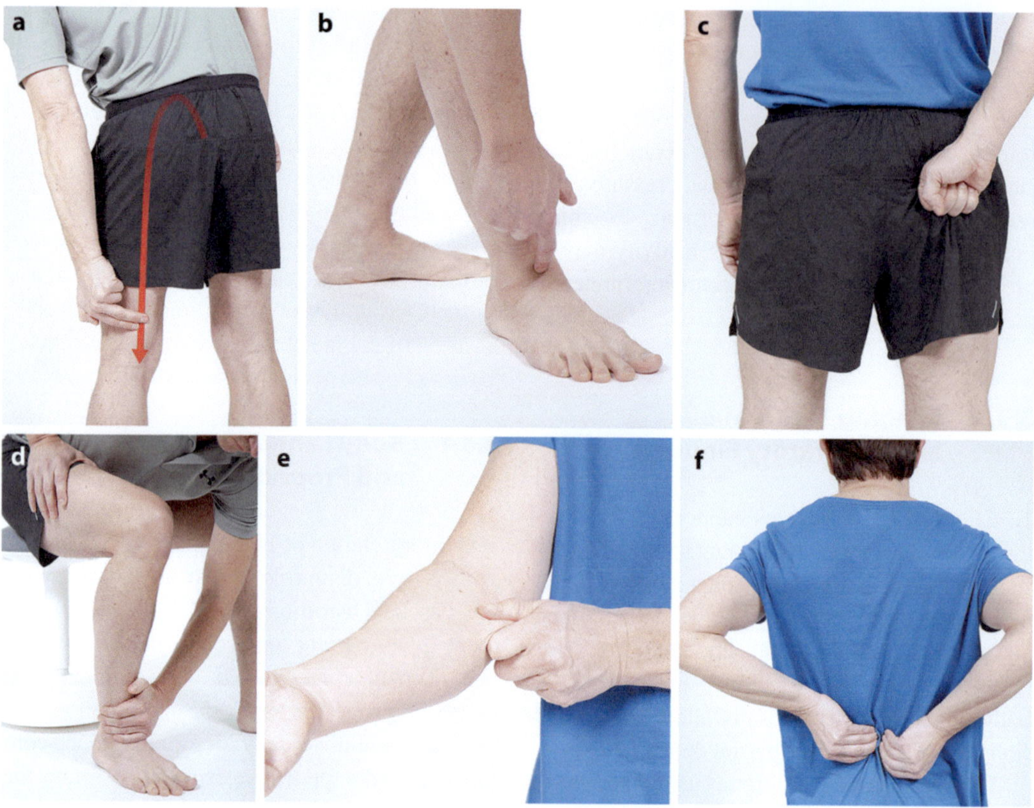

Fig. 3.7 Typical body language for the six fascial distortions. Gestures for a posterior thigh triggerband (**a**). Gesture for a continuum distortion at the anterior ankle, the so-called AACD (**b**). Body language for a herniated triggerpoint at the buttock, bullseye HTP (**c**). Typical hand position as an indication of a folding distortion at the lower leg or ankle (**d**). Pinching the soft tissues of the elbow as an indication of a cylinder distortion (**e**). Pressing with the fingers in the center of the back as a typical gesture for a tectonic fixation (**f**). (© Anker 2022)

on fascial distortions, which integrated body language as a criterion for assessment and treatment.

Background Information
Typaldos considers the continuous fascia to be a tension receptor that involves all structures of the body. The fascia provides information about changes in tension, which are integrated in the central nervous system and support the patient's self-perception. From this, the hypothesis is derived that body language reflects tension information from within the patient's body. From the perspective of the Fascial Distortion Model, its interpretation makes it possible to use the patient's proprioception for the diagnosis of fascial deformations. This opens up an insight into the patient's individual problem, shaped by their own perception, which can neither be replaced by technical diagnostic means nor by a detailed medical history.

As described in the first chapter, fascia plays a central role in proprioception, nociception, and interoception (see 1.1.1.1). To what extent body language reflects these mechanisms, however, has not yet been clearly demonstrated. In contrast, the reliability of interpreting body language does seem to be present. Different therapists reliably interpret the gestures presented by patients [1, 2].

3.4.2   Gesture Vocabulary of the Fascial Distortion Model

The interpretation of body language allows conclusions to be drawn about the type and location of specific fascial distortions and, in certain cases, facilitates the selection of an effective treatment technique for the respective deformation.

Each fascial distortion can be assigned a specific body language pattern. These patterns are universal, as they relate to the human body, and can be observed across a wide range of cultures. In conventional medical diagnosis, these patterns have no points of reference, which is why conventional medicine pays little attention to body language.

- Triggerbands: dynamic stroking with the fingertips along a linear pathway.
- Herniated triggerpoints: pressing with several fingers, the thumb, or the knuckles into the protrusion area.
- Continuum distortions: pointing with the fingertip at a spot (applies to both everted and inverted continuum distortions).
- Folding distortions: placing the hand on the affected area or grasping a joint (applies to both unfolding and refolding distortions).
  - Specifically for refolding distortions: stroking with fingers horizontally across the joint (according to Typaldos, about half of all patients with refolding distortions show this gesture).
  - Specifically for folding distortions in the area of the interosseous membrane: pushing several fingers between two parallel bones (additionally, deep rubbing may be visible) or grasping both bones.
  - Specifically for folding distortions of the muscle septa: pushing several fingers between two soft tissue areas or pulling on the soft tissues.
- Cylinder distortions: dynamic wiping, kneading, and rubbing with the fingers or the hand.
- Tectonic fixations: self-mobilization of a jointed area with the hands or through active movements.

3.4.3   The Practice of Interpreting Body Language

Body language occurs spontaneously and should be provoked by therapists as little as possible. It can be observed particularly well when the patient feels unobserved or is distracted (for example, during movement tests or treatment when symptoms are elicited).

The interpretation of body language is a continuous process that takes place throughout the entire diagnosis and treatment. Gestural language is a dynamic phenomenon, which often appears only for a brief moment and can change in expression according to the course of treatment. This is evident, for example, in chronic complaints, where the patient is initially unable to precisely localize the area of discomfort and the gestures used appear blurred and diffuse (comparable to the body language seen in cylinder distortions). However, the more chronicity can be reduced by resolving adhesions, the clearer and more precise the gestures presented by the patient become.

When analyzing the gestural signals that Typaldos describes as indicative of specific fascial distortions, two basic categories can be distinguished. FDM body language can be divided into non-verbal signs that are indicated either (1) with the fingertips or (2) with the surface of the hands and fingers. The pointing fingers or hands can (A) remain static on the skin or (B) move dynamically across the skin. These two distinctions (1–2 and A–B) can be helpful in interpreting body language (fig. 3.8). As already mentioned, it is often only brief moments in which patients communicate non-verbally in such a way that information relevant to the FDM diagnosis can be derived. In addition, patients repeatedly make gestures that are not visible to the therapist, e.g. when the patient and therapist are facing each other and the patient reaches for their back. Nevertheless, the therapist can at least see part of the gesture and, using the simple criteria (1–2 and A–B), can still interpret the gesture well.

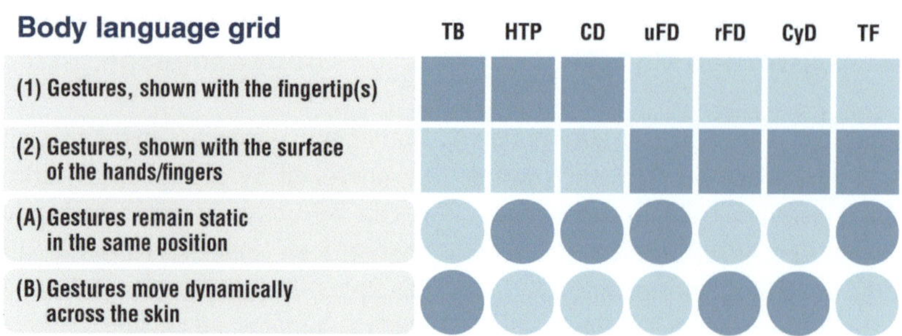

FDM body language can be divided into non-verbal signs that are indicated either **(1)** with the fingertips or **(2)** with the surface of the hands and fingers. The pointing fingers or hands can **(A)** remain static on the skin or **(B)** move dynamically across the skin. These two distinctions (**1-2** and **A-B**) can be helpful when interpreting body language

Fig. 3.8 Body language grid. (© Anker 2022)

In clinical practice, the following tips can facilitate the interpretation of body language and help maintain an overview during diagnosis:

- Body language is an indication of certain fascial distortions, but not every observable gesture can immediately be equated with the existence of a fascial distortion. It is necessary to establish a context between the body language, the subjective complaints, and their mechanism of injury. This also makes it easier to recognize the gestures that are relevant to the specific therapeutic situation.
- Body language can appear contradictory, for example, when patients gesture very strongly and therapists try to interpret every single sign. Repeated and targeted questioning by therapists about the location of symptoms can also be disadvantageous. This provokes gestures that provide more information about the location of symptoms than about fascial distortions. In addition, not all gestures that patients indicate can generally be deciphered or clearly assigned to specific fascial distortions.

In this context, it is advantageous to focus the diagnosis on the overall picture of the individual problem. In such cases, it is advisable to primarily interpret a specific part of the body language that occurs when the patient feels unobserved, or to wait for the moment when the patient intuitively and without prompting, presents body language.

- The interpretation of body language is an exceptional diagnostic tool, which most therapists quickly internalize once they become familiar with it. However, this can lead to this part of the FDM diagnosis being overemphasized and all therapeutic actions being made dependent on it.

In this context, it should be emphasized that body language does not determine whether certain fascial distortions can be treated. The reverse is also true: even if no body language is observable, fascial distortions can be diagnosed and treated based on anamnesis and examination.

3.4.4 Localization of Fascial Distortions Through Body Language

The FDM fundamentally assumes that body language indicates the location of the fascial distortion. Furthermore, there is usually a local correspondence between the fascial distortion and the respective symptoms. Therefore, therapy can usually be initiated at the site where the patient localizes the symptoms. (A typical example of this is a continuum distortion, in which the patient's gestures correspond with the relevant symptoms, the location of the distortion, and the site of local treatment).

However, the Fascial Distortion Model also describes the possibility that fascial distortions can have remote effects or, through impairment of fascial metabolism, can trigger diffuse symptoms. Consequently, therapists must distinguish between gestures that localize symptoms and those that indicate the site of the fascial distortion. This can mean: a fascial distortion isn't necessarily present everywhere the patient indicates a symptom through body language.

Correspondingly differentiated observations can also play a role during treatment. It may occur that after the correction of a fascial distortion, supposed additional distortions the patient had indicated with gestures disappear without treatment. At first glance, it appears as if some fascial distortions resolve without correction of the fascial architecture. However, such phenomena can also be explained by the fact that the localization of symptoms and fascial distortions cannot always be equated.

> **Practical Tip**
> The challenge of distinguishing between local effects of fascial distortions and remote effects can be managed with the following pragmatic approach:
>
> 1. The first instance should be the diagnosis according to all four diagnostic criteria. This helps avoid premature diagnostic conclusions and makes it much easier to classify the observed body language.
> 2. According to the working hypothesis, local treatment is started in accordance with the respective fascial distortion. The effect on the patient (and also on their body language) is observed.
> 3. Depending on the dynamic development during the course of therapy, two reactions can be distinguished:
>   - The course of therapy meets expectations. The local treatment approach is continued, or the location of treatment is adapted to the dynamic development of the body language.
>   - Therapeutic success does not occur or is insufficient. The diagnostic process must be revisited. The interpretation of gestures temporarily takes a back seat, and the analysis of information from the patient's history and examination determines the diagnostic process. Through this reorientation, body language often gains clarity and completes a coherent hypothesis.

3.4.5 Adjustment of Treatment Based on Body Language

As previously mentioned, body language can provide clues for distortion correction. Just as the stroking finger movement in the body language of a triggerband, treatment with the triggerband technique also involves a forceful stroking along the same pathway. Similar correlations can be observed with the herniated triggerpoint, continuum distortion, and cylinder distortion, and to some extent with the folding distortion.

Body language can be interpreted as a rudimentary form of self-treatment. Especially in the treatment of acute injuries, the patient's body awareness appears to be so heightened that a form of treatment can be directly derived from the observable body language. This should not be misunderstood as a recommendation to downplay other diagnostic criteria. The intention here is merely to emphasize the wealth of information that can be derived from gestures for therapy.

The following correlations can be observed:

- *Triggerbands*
  - Direction of the gesture:
    In practice, better treatment outcomes are observed when the correction is performed in accordance with the direction of the body language.
  - Depth of the gesture (as an indication of tissue localization):
    Depending on the tissue depth of the triggerband, patients use more or less pressure

to perform stroking movement with their fingertips. Accordingly, palpation and the force applied for correction can be adjusted.

- Position or posture in which the body language is displayed:
  Gestures are often displayed in a specific position or posture. This may indicate increased pre-load of the triggerband, which is why this position is also suitable for treatment.

- *Herniated triggerpoints*
  Here, too, we observe gestures that indicate different tissue depths. It may be beneficial to adapt palpation and treatment to this specific body language.

- *Continuum distortions*
  Patients typically use a fingertip to indicate the deformation. Often, a specific body position is also suggested in which the continuum distortion causes symptoms. Generally, treatment in this position is advantageous if precise palpation is possible. Furthermore, it has been observed that when several continuum distortions are present in one area, patients indicate the distortions with all five fingertips simultaneously.

- *Folding distortions*
  In addition to the hand gesture, relieving body postures are often visible, which, depending on the subtype of the folding distortion, lead to traction or compression in the affected area. This ranges from unloading a leg in unfolding distortion of the knee to deliberately supporting oneself on the elbow in refolding distortion of the shoulder. These behaviors can be incorporated into the diagnosis and treatment of folding distortions. Moreover, such behaviors provide a visible sign of treatment success, as they disappear after successful correction of the fascial distortion.

- *Cylinder distortions*
  Various types of body language have been described, which can be interpreted as indications of the most efficient treatment approach as follows:

  - The broader the gesture, the more effective are broad treatment techniques.
  - A kneading or pinching gesture may indicate a stuck and strongly constricting cylinder distortion.
  - A diffuse gesture may possibly be interpreted as an indication of the jumping pain phenomenon typical of a cylinder distortion.

- *Tectonic fixations*
  Body language related to tectonic fixations can be interpreted less specifically. In many cases, the diagnosis of this distortion is based more on the anamnesis and objective testing than on the interpretation of gestures. Exceptions are certain body regions in which Typaldos describes typical behaviors: for example, it is an indication of a tectonic fixation of the shoulder if, when abducting the arm laterally, the patient increasingly lifts it forward instead of moving the arm in a straight line overhead. In the case of a tectonic fixation in the lower back or hip region, patients support themselves with both hands on their pelvis, sometimes additionally rotating the upper body to the right and left or pressing both hands into the center of the lower back.

3.5   The Role of The Patient

The way in which the Fascial Distortion Model analyzes and interprets complaints using the four diagnostic criteria also changes the role of patients. They are experts on their own complaints and are therefore integrally involved in the process of diagnosis and treatment.

Background Information
When Typaldos discovered and successfully corrected the first triggerband in 1991, he did so at the request and guidance of a patient. She was able to describe in detail where her complaints were located, how they felt, and which

treatment method seemed promising from her perspective. Although Typaldos was initially skeptical as to whether a patient without medical knowledge could accurately assess the situation, he followed her description and was subsequently able to sustainably resolve her problem.

Based on this event, Typaldos realized that the subjective perception of pain and functional limitation is much more than just the individual experience of an impairment. Rather, the symptoms patients describe verbally and nonverbally can be interpreted as direct indications of fascial distortions, and therefore point to effective treatment methods. This fundamentally changed his view of the patient's role. The analysis and integration of a patient's subjective perception, their ideas about the cause of the complaints, and how these could be resolved, subsequently became a driving force in the development of the Fascial Distortion Model. In that sense, many of Typaldos' patients had a significant influence on the FDM.

Although this approach may seem unconventional in today's often highly technological and evidence-based medicine, and appears to turn the hierarchy between the therapist as the expert and the patient as the recipient of treatment on its head in clinical practice, it offers tangible advantages. Apart from the appreciation it shows to the patient, it primarily eliminates a blind spot in modern medicine—namely, recognizing the patient's role as an expert on their complaints, and utilizing their knowledge for treatment.

3.5.1 Patients as Experts on Their Complaints

The focus of medicine on objective and measurable findings is understandable given the prevailing biomedical model, but it tends to downplay the individual perception of subjective complaints. Not infrequently, patients undergo surgery or are treated with medication solely based on their X-ray images and not on the overall clinical picture. In contrast, the Fascial Distortion Model bases its diagnostics primarily on the patient's verbal and nonverbal description of the problem.

All of us are familiar with the situation: when in pain, we instinctively treat ourselves by massaging, pressing, or stretching the affected tissue. We also often have a precise idea of what triggered the complaints and whether they are severe enough to require medical treatment, or if home remedies or simply waiting will suffice. Although this instinctive behavior does not always lead to the desired result, it is remarkable that these phenomena are hardly considered in conventional medical diagnostics and therapy. In contrast, imaging techniques and laboratory findings are given great importance, even though they often do not significantly influence the choice of optimal treatment strategy, but rather serve to rule out serious pathologies.

After a medical examination, there are usually two possibilities in practice: either the complaints can be attributed, in line with the patient's clinical picture, to a conventionally defined diagnosis, or the pattern of complaints cannot be clearly classified. In the first case, a logical treatment can be derived; in the second, nonspecific therapies are often used, or the patient is sent home without a diagnosis, supposedly healthy. Integrating and utilizing the patient's perception has the advantage, in both cases, of capturing the symptomatology more precisely. In the first case, this expands the medical diagnosis and helps select an optimally tailored treatment strategy. In the second case, using the patient's subjective perception makes it possible to create a practical and verifiable concept of the complaint causes when this is not possible from a conventional medical perspective.

The FDM recognizes that the patient is the expert on their own complaints. Their verbal description of the problems and their intuitive behavior in response to those complaints are irreplaceable pieces of information that, together with other clinical findings, enable an FDM diagnosis.

3.5.2 Definition of Treatment Goals

The Fascial Distortion Model and the Typaldos Method focus on the *restoration of functional limitations.* The patient describes these during the anamnesis, not only by reporting symptoms but also by describing the activities triggering the symptoms. From this, a functional treatment goal can be derived.

It is important that the patient formulates the treatment goal as concretely as possible. General pain relief is often too vague and, in some cases, not achievable, even if it's the desired outcome. It is better to assess the effectiveness of a treatment based on everyday activities that are important to the patient. Some patients are initially surprised when their therapist asks them to describe in detail what a successful therapeutic outcome would look like for them. However, this is important to a patient's involvement in the therapy process.

> **Background Information**
> The FDM accepts the patient's treatment goals, even if these seem difficult or impossible to achieve from a conventional medical perspective. The unwavering focus on the patient's functionality and their perception of the problem puts the FDM and the therapist to the test. In contrast to the common assumption that various causes of complaints, such as degenerative processes, are irreversible and that the patient must therefore accept certain complaints, the FDM assumes the plasticity of the fascia. It emphasizes the possibility that fascial distortions and their symptoms can, in principle, be corrected at any time. The focus of conventional medicine on anatomical-structural changes instead of the patient's functional capacity can, however, lead to manual treatment strategies appearing pointless and therapists becoming discouraged in cases of acute injuries or complex chronic problems. Here, the FDM goes a step further.

3.5.3 Assessment of Treatment Success

Fascial distortions being corrected will lead to an immediate functional improvement that can be clearly perceived by both the patient and the therapist. In particular, the patient's assessment of the treatment outcome is crucial, as they, being the expert on their complaints, can best judge the extent of improvement. Although experienced therapists can detect positive changes in functionality through various, often subtle, parameters, we must accept that complaints are perceived individually, and that the treatment goal is to improve the patient's situation. In addition, as therapists, we must acknowledge that after a treatment session, we are no longer confronted with the patient's symptoms, but the patient (and their environment) certainly is. It is therefore difficult to understand why, as a rule, it is the therapist who is called upon to assess the effectiveness of a therapy instead of the patient.

References

1. Anker S (2011) Interrater reliability in evaluating the body language based on the fascial distortion model (FDM) [thesis]. Vienna School of Osteopathy, Danube University Krems—Centre for Traditional Chinese Medicine and Complementary Medicine, Vienna
2. Stechmann K (2011) Interrater-reliability of distortion-classification using body language within the fascial distortion model (FDM) [thesis]. University of Applied Science and Arts, Hildesheim

Based on the idea of correcting fascial distortions according to their individual formation and development, Typaldos came up with treatment concepts for each of the six deformations. He tested their effectiveness and practicality in clinical practice and optimized them until they met his own standards and those of the patients being treated. Over time, this led to the development of a repertoire of proven manual techniques and therapeutic measures, which Typaldos summarized under the term Typaldos Manual Therapy (TMT). After his death in 2006, the term "Typaldos method" became more common.

Overall, the state of knowledge established by Typaldos regarding the treatment of fascial distortions at the time of his death remains valid today, and has only been expanded in certain details. For this reason, the curriculum of the European Fascial Distortion Model Association (EFDMA) for the training in "FDM and Typaldos method" is fundamentally based on these therapeutic concepts.

The second part of this book now addresses these treatment approaches. First, the course of treatment according to the Typaldos method is explained, and the characteristic elements of the correction of fascial distortions are described. Subsequently, the fundamental maneuvers and techniques for each of the six fascial distortions and their subtypes are discussed.

Typaldos Method 4

The goal of the Typaldos method is to correct fascial distortions through mechanotherapeutic means. This principally involves the application of therapeutic manipulations and the use of mechanically acting therapeutic devices.

Both static and dynamic pressure or traction techniques are used on the soft tissues, as well as manual techniques that induce traction, compression, or gliding movements in jointed areas. Impulse manipulation plays a special role, particularly for the treatment of folding distortions and tectonic fixations.

The triggerband technique, the herniated triggerpoint technique, the continuum technique, and the techniques for correcting cylinder distortions are typical, standardized procedures of the Typaldos method. In contrast, the correction of folding distortions and tectonic fixations is based on treatment maneuvers already established in manual therapy, which are specifically adapted for the treatment of these distortions.

The techniques of the Typaldos method correct fascial distortions in a direct manner. They are oriented toward reversing the deformation of the tissue according to the respective mechanism of injury. For this, a vector specific to each distortion is necessary, the application of which leads to the disappearance of the fascial distortion.

A key term in the treatment of fascial distortions is the "release," a yielding of the tissue as a result of the applied manual technique. This treatment response is associated with many techniques of the Typaldos method and enables the precise adjustment of the applied vectors to the patients. A release confirms the effectiveness of a manual technique, but does not necessarily correlate with the resolution of the patient's problem.

According to the basic principles of the Fascial Distortion Model, any therapeutic procedure can be examined for its potential corrective effect on fascial distortions, even if it is not anchored in the Typaldos method. This also applies to therapeutic approaches that, at first glance, are not associated with a mechanical effect on the body (for example, the FDM describes a mechanical effect of certain pharmacological therapies).

4.1 Indications and Contraindications

In principle, the use of the Typaldos method is indicated when patients experience pain or loss of function that can be explained by the Fascial Distortion Model. The goal is to resolve these complaints as immediately, sustainably, and objectively as possible.

The Typaldos method has proven effective particularly for complaints of the musculoskeletal system. Originally, it was soft tissue injuries such as strains or sprains and their nonspecific treatment in medical practice that motivated Typaldos to develop new treatment concepts. Accordingly, the FDM and the Typaldos method were successfully tested from the outset in the field of acute orthopedics. In particular, *complaints resulting from physical trauma or overuse* can often be reduced with just a few manual techniques, making immobilization, pharmacological treatments, or, in some cases, even surgical interventions unnecessary.

The Typaldos method can also be advantageous in the treatment of *chronic, persistent complaints* of the musculoskeletal system, for example after a long-standing injury. The perspective of chronicity as a result of fascial adhesions opens up treatment options for a range of problems which are hardly amenable to sustainable therapy from a conventional medical standpoint.

Good results have also been observed in *postoperative rehabilitation.* The Typaldos method's focus on functional restoration helps shorten rehabilitation times and accelerate the return to everyday activities.

The Typaldos method can be applied in the field of neurology as well. *Symptoms such as numbness, muscle weakness, or coordination disorders* can be interpreted by the FDM as the result of certain fascial distortions. This expands the conventional, neurologically oriented understanding of such symptoms, and opens up possibilities for resolving these complaints through manual therapy.

> **Background Information**
> In his medical practice, Typaldos also treated patients with complaints involving internal organs using manual methods. He described good results in cases of renal or biliary colic or certain types of abdominal pain. He postulated theoretical concepts for the treatment of asthma or cardiological diseases, was convinced that the FDM could be used successfully in these areas in the future, and that new therapeutic concepts could be developed from its

> principles. However, since his death, there have been no significant advances in this field, and the Typaldos method has been used almost exclusively for the treatment of the musculoskeletal system.

However, there are contraindications and limitations for the use of the Typaldos method and for the application of certain manual techniques.

The most important general contraindication is the lack of patient consent for the treatment.

This is important because some techniques of the Typaldos method are performed with strong, sometimes painful pressure on the tissue, or involve manipulation techniques using thrust. Side effects such as hematomas, muscle pain, or autonomic symptoms may occur temporarily. Therefore, the patient must be informed in advance about such treatment effects so that they can decide for or against the treatment or the use of specific techniques. If the patient does not understand this information (such as in the case of patients lacking legal capacity), the use of the method should be reconsidered. In addition, the therapist must independently assess whether the patient can tolerate potential side effects in view of their general condition.

> **Background Information**
> No form of manual therapy can completely rule out the possibility that serious medical problems (such as bone fractures or the dislodgement of blood clots) may occur as a result of certain manual techniques. Although such side effects are very rare, any risk to the patient must be considered by the therapist. The therapist must weigh which techniques can be safely used with any given patient in specific situations. This assessment is based on medical criteria as well as a detailed understanding of the full range of Typaldos method techniques.

Another general contraindication is the *lack of explainability of the symptoms* by the FDM or *insufficient medical evaluation* prior to treatment. Although the FDM provides an independent explanatory model for pain and functional limitations, this does not automatically mean that conventional considerations regarding the cause of complaints are irrelevant in individual cases. Typaldos described that his method could replace existing therapeutic concepts in certain cases, because it was more effective. In other cases, the Typaldos method is used complementary to conventional medical treatment, as it can address the symptoms but not their underlying cause. For example, in rheumatic diseases, functional improvements can be achieved. However, the fundamental rheumatic problem cannot be corrected with the Typaldos method.

Background Information
In clinical practice, patterns of complaints regularly occur that are inadequately explained from a conventional medical perspective. For Typaldos, these situations were predestined for analysis according to the Fascial Distortion Model, in order to develop new treatment concepts. However, this must be distinguished from the use of the Typaldos method based on insufficient medical knowledge and the resulting misjudgment of the problem.

A number of pre-existing conditions or physical states can be contraindications for manual therapy in general. They may also limit the use of certain techniques of the Typaldos method in the affected region, as their mechanical forces may pose incalculable risks for the patient. The following list of medical diagnoses serves as a guideline for cases in which caution should always be exercised:

- Known aneurysms
- Tumor diseases and their treatment
- History of stroke
- Vasculitis or vascular occlusions

- Severe cardiovascular diseases
- Generalized infections and inflammations
- Unclarified fractures or osteoporosis
- Open wounds, burns, fresh scars in the treatment area, as well as conditions that generally reduce the resilience of the skin and bodily tissues
- Pregnancy (especially up to the 4th month of pregnancy)
- Neuropathies
- Connective tissue diseases
- Mental illnesses
- Use of high-dose pain medications (especially corticosteroids)
- General state of weakness

(Contraindications for specific manual techniques are further described in the respective chapters on treatment techniques.)

Background Information
The way in which the Typaldos method is applied in practice depends, not least, on the *profession of the therapist*. Typaldos aimed to establish the FDM in medical practice. He therefore specifically addressed physicians in his teaching, as their professional training and legal status made them particularly suited to implement a novel treatment concept in their clinical practice.

After his death, this focus largely dissolved. Today, it is especially manual therapists, even those without a medical background, who are interested in training in FDM and the Typaldos method. Therefore, professional legal issues may need to be considered to determine who is permitted to apply these treatment techniques, and in what form. (This applies, for example, to the area of thrust manipulations in the cervical region, which are firmly anchored in the Typaldos method. However, from a legal perspective, not every non-medical professional group is unconditionally permitted to perform them).

4.2 Diagnostic Process and Treatment of Fascial Distortions

The Typaldos method describes a therapeutic process in which diagnosis and treatment are closely intertwined. This means that the diagnosis of fascial distortions is not a process that is completed prior to treatment or can be completely separated from it. Rather, the therapeutic process can be described as a dynamic procedure in which diagnosis and treatment mutually influence each other. The FDM diagnosis serves as a case-specific, adaptable guideline for treatment with the Typaldos method, not as a preliminary determination of a medically recognized pathology (fig. 4.1).

The clinical practice of the Typaldos method proceeds in three steps, which are repeated until the optimal treatment outcome is achieved:

- Analysis of the individual symptoms and functional impairments based on the Fascial Distortion Model
- Treatment of the underlying fascial distortions using the Typaldos method
- Assessment of functional improvement

Prior to treatment, a *treatment goal* should be defined. It is advantageous to use specific functions, such as everyday movements or athletic activities, as benchmarks for improvement. For example, a treatment goal for a patient with painful restriction of movement in the shoulder may not only be to achieve general freedom from symptoms, but to demonstrate this during specific activities (e.g. lifting a weight overhead).

As described in the third chapter, it is fundamentally the patient's responsibility to define the treatment goal. The therapist, on the other

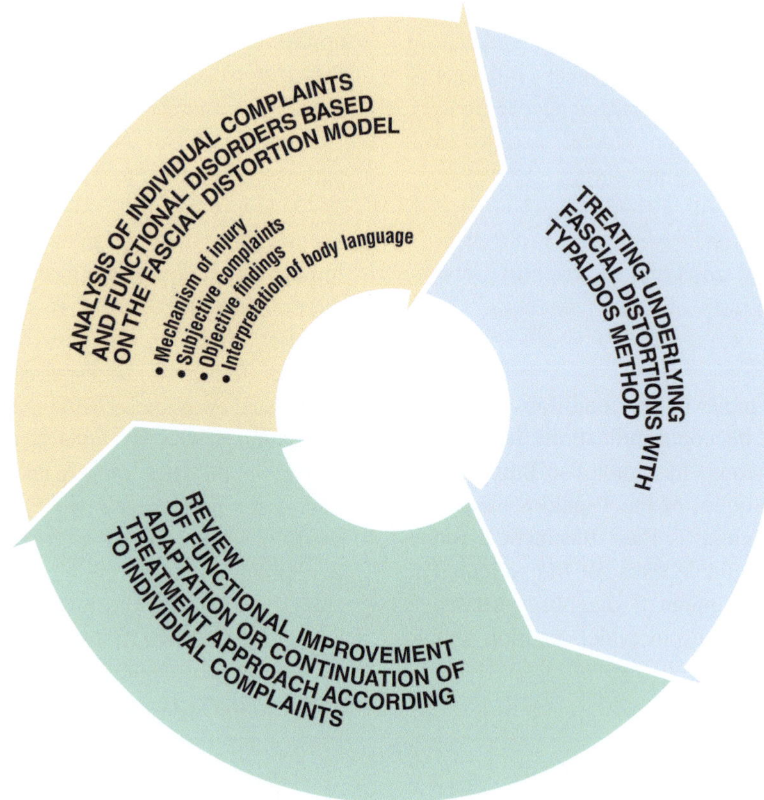

Fig. 4.1 Process of diagnosis and treatment in the Typaldos method. (© Anker 2022)

hand, must assess to what extent the patient can move closer to their goal through the use of the Typaldos method. In addition, the therapist defines intermediate goals based on their experience and knowledge, making it possible to evaluate the effectiveness of individual treatment steps.

Before manual treatment, the patient must be informed about the relevant treatment effects and side effects:

- Depending on the fascial distortions to be corrected, the treatment may be painful and may lead to skin redness or bruising.
- The release of adhesions in the context of a chronic problem may additionally lead to an initial worsening of symptoms and autonomic complaints after treatment. These may persist for several days.
- Certain manual techniques (such as impulse manipulations) carry specific risks, about which the patient should be informed.

After treatment, the following recommendations are helpful for patients:

- It is beneficial to actively move the treated area and to immediately integrate the achieved functional improvements into daily life and sports.
- The application of direct heat (such as hot baths) is not recommended for up to 48 hours after treatment, as it may worsen the aftereffects of the distortion correction. The use of cooling bandages or ice massages, on the other hand, may have a pain-relieving effect.
- If new, unexpected, or increasing symptoms occur, it is advisable to contact the treating therapist.

This process of diagnosis and treatment also assists in deciding whether the Typaldos method should be used as a stand-alone treatment or in combination with other therapies to achieve the treatment goal. If the Typaldos method results in a sustained improvement in function, conventional medical explanatory models and the associated therapeutic measures for the respective condition become less relevant. If this effect does not occur despite appropriate application of the treatment, then either the Typaldos method is insufficient for the specific condition, or the interpretation of the symptoms according to the FDM is not adequate in the individual case to arrive at an effective treatment strategy.

Background Information

In his textbooks, Typaldos describes, in addition to the fundamental interconnection of FDM diagnosis and fascial distortion correction, treatment protocols for specific symptom patterns in certain body regions. For example, he advocates a step-by-step guide for the treatment of ankle sprains (fig. 4.2) or for the correction of shoulder movement restrictions (see 6.1). In flowcharts, he outlines sequences of simple tests and the resulting treatment steps. These instructions are particularly helpful when therapists have little experience with clinical application. They illustrate Typaldos's intention to make his method easy to apply in medical practice, even when the time available for treating individual patients is limited. Even more important, however, is to understand the underlying concept. Every clinical presentation can be broken down into individual symptom components (e.g. specific types of pain or movement restrictions). These components can be corrected in a particular order that has proven effective in clinical practice. This allows the Typaldos method to be applied analytically and in a reproducible manner.

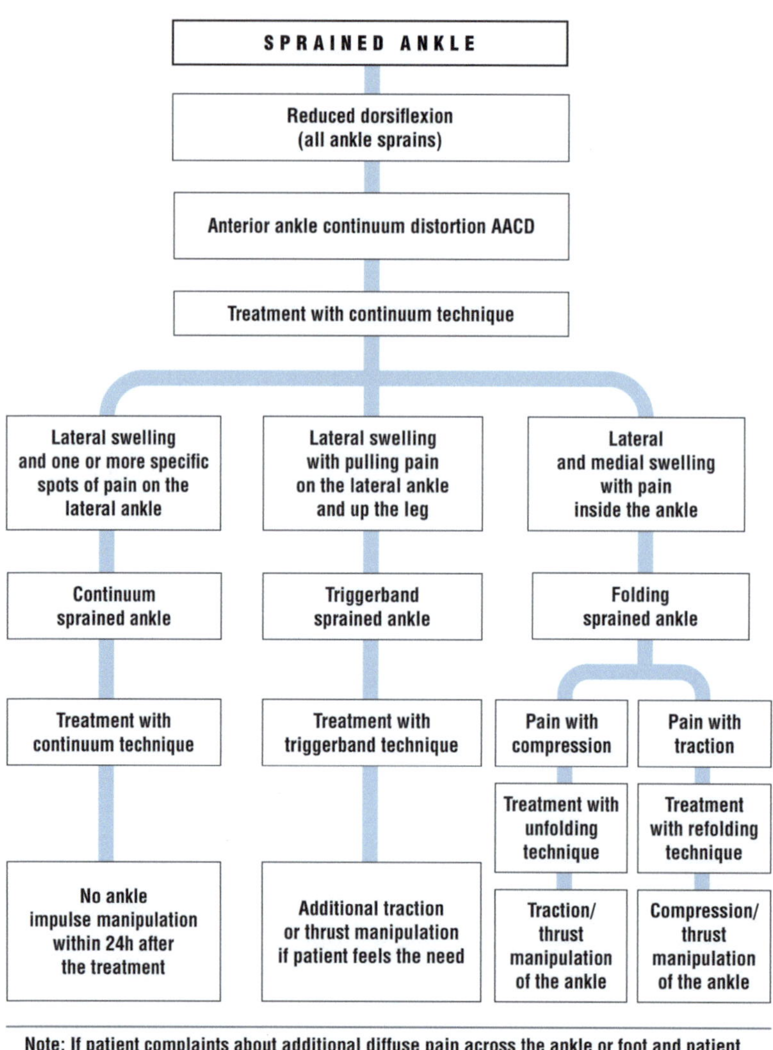

Fig. 4.2 Flowchart for acute ankle sprains [1]

4.3　Qualities of Treatment Techniques

For each fascial distortion, there are specific treatment guidelines and procedures aimed at correcting them. Mastery of these fundamental techniques is a prerequisite for the appropriate application of the Typaldos method and enables the theoretical concept of the Fascial Distortion Model to be implemented in clinical practice.

4.3.1　Finesse and Force

Typaldos describes the treatment techniques of the Typaldos method as fundamentally more precise and forceful than standard manual therapy maneuvers. More precise, because each technique is adapted to the tissue being treated, its deformation, and the patient's clinical presentation. More forceful, because it often requires greater use of force by the therapist to correct fascial deformations. (In this context, Typaldos was initially surprised that acute injuries and their associated symptoms responded particularly well to the application of direct, vigorous techniques).

It is important to understand that force cannot replace precision; on the contrary, greater precision usually requires less force.

4.3.2   Pain in the Treatment of Fascial Distortions

The treatment of fascial distortions can be painful for patients. Depending on the type of fascial distortion, pain provocation serves different functions:

- Certain fascial distortions are tender to pressure, which allows their precise localization on the body.
- Pain and its reduction can confirm the effectiveness of a manual treatment.
- Increasing pain, on the other hand, is an indication of imprecise or improper treatment, or of contraindications.

Performing a painful treatment is a challenge for both the patient and the therapist. It is important for the patient to be informed about possible pain reactions before the treatment, and to be able to give consent to the treatment or withdraw it during the procedure. For the therapist, the challenge lies in treating beyond the patient's pain threshold while still maintaining sensitivity to the patient and their tissues.

The provocation of pain within the framework of the Typaldos method is clearly defined:

- The pains familiar to the patient are triggered during palpation and correction of a triggerband, a herniated triggerpoint, and a continuum distortion. In the treatment of these three fascial distortions, the typical pain is deliberately reproduced, as this confirms the correct application of the manual technique. Depending on the type and location of the distortion, these may be easily tolerable for the patient or perceived as borderline intense.
- With successful treatment of herniated triggerpoints or continuum distortions, these symptoms subside during the manual treatment. In the correction of triggerbands, they are provoked along the entire course of the fascial twist up to its endpoint.
- In the diagnosis of folding distortions, cylinder distortions, or tectonic fixations, the typical pains may occur during provocation tests. Treatment of cylinder distortions or tectonic fixations can also be perceived as uncomfortable or painful, depending on the manual technique used. However, the aim of these techniques is not to reproduce the patient's individual symptoms. The correction of a folding distortion is painless if the direction of the manual treatment is aligned with the mechanism of injury. Pain provocation should therefore be interpreted as a prompt to adjust the applied manipulations accordingly.
- The amount of force applied in a technique fundamentally depends on the distortion being treated. Depending on the depth of localization and the type of deformation, more or less force may be required to reach the distortion on the one hand, and to correct it on the other. The pain provoked by certain manual techniques can only be reduced to a limited extent. However, skillful palpation can avoid unnecessary stress to tissues outside the fascial distortion.
- How patients react to the provocation of pain varies individually. Pain reactions such as *muscle spasms or the appearance of a withdrawal reflex* should always be noticed by the therapist, and the treatment should be adjusted immediately. It can be helpful to encourage the patient to relax and breathe calmly. If the patient cannot tolerate the correction technique, the therapist must stop and choose an alternative treatment. It is therefore advisable to invest time in explaining

the treatment so that the patient understands why and in what context certain manual techniques may be painful. If the patient understands a painful treatment as a necessary maneuver of limited duration over which they retain control, they can accept it more easily.

- The therapist also has a significant influence through their behavior on how the patient interprets the treatment. *Calm, focused work,* precise palpation, and sensitivity to the sometimes subtle pain reactions of the patient, such as sweating or a change in breathing, help to build a foundation of trust. Furthermore, the therapist can involve the patient in the treatment by asking for feedback regarding the development of pain. This information, in turn, helps the therapist to better assess the progress of the treatment and adjust the manual technique if necessary.
- Immediately after the correction of a pain-inducing distortion, the pain itself and the symptoms triggered by the manual treatment may persist for a short time. Through *active movement after the treatment*, these should resolve quickly, allowing the patient to verify the outcome of the treatment. Regardless of this immediate reaction, soft tissue pain as a side effect of the treatment may persist for hours to days. (This is explained in detail in the chapter on the treatment of the six fascial distortions).

Background Information

Painful manipulations are frowned upon in many manual therapy methods and, for some therapists, exceed the acceptable limits of treatment. Ethical concerns regarding the patient are cited, and such manipulations are considered an incalculable risk for the treatment, for which the therapist cannot or does not wish to assume responsibility.

Typaldos held the opposite view on this issue. He considered it ethically unacceptable not to adequately treat patients with severe symptoms due to fascial distortions, even if this temporarily caused pain. The success of his treatments reinforced this view and his confidence in the effectiveness of his model. He accepted his responsibility as a physician to take personal risks and make the greatest possible effort for the well-being of the patient, even though he repeatedly described this obligation as a burden.

4.3.3　Implementation of Treatment Techniques

The thumb is the tool of choice used to perform corrections of triggerbands, herniated triggerpoints, continuum distortions, and certain cylinder distortions. It possesses great adaptability in terms of adjusting to various angular positions relative to the tissue being treated, and it also provides good stability and strength to generate the necessary intensity for the treatment.

Practical Tip

At the beginning of practicing the Typaldos method, therapists may experience fatigue in the thumb area. Initially, it may also seem difficult to find an optimal, stable treatment position. Experience shows that these problems disappear with appropriate training of the techniques. In this context as well, the principle of finesse and force should be followed: only a correctly positioned thumb should be used with force.

The use of aids as a substitute for the thumb during treatments, such as massage sticks, is not recommended, as they carry certain risks: They make it more difficult to dose the applied force and more importantly reduce the ability to sense both the individual tissue quality and its changes during treatment.

The use of lubricants such as massage oils is also not recommended. They reduce the sometimes necessary friction on the skin (especially important in the triggerband technique or the various cylinder techniques). Apart from that, they make it more difficult to establish a firm and targeted contact with the fascia to be treated, which is fundamentally disadvantageous for all techniques of the Typaldos method.

The treatment of folding distortions, certain types of cylinder distortions, and tectonic fixations is performed with the whole hand (palm). Within the respective technique, the hand must be positioned precisely and applied with appropriate force. Especially with impulse techniques, a comfortable, broad, and pain-free positioning of the hand can be crucial for success.

For certain types of distortions, therapeutic devices such as *cupping glasses or inversion tables* may be used if their specific mechanical effects cannot be achieved by hand or thumb. Another advantage of such aids is the possibility of home use by the patients themselves.

> **Practical Tip**
>
> In general, it should be noted that the positioning of both the patient and the therapist is important for the implementation of the treatment.
>
> A stable stance, a favorable alignment of one's own body in relation to gravity and to the area of the body being treated are prerequisites for applying the corresponding correction vectors with minimal effort. Concentration and attentive work further enhance effectiveness.

4.3.4   Adaptation of Treatment Techniques

In general, each treatment technique is adapted to the fascial distortion, its symptoms, and the patient. The following observations can be made in clinical practice:

- As already mentioned, certain techniques reproduce the typical pain in the patient, which must, however, always be tolerable for the patient and their tissue.
- The more chronic a problem, the more intensive the initial treatments in order to free the tissue from adhesions.
- The more recent an injury, the more targeted and focused the therapy. This does not mean that forceful techniques cannot be used in these cases. Especially with recent injuries, however, treatment should be performed with maximum precision to avoid unnecessary strain on the injured tissue.
- Typaldos describes that the dynamics of fascial distortion development can also be reflected in treatment. Complaints that have developed over a longer period often also require more time for correction than symptoms that appear abruptly, which can often be resolved just as quickly.
- The general condition of the patient can also play a role in how forcefully the therapist can work on the patient. This mainly concerns the number of techniques applied in a single therapy session. In case of doubt, it is better to apply a few maneuvers with adequate intensity than to overwhelm the patient with an excessive number of correction techniques.
- Therapy should be ended when the potential for improvement in the respective treatment session has been exhausted. In addition to the therapist's assessment, the perception of (non-verbal) signals from the patient is also important in this context. For example, pay attention to withdrawal behavior or statements about future treatment sessions as signs that further manual treatment is no longer tolerable or meaningful for the patient.

4.3.5   Treatment Sequence

If several fascial distortions are responsible for a clinical picture, they are corrected step by step, thereby gradually resolving their symptoms.

Fascial distortions can influence each other, and their correction can be associated with interactions. Therefore, the order in which the therapist treats the diagnosed distortions can be important:

- *As a general rule, it is recommended to first perform the clearly painful techniques.* This means that triggerbands, herniated triggerpoints, and continuum distortions should be treated before folding distortions, cylinder distortions, and tectonic fixations. However, this recommendation is relative for experienced therapists, who can assess which distortion should be prioritized in the individual treatment situation. For example, the treatment of a folding distortion may appear particularly promising, so the therapist may perform this at the very beginning of the treatment.
- The distinction between everted and inverted continuum distortions influences the treatment sequence in that, after correcting an everted continuum distortion, impulse manipulations in the affected region should be avoided for 24 hours. The induced traction effect on the transition zone could, in turn, draw more minerals from the bone into the transition zone. This would counteract the effect of the continuum technique. In the case of inverted continuum distortions, however, this does not matter, as in that case, an increase in mineral concentration in the transition zone is actually desired. *Since the clinical distinction between the two subtypes is difficult, if not impossible, we recommend applying the continuum technique and impulse manual treatment at different times.* This is especially true for recent injuries with symptoms that can be attributed to continuum distortions.
- *It may be advantageous to treat existing cylinder distortions at the end of the therapy session,* unless their symptoms are so dominant that they cannot be postponed or hinder the treatment of other distortions.

4.4 Success and Failure with the Typaldos Method

In general, treatment success is characterized by the sustainable resolution of the patient's problem. Improvement should be achieved as quickly as possible and with as little treatment pain and as few side effects as possible.

In order to assess the success of a treatment, it is important to know how fascial distortions respond to their correction (this is explained in detail in the fifth chapter). Additionally, the origin of the symptoms also influences the extent to which therapeutic success can be achieved:

- For acute symptoms that have occurred without warning (such as an ankle injury or a blockage in the back), the goal of therapy is to achieve a clear improvement during the very first treatment session. Ideally, this effect remains stable. However, some patients report that after successful treatment, the symptoms reappear, sometimes with an intensity comparable to the status before therapy. This does not necessarily indicate therapeutic failure. In such a situation, the patient should be reassured and encouraged to stay active and avoid applying direct heat. Follow-up therapy should be delayed for at least 24 hours, as experience shows that after this period, the treatment effect can be assessed most clearly. This approach also minimizes the risk of treating symptoms caused by tissue irritation that would resolve on their own with a little patience.
- For chronic symptoms (such as chronic frozen shoulder), the course of therapy can be more prolonged. The first step is to release adhesions, which often leads to side effects such as pain or hematomas. These side effects can last up to 24 hours, and in rare cases, several days. The patient should be informed that these reactions should decrease with each subsequent treatment. After an average of three therapy sessions, the first stable results should be visible. If possible,

the patient should also remain as active as possible in that case and avoid applying direct heat. However, if these side effects do not subside over the course of several therapy sessions, the therapist should reconsider the diagnosis or the application of the technique.

- Overuse syndromes (such as Achilles tendon complaints) usually develop over a longer period and lead to a reduction in the tissue's load-bearing capacity. Therefore, it is not to be expected that a single treatment will completely resolve the problem; rather, several sessions will be necessary. The patient should continue to actively move the affected area, but not subject it to maximum load. A simple guideline in this context is that tolerable, pulling pain during activity is acceptable as long as it does not persist for hours after the activity or is accompanied by additional nocturnal pain.

> **Practical Tip**
>
> Apart from that, the following point should be noted: many patients have been suffering from their symptoms for a long time and therefore tend to constantly test whether the pain is still present. This behavior is rather unfavorable. The patient should give themselves some time to assess the effect of the treatment. It is therefore advisable to agree with the patient on a time frame for the therapy at the beginning of treatment, after which a summary of the treatment effect can be drawn. Three to six weeks is a realistic period for this.

4.4.1 Analysis of Treatment Failures

If the expected positive treatment effects do not occur, the therapist should reconsider their treatment concept within the framework of the Fascial Distortion Model. The following points serve as guidance:

- *The plausibility of the diagnosis*
  From the perspective of the Fascial Distortion Model, a diagnosis is plausible if it offers a credible explanatory model for the patient's problem and subsequently enables a practically applicable therapeutic concept. When formulating a working hypothesis, symptoms can be interpreted in different ways. Therefore, it matters how much weight the therapist gives to individual diagnostic details. In practicing the Typaldos method, several working hypotheses are often possible, and the therapist must weigh which approach offers the *best effect with the lowest risks and side effects*. If a clear diagnosis of fascial distortions cannot be made, further conventional medical clarification may be indicated.

- *Proper execution of the technique*
  The manual techniques of the Typaldos method appear simple and easy to learn at first glance. The effectiveness of the method allows even beginners to achieve initial treatment successes quickly. Nevertheless, it is worthwhile to invest time and effort in mastering the individual techniques. An experienced therapist knows the possible sources of error in a manual technique. Through detailed knowledge of manual techniques and their adaptation to the patient, they cause less tissue irritation and can resolve fascial distortions with a few targeted manipulations. Achieving this skill requires an interest in further developing one's expertise in manual therapy. Practical experience and a critical approach to successes and failures in treatment are also helpful. Of particular importance in this context is the amount of force applied by the therapist during treatment. Each technique must reach the deformed fascia while sparing the surrounding tissue. Therefore, it is advisable to first palpate and examine the distortions in a targeted and sensitive manner before applying significant force, but not to act hesitantly during manual correction. Otherwise, the tissue is often only irritated, and the actual distortion is not corrected due to insufficient force.

- *Immobilization, heat, and related factors*
  Immobilization and restriction of movement are commonly used therapeutic measures in the treatment of the musculoskeletal system.

The Typaldos method views such a priori measures critically, as they can have side effects that may prevent therapeutic success or mask treatment failure.

For example, constrictive bandages can exacerbate existing cylinder distortions. Lack of activity is known to increase the risk of chronic triggerbands or the development of a tectonic fixation after an injury. For this reason, we recommend that patients remain active and immediately incorporate the functional improvements achieved in therapy into daily life and sports. If the patient fails to do so, any remaining fascial distortions impairing function must be corrected. If the patient does not remain active despite being able to, this can hinder the restoration of load-bearing capacity. (The same applies in reverse, of course, if the patient overexerts themselves despite severely limited function, thereby causing additional fascial distortions and symptoms.)

Background Information

In his books, Typaldos advises against the direct *application of heat* to the affected area and also cites this as a possible cause of treatment failure. In his view, heat can cause existing triggerbands to potentially adhere and generally makes the correction of fascial distortions more difficult. The only exception is tectonic fixations, which respond positively to heat applications.

However, patients tend to generally use heat packs or hot baths for pain and experience this, at least initially, as relieving and pleasant. This contradiction can be partially resolved by the following distinctions:

- The application of heat temporarily reduces pain and muscle spasms. However, it does not correct the underlying fascial distortion and therefore rarely provides lasting relief.

- General heat therapy should be distinguished from the application of direct heat. The negative effect of moist-hot compresses or hot baths observed in clinical practice is usually more pronounced and less predictable than that of moderate sauna sessions or direct sun exposure.

- The direct application of heat may be an option before treating tectonic fixations or, in exceptional cases, chronic trigger bands. It improves the elasticity of fascial structures and can facilitate the release of adhesions. However, after treatment, within a time window of up to 48 hours, the application of heat is not advisable. For one, the vigorous manual treatment of the tissue can cause irritation, which may be exacerbated by heat. In addition, adhesions that have been broken up by treatment tend to re-adhere if the metabolism is further stimulated by heat application.

- According to Typaldos, ultrasound applications also have a heating effect, which can make the treatment of fascial distortions more difficult.

4.4.2 "Stay in the Model"

With the FDM, Typaldos defines a framework within which a therapist can examine the relationships between symptoms, fascial distortions, and their correction using specific techniques. The instruction to continue analyzing the problem within this framework, even in the case of unsatisfactory treatment outcomes, is described by Typaldos with the phrase "Stay in the model".

Failures should not reflexively lead to abandoning the use of the Fascial Distortion Model or the Typaldos method. On the contrary, failures can serve as motivation to develop an even more detailed understanding or to create individual and creative therapeutic solutions based on

FDM principles. For example, it may be helpful to involve the patient and ask for their perspective on the problem, as they are the expert on their own symptoms.

If the expected therapeutic successes do not occur, therapists are often inclined to simultaneously apply treatment approaches outside of FDM. However, this prevents the therapist from drawing any conclusions about which form of therapy is effective. It is better to agree with the patient on a time frame during which treatment is carried out consistently according to FDM principles. If no improvements occur, a change in the therapeutic concept should be considered.

However, "Stay in the model" can also be interpreted to mean that the Typaldos method can or must be adapted if clinical practice requires it. As long as these adaptations and extensions can be logically argued on the basis of the Fascial Distortion Model, and thereby improve the chances of sustainably resolving fascial distortions and therefore the patient's symptoms, a variety of therapeutic approaches can be integrated into the treatment. The Typaldos method represents a coherent, yet evolving concept for the treatment of fascial distortions.

Reference

1. Typaldos S (2002) Clinical and theoretical application of the fascial distortion model within the practice of medicine and surgery. 4th edn. 209. Orthopathic Global Health Publications. Brewer, ME

Treatment of the Six Fascial Distortions

5

The manual techniques and therapeutic approaches for treating the six fascial distortions are the essential elements of the Typaldos method. The execution of the individual techniques, as described in the following sections, has proven effective, and it is advisable for therapists to use this guidance as a reference.

Nevertheless, we must not forget that, ultimately, the therapeutic goal pursued by the technique is decisive, and the manual technique itself is merely a means to an end. Therefore, the Typaldos method should not be accepted as dogma. Rather, it provides the foundations necessary for implementing the Fascial Distortion Model with manual treatment approaches. Each technique can and must be adapted to the patients being treated and to their specific problems.

In the following sections, this book will focus on the explanation of:

- the triggerband technique as the standard for the treatment of triggerbands,
- the herniated triggerpoint technique as the method of choice for correcting herniated triggerpoints,
- the continuum technique for the treatment of continuum distortions,
- the principles of correcting folding distortions at joints, in the area of the interosseous membrane and the muscle septa,
- the basic treatment approaches for correcting cylinder distortions, and
- the therapeutic considerations for resolving a tectonic fixation.

Additionally, in each of these six sections, the application of these manual techniques on various body regions is demonstrated. Based on the respective treatment indication, selected manipulations are explained step by step. Photographs and schematic illustrations of the corrections support the communication of the mechanotherapeutic considerations behind the techniques. Additional information on adapting the manual techniques and cross-references to other treatment methods can be found in the practical tips.

Background Information
A detailed understanding of these techniques and manual skills is a prerequisite for successfully applying the Typaldos method in clinical practice. Even though theoretical information cannot replace practical instruction by experienced FDM instructors, in-depth knowledge of the execution and application of the Typaldos method is of crucial importance. This enables therapists to adapt the manual techniques to their own abilities and possibilities without losing sight of their purpose and function, with detailed

knowledge still being the best prerequisite for treating as precisely as possible. This reduces the physical effort required by the therapist and makes the distortion correction more tolerable for the patient.

5.1 Treatment of Triggerbands

Triggerbands are twists of band-like fasciae resulting from damage to stabilizing crosslinks. They lead to a mechanical shortening of the affected tissue and, during wound healing, tend to form adhesions and, subsequently become chronic (see 2.1).

It follows that every treatment intervention for a triggerband, regardless of the therapeutic means, pursues three goals:

- Release adhesions (in chronic triggerbands)
- Untwist and align fibers of the deformed band-like fascia
- Seal the triggerband

Typaldos experimented with various therapeutic approaches to correct triggerbands. For example, he used stretching techniques or treatment methods from classical osteopathy to restore the optimal form of the band-like fasciae.

However, these applications only partially addressed the entire mechanical problem of triggerbands. As a result, the manual triggerband technique emerged as the standard procedure of the Typaldos method. With its help, adhesions can be released, twisted fibers aligned and simultaneously brought closer together.

5.1.1 Triggerband Technique

This manual correction technique for a triggerband can be applied regardless of its location on the body or the specific form of fascial twisting. It is performed in three steps:

- Determination of the triggerband course
- Palpation of the triggerband starting point
- Untwisting and sealing of the triggerband

5.1.1.1 Determination of Triggerband Pathway

In principle, triggerbands can occur anywhere in the body in the area of band-like fasciae. Despite the individual courses of triggerbands, clinical practice shows a clustering of certain triggerband locations, which are associated with typical complaint patterns.

For many body regions, Typaldos describes such pathways with defined starting and end points in the area of the crossbands (connective tissue structures oriented transversely to the triggerband, e.g. retinacula in the area of joints; fig. 5.1a). Knowledge of these typical courses serves as a rough guide for their treatment. However, the exact location of the triggerband is determined by the patient's verbal description and, above all, by their typical gestures (fig. 5.1b and c). They can pinpoint the triggerband precisely, so that the therapist can then palpate the area specifically in search of the twist.

5.1.1.2 Palpation of Triggerband Starting Point

The starting point is the location in the tissue where the twist in the fascial band begins. It is important to start the treatment at this point. This allows for complete correction of the twist, thereby reducing the risk of recurrence.

Unlike the general course of the distortion, the starting point of the twist usually cannot be determined precisely from the patient's body language, so the therapist must identify it by palpation.

The starting point is located in the area of a crossband or an extension of the triggerband course, as indicated by the patient. Typaldos describes its palpatory quality as a sensitive roughness or thickening in the fascia.

To feel the starting point, the therapist repeatedly pushes the tip of her thumb through the tissue until she can perceive a resistance (fig. 5.2a and b). The patient confirms correct palpation, as the typical pain associated with the

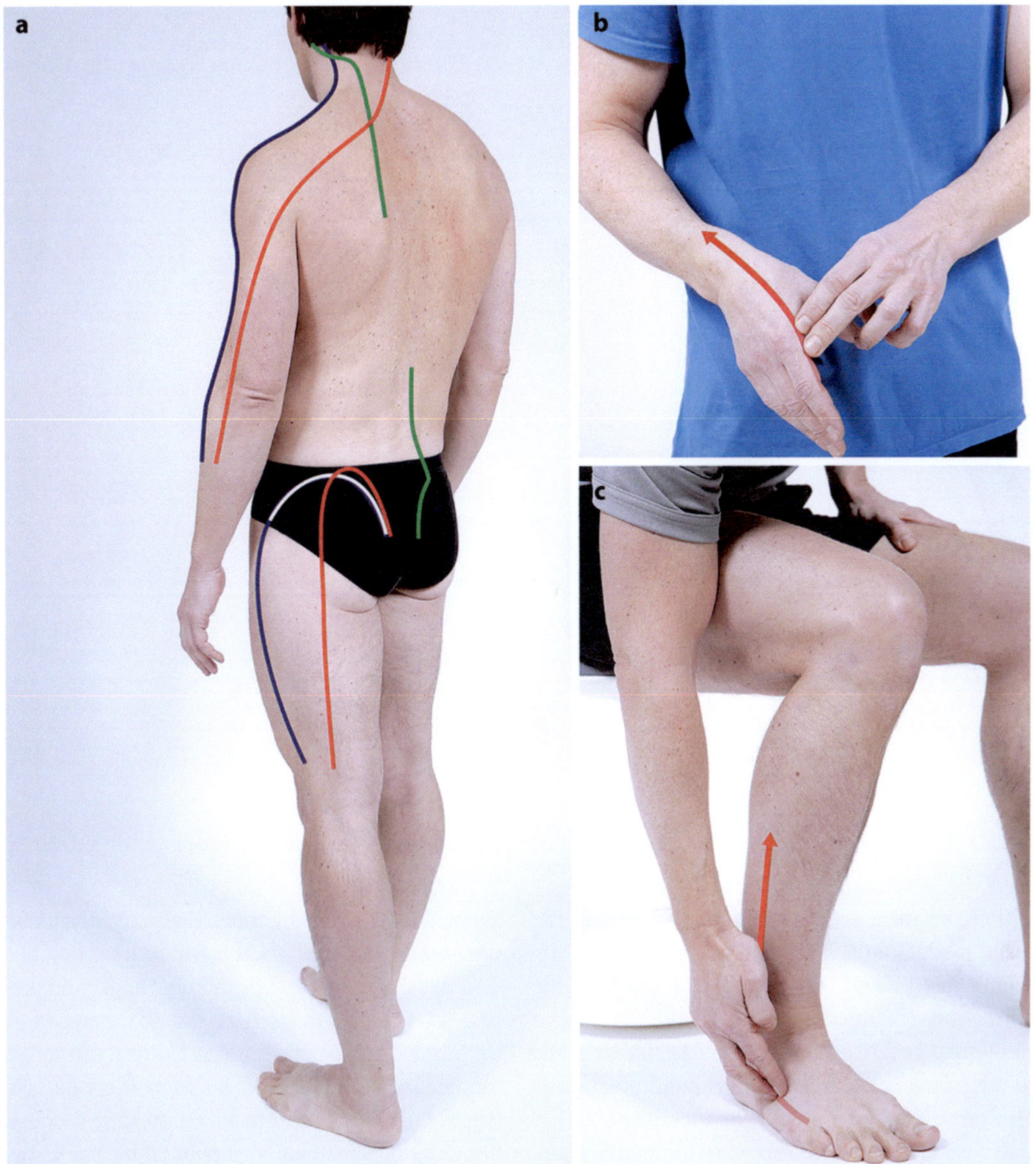

Fig. 5.1 Triggerband pathways. Typical courses in the lower back and star triggerband (green), in the posterior thigh and posterior shoulder (red), as well as in the lateral thigh and anterior shoulder (blue) (**a**). Triggerband body language at the index finger and forearm (**b**). Triggerband body language at the lateral ankle (**c**). (© Anker 2022)

triggerband can be provoked for the first time at the starting point.

5.1.1.3 Untwisting and Sealing of the Triggerband

Once the starting point has been identified, the actual correction of the distortion begins. The therapist mobilizes the twist in the fascial band, untwists the deformed fibers, and brings them closer together along the entire course. This seals the triggerband, and the fascia regains its original length.

The therapist pushes the twist away from the starting point along the entire course to its endpoint with her thumb, as if ironing out the distortion (fig. 5.3a and b). A palpable mobilization of the fascial twist occurs—a kind of yielding of the tissue—which the therapist aims to achieve.

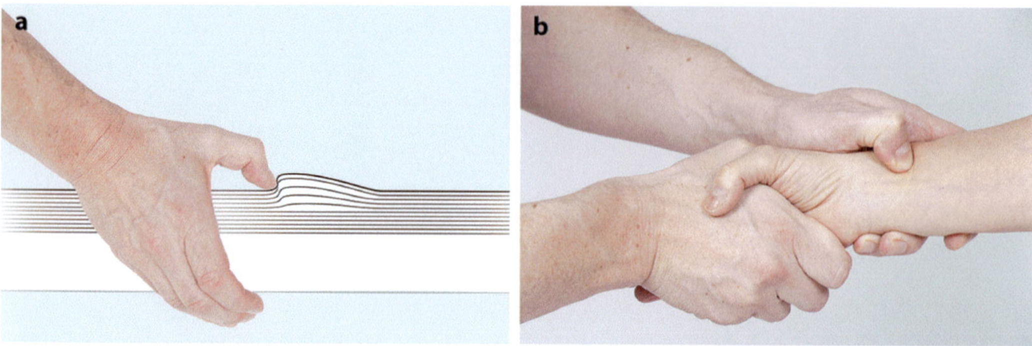

Fig. 5.2 Palpation of the triggerband starting point. Illustration of palpation (**a**). Positioning of the thumb tip for palpation and correction (**b**). (© Anker 2022)

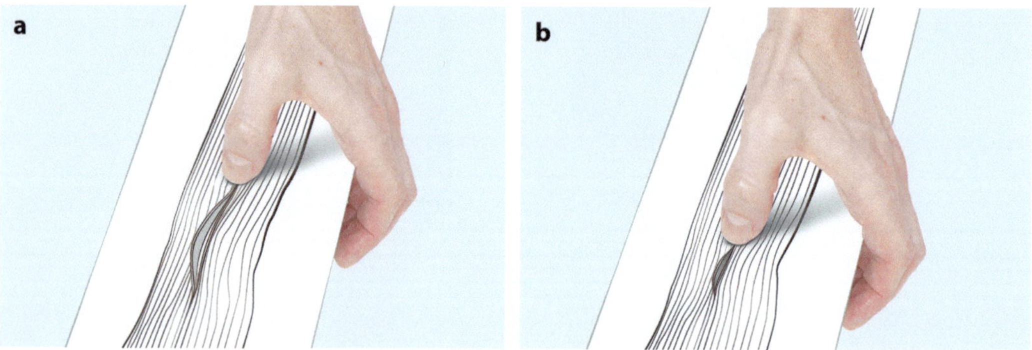

Fig. 5.3 Illustration of the triggerband technique. Start of the treatment (**a**). Increasing closure of the triggerband (**b**). (© Anker 2022)

For the maneuver, the thumb is flexed at the distal phalanx at a right angle, and the tip of the thumb just behind the fingernail is used for the correction. It is recommended to slightly extend the wrist, as this optimizes the transfer of force to the tissue being treated. This hand position is also more joint-friendly for the therapist.

To generate the force necessary for mobilization, the remaining fingers of the hand should be used for support, for example by counterbalancing the thumb pressure or stabilizing the tissue to be treated. If necessary, the second hand or thumb can also be used to assist. On the one hand, the skin in the area of the triggerband can be pre-tensioned, which can reduce the treatment pain caused by friction on the skin (fig. 5.4a). On the other hand, the treating thumb at the distal phalanx can be supported by the second thumb or the thenar eminence (fig. 5.4b).

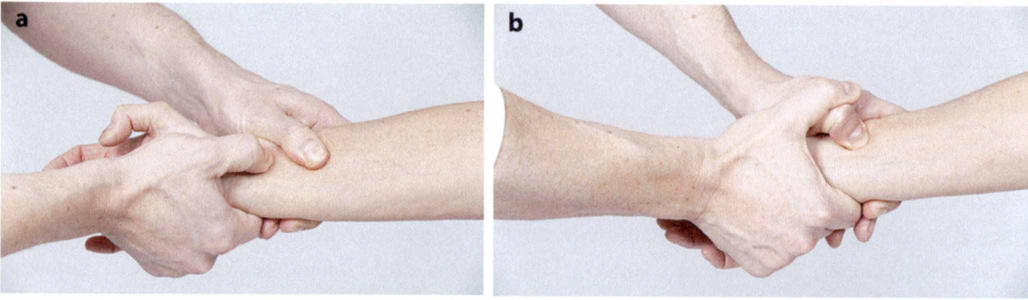

Fig. 5.4 Modification of the triggerband technique. Pre-stretching the skin in front of the treating thumb (**a**). Grip variant with support from the second thumb (**b**). (© Anker 2022)

The hand grip must be continuously adapted to both the anatomical conditions and the symptoms presented by the patient in order to correct the twist as precisely as possible. For this, constant palpation of the fascial twist (and its palpable mobilization) during the correction is necessary. The angle at which the therapist's thumb presses on the triggerband is adjusted accordingly.

If the triggerband technique follows the exact course of the distortion, the typical symptoms are elicited throughout the entire treatment (albeit with varying intensity). It is important to distinguish between nonspecific pressure pain and the provocation of the pulling-burning pain of the triggerband, which the patient immediately recognizes. In this sense, the patient can also be asked during the treatment to confirm the location ("Is this the correct pathway?"), as these symptoms only disappear at the endpoint of the twist.

> **Practical Tip**
> Pain provocation does not necessarily correlate with the amount of pressure applied by the therapist. For example, treatment of superficial triggerbands can be very painful for the patient, even though only minimal pressure is required for correction.

Through the triggerband treatment, the twist and therefore the symptoms shift along the pathway. As a result, triggerband symptoms can appear to move dynamically along the course up to the endpoint of the twist. In this context, several phenomena can be observed:

- If the pain suddenly subsides, then either the endpoint of the distortion has been reached, or the therapist has lost the triggerband twist during the course of treatment. In the latter case, she must reposition her thumb a few centimeters back to relocate the twist of the triggerband— also with guidance from the patient—and continue the treatment to the endpoint.

- If the therapist does not correct the distortion all the way to the endpoint, the twist (and the symptoms it causes) may persist, possibly in a different location. Typaldos gives the example of a patient with a triggerband at the shoulder, running from the forearm to the occiput. If the distortion is only partially corrected, shoulder pain may be reduced, but new neck pain may occur. To prevent this, the entire course must be treated up to the endpoint.

- Some patients experience pain along the entire course of the twist up to the endpoint when local pressure is applied to the triggerband. Typaldos describes this as the *headlight effect,* a phenomenon that typically occurs with triggerbands and can also be interpreted as confirmation of the diagnosis.

From palpable nodules of various sizes, to wavy or cord-like changes, to grain-of-salt-like roughness in the tissue—this is how Typaldos describes what triggerbands can feel like to therapists (fig. 5.5a–c). These subtypes require different amounts of force necessary for mobilizing the deformation. For example, acute twists require less force than nodule- or pea-like triggerbands to be released step by step. However, the technique itself remains the same.

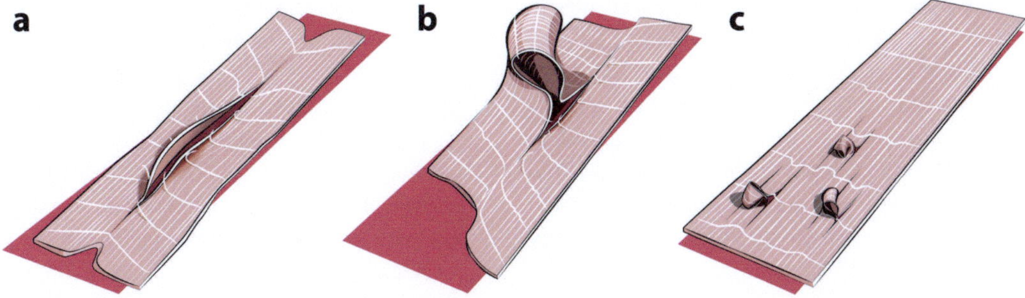

Fig. 5.5 a to c: subtypes of triggerbands. Acute twist (**a**). Nodule (**b**). Grain-of-salt-like triggerbands. (© Anker 2022)

An exception is the so-called *grain-of-salt technique* (see sect. 5.1.5.5). This variant is particularly effective for triggerbands on the fingers, toes, or face, which can be perceived as a grain-of-salt-like, several millimeter wide track in the tissue. For this technique, both thumbs are alternately, and slightly offset, pushed along the course of the triggerband. The goal is to mobilize the tiny, palpable irregularities of the grain-of-salt-like triggerband until the resistance in the tissue is reduced.

▶ In addition to the triggerband subtype, the location and the extent of existing adhesions also influence the triggerband technique:

- Deep-seated triggerbands generally require more force to even reach the area of the twist.
- Chronic triggerbands must first be freed from adhesions before correction of the twist is possible. Typaldos refers to this as returning chronic triggerbands to their acute state (meaning without adhesions). For this, the triggerband technique is applied with increased force (and usually repeatedly), which can result in side effects such as skin irritation or bruising after therapy. Several therapy sessions may be necessary to resolve adhesions as effectively as possible.

The triggerband technique can be adapted to patients and their specific problems in various ways:

- It is important to select the *treatment direction* according to the gestures of the patients, and to treat the triggerband in the direction indicated. In clinical practice, this results in a more effective correction. In any case, the treatment direction should be adjusted if the expected therapeutic effect is insufficient.
- The *pressure intensity* with which a patient traces a triggerband pathway into the tissue can also provide information about the required treatment strength. Superficially indicated twists require less force to reproduce the patient's symptoms than triggerbands that are indicated with strong pressure.

- Another way to adapt the technique is to *treat the triggerband in a functional, pre-stretched, or weight-bearing body position*. Many patients intuitively describe such a posture, as it triggers the typical pulling-burning pain. For the therapist, this offers the advantage of being able to palpate the triggerband more easily. However, the therapist must adapt to this position, which may make the treatment more physically demanding for them.
- The *speed* at which a triggerband can be treated depends on the tissue's response. The more easily the twist can be mobilized, and the more the tissue resistance yields, the faster the therapist can move their thumb through the tissue. In cases of persistent adhesions, correction therefore often proceeds more slowly.

5.1.2 Treatment Effects of the Triggerband Technique

The better the deformation of the fascia can be reduced, the more the symptoms are immediately alleviated. Ideally, this goal would be achieved with a single targeted correction.

If several treatment steps are necessary, the following parameters may be helpful:

- If triggerbands primarily restrict mobility, correction is performed in the pre-stretched position of the distortion. This means that the affected body segment is first moved to the limit of its range of motion, and the correction is performed under this pre-stretch. Subsequently, the pre-positioning is adjusted according to the therapeutic effect, and the technique is repeated until the maximum result for this treatment session is achieved.
- If pain management is the primary focus, the patient can be asked to assume the pain-inducing position before the twist is corrected. The advantage again lies in the pre-stretching of the triggerband, which facilitates its palpation and treatment. In addition, the patient can more easily compare the treatment effect before and after the application of the triggerband technique. The following outcomes may occur:

- If the pain disappears completely after the initial treatment, no further use of the triggerband technique is necessary.
- If there is improvement but not complete resolution of symptoms, treatment can be continued.
- If the patient describes altered symptoms, further treatment should be adjusted accordingly. For example, it can be observed that the location of symptoms changes after the first application of the technique. This should be addressed in the next correction step.
- If there is no treatment effect at all, the working hypothesis must be reviewed.

5.1.3   Side Effects and Contraindications of the Triggerband Technique

Open wounds, burns, or skin injuries in the area of the triggerband preclude the use of the triggerband technique.

In principle, a therapist must assess before treatment whether the tissue to be treated can withstand the corrective force applied. Parchment-like skin in elderly patients or inflammatory skin diseases may be contraindications in this context. The use of the technique should also be carefully considered in patients with increased tendency to bleed.

Redness and warmth of the skin as well as *soft tissue pain* are possible side effects of the triggerband technique. In addition, especially when treating chronic triggerbands, *hematomas* may occur. Patients should be informed of this prior to treatment. Even though these symptoms are neither dangerous nor persistent, bruising in particular is, from a legal perspective, a form of bodily harm. For this reason, patient education is especially important.

Immediately after the triggerband technique, pain may occur as a result of manual treatment of the tissue. It is therefore recommended to ask patients to move actively after each correction step and to observe whether and how these symptoms develop:

- If active movement reduces the treatment-related pain and a positive treatment effect is observed, therapy can be continued.

- If active movement does not reduce the pain, a short treatment break may be necessary. Cooling packs can further soothe the tissue. If the symptoms subside as a result, therapy may possibly be continued. However, it is usually more sensible to postpone further correction of the triggerband to the next treatment session. This avoids misinterpreting the induced side effects as symptoms of further fascial distortions and treating them. This would not lead to improvement, but only to additional irritation of the tissue.
- The same applies if, after repeated manual treatment, patients are no longer able to assess whether improvement has occurred or not. Such a reaction may indicate that further triggerband corrections should be temporarily withheld and continued in the next therapy session.
- If active movement immediately after treatment increases the pain, it must be assumed that the correction of the triggerband has failed. The working hypothesis may also need to be reconsidered, as triggerbands generally respond positively to treatment.

After treatment of chronic triggerbands, the so-called *hit-by-a-truck effect* may occur, which results from the release of adhesions. This is typically characterized by soft tissue pain, fatigue, autonomic symptoms such as nausea or hypotension, and hematoma formation. These side effects can last up to 48 hours, in rare cases several days. During that time, repeating the triggerband treatment is not advisable.

> **Practical Tip**
> Severe side effects should not be misinterpreted as an indication of the particular effectiveness of a treatment. The Typaldos method accepts side effects during the correction of chronic triggerbands if a lasting improvement can be achieved in the further course of treatment. Accordingly, such reactions should occur less frequently in subsequent treatments, as the adhesions of the triggerband are increasingly resolved.

5.1.4 Additional Measures for the Treatment of Triggerbands

In general, *active movement* is a factor that can positively support the correction of a triggerband. The associated mobilization of the tissue can help release adhesions and reduce the twist in the band-like fascia. For that reason, patients should move the affected area, either through daily activities or targeted exercise programs. If the latter are used, activating training programs are preferable to static stretching. This is especially true following triggerband treatment and in cases of chronic complaints, where adhesions are usually insufficiently resolved by stretching alone.

In contrast, immobilization does not offer a way to counteract fascial deformation and is therefore avoided as a form of treatment as much as possible. In clinical practice, there is also an increased risk of adhesion formation or loss of function due to non-use of the affected body part.

After successful correction of an acute triggerband, *there is no need for further protection.* If the functional limitation is resolved by realigning the fascial fibers, patients can resume normal use of the affected area in daily life. This re-exposes the tissue to appropriate movement and loading stimuli, thereby supporting the complete regeneration of the band-like fascia.

For chronic triggerbands, the approach after treatment must be considered in a more differentiated manner. Adherent twists cause a stronger roadblock effect, leading to reduced resilience of the affected tissue. Consequently, the load-bearing capacity of the area improves only gradually, as the triggerband correction normalizes metabolism in the affected region, and the tissue gradually regains its original quality.

The use of *ice packs* after triggerband correction can be effective for two reasons. On the one hand, cold therapy can alleviate tissue irritation caused by the treatment, on the other, bleeding into the tissue, which may be caused by forceful release of adhesions, can be stopped.

> **Background Information**
> In his books, Typaldos describes the adverse effect of heat as a therapeutic agent. According to his experience, the application of direct heat, such as hot showers, baths, or heat packs, tends to cause triggerbands to become chronic, making subsequent treatment more complex. In clinical practice, it is observed that no direct heat should be applied for up to 48 hours after treatment, as tissue pain triggered by the intervention may be intensified and the treatment outcome compromised.

In addition to the triggerband technique, Typaldos describes further therapeutic measures to influence triggerbands:

The *muscle energy technique* is a classic osteopathic mobilization technique in which the joint to be treated is positioned at the movement barrier and the patient actively performs an isometric muscle contraction against a defined resistance provided by the therapist. According to Typaldos, this can mobilize both the twist in the fascial band and any adhesions.

Thrust manipulation techniques can have a positive effect on acute, periarticular, and wave-like triggerbands. However, they are usually ineffective for chronic triggerbands.

Certain *medications* can alleviate the typical symptoms of triggerbands. Locally injected or orally administered steroidal anti-inflammatory drugs are used for this purpose. From the perspective of the Fascial Distortion Model, their effect is not due to their anti-inflammatory action, but rather their effect on the fascial continuum: the roadblock effect caused by triggerbands is partially responsible for the pulling, burning discomfort. Steroids mobilize minerals from the bone into the soft tissue area. This compensates for the local undersupply of the fascia caused by the roadblock effect, thereby reducing these symptoms. However, it is unclear to what extent this pharmacological treatment influences the twist in the fascial band. In the context of adhesions, it is conceivable that an injection of anti-inflammatory drugs causes a local increase in volume, thereby mechanically mobilizing adhesions. Additionally, patients move the affected area more due to pain reduction. Despite these mechanisms, clinical practice often shows that the effect of chemically acting medications on mechanically induced triggerbands is insufficient or only temporary.

Adhesions that develop in connection with triggerbands can, in certain cases, also be severed by a *surgical intervention*. This option may be considered if the adhesions are not accessible to manual correction (such as adhesions in the knee joint after ligament injury or surgery). As a result, other twists in the band-like fascia may be more easily reduced due to improved mobility.

> **Background Information**
> Typaldos also describes a similar therapeutic approach in connection with triggerbands in the area of blood vessels. Specifically, in cases of flow disturbances, he suspects triggerbands and cylinder distortions that could narrow the vessel diameter. These restrictions could be resolved by special surgical laser procedures, which release the associated adhesions.

5.1.5   Treatment Examples

The following section presents the treatment of commonly occurring triggerbands. Their typical location is shown in the photos as a red line. However, it is important to understand that the course of a triggerband can be highly individual, and therefore the correction must be adapted according to the patient's feedback.

5.1.5.1 Star Triggerband Technique

> **Background Information**
> Typaldos refers to this course as the "star among triggerbands" because it was the first fascial distortion he treated.

Indications

- Pulling, burning pain and movement restrictions of the upper back and neck; tension headaches
- Possible mechanism of injury: mechanical trauma (e.g. whiplash or neck strain); gradual onset due to overuse with a tendency to become chronic
- Typical body language: dynamic stroking with the fingers along the posterior neck or in the area of the shoulder blade

Course and Treatment

- The typical starting point is in the area of the shoulder blade or the middle ribs. The triggerband ends either at the ipsilateral or contralateral mastoid.
- Treatment is performed using the triggerband technique. A stable, forward-leaning position of the patient is recommended to pre-stretch the triggerband and allow for appropriate pressure to be applied (fig. 5.6a and b).
- Typaldos usually describes the star triggerband as nodular, so that forceful application of pressure is often necessary to mobilize the twist.

Practical Tips

- Typaldos describes that an additional folding distortion of the intercostal membrane ("star folding distortion") is often found and can be corrected in the area of the starting point of the triggerband (see sect. 5.4.5.5).
- According to the body language, the treatment direction can also be reversed. In patients with headaches, treatment from the head toward the shoulder blade is recommended.

5.1.5.2 Triggerband Technique on the Lateral Ankle

Indications

- Pulling-burning pain, restricted movement, and swelling of the lateral ankle or along the entire triggerband pathway

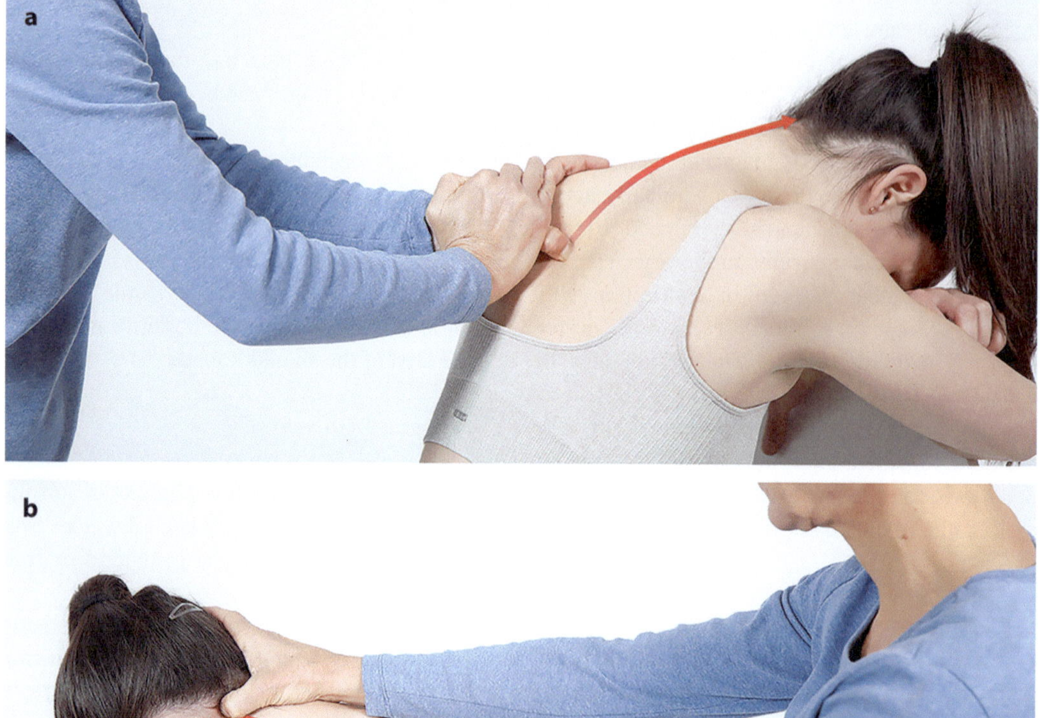

Fig. 5.6 Star triggerband technique. Starting point between the shoulder blade and the thoracic vertebrae (**a**). End point at the occiput or mastoid (**b**). (© Anker 2022)

- Possible etiology: often traumatic, as part of an ankle sprain
- Typical body language: dynamic stroking with the fingers along the triggerband pathway

Course and treatment

- The starting point is usually at the metatarsal bones of the 4th or 5th ray (fig. 5.7a). The triggerband typically runs posterior to the lateral malleolus, deep along the posterior aspect of the fibula, up to the mid-calf.

- Treatment is performed using the triggerband technique with the patient seated or lying down. During the course of therapy, a standing position is also possible.
- In the area of the lateral malleolus, the direction of pressure must be adjusted to follow the course along the posterior aspect of the fibula (fig. 5.7b).

Practical tips

- Around the lateral ankle, persistent adhesions frequently occur, resulting in ongoing pain, restricted movement, and swelling.

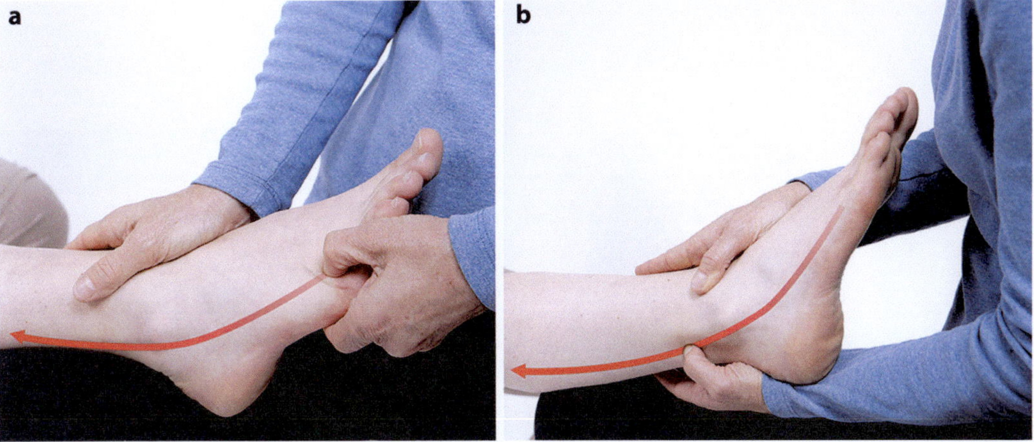

Fig. 5.7 Triggerband technique at the lateral ankle. Palpation of the starting point in the area of the metatarsal bones (**b**). Adjustment of the direction of pressure at the fibula (**c**). (© Anker 2022)

- A stroking body language below the lateral malleolus can also be interpreted as an indication of a refolding distortion of the interosseous membrane of the lower leg (see sect. 5.4.6.2). This can occur in inversion injuries as well. In such cases, patients usually describe deep load-dependent pain. However, the suggested triggerband pathway cannot be provoked as painful by palpation.

5.1.5.3 Triggerband Technique on the Anterior Shoulder

Indications

- Restriction of shoulder movement in various directions; pulling-burning pain in the area of the anterior shoulder, down to the elbow or up to the neck; nocturnal pain in the shoulder region
- Possible mechanism of injury: mechanical trauma to the shoulder (e.g. a fracture or strain of the shoulder) or overuse of the shoulder region
- Typical body language: dynamic stroking with the fingers along the triggerband pathway

Course and treatment

- The typical starting point is about one hand's width below the antecubital fossa (sometimes even further towards the wrist). The triggerband ends at the ipsilateral mastoid process.

- Treatment is performed using the triggerband technique with the patient seated. If triggerbands lead to restricted shoulder movement, treatment at the end range of motion is recommended.
- After palpating the starting point (fig. 5.8a), the twist is pushed through the antecubital fossa along the upper arm towards the shoulder fFig. 5.8b). The treatment thumb rolls over the clavicle to continue the correction just behind it, laterally along the neck to the ipsilateral mastoid process (fig. 5.8c).
- Pre-positioning the shoulder to pre-stretch the fascial band is particularly important. This helps to mobilize the twist with sufficient force up to the clavicle (fig. 5.8d).
- During the course of treatment, the treatment thumb is often switched to generate sufficient counterpressure with the remaining fingers.

Practical tips

- In some cases, the triggerband runs from the shoulder along the clavicle to the sternum (instead of toward the head). In this course, the mobility of the clavicle may be impaired. The same can be caused by another typical triggerband at the shoulder: The *shoulder-mastoid triggerband* starts at the acromioclavicular joint and runs along

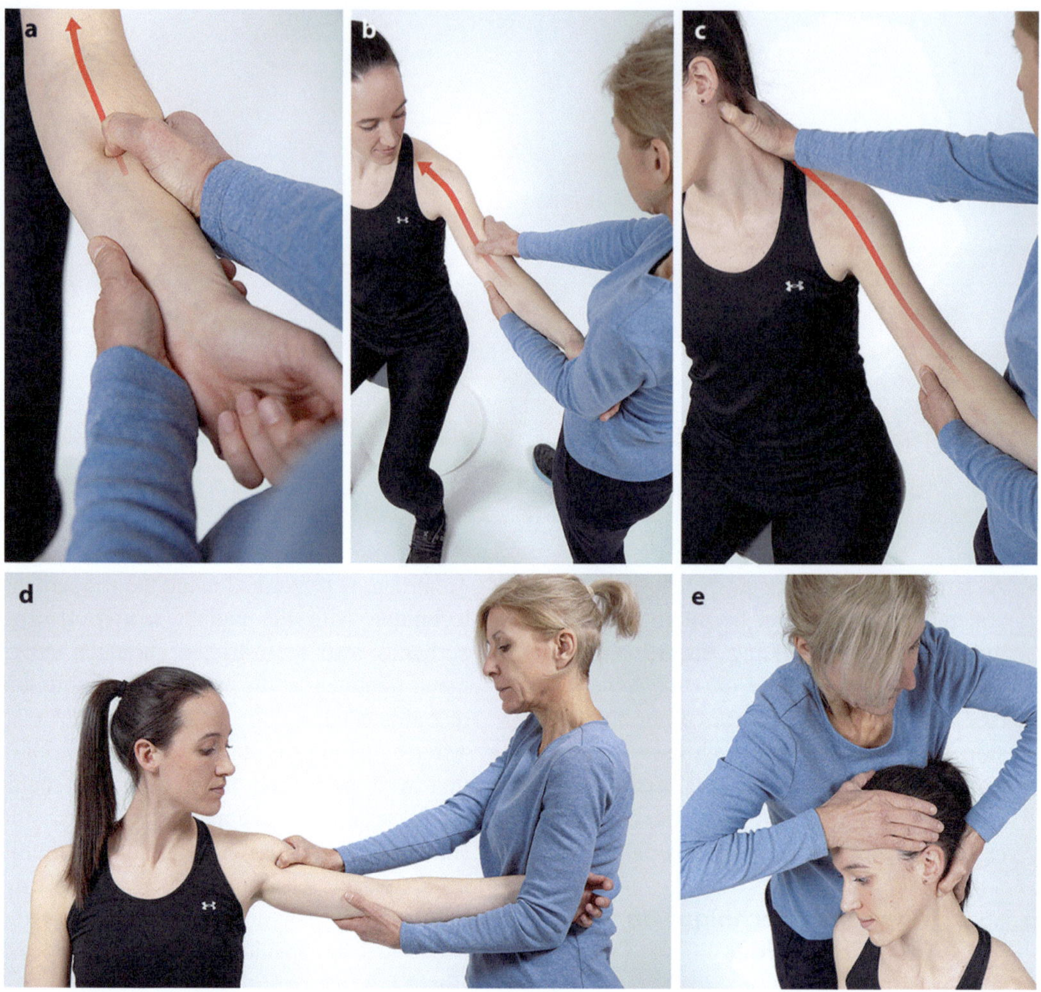

Fig. 5.8 Triggerband technique at the anterior shoulder. Starting point at the forearm (**a**). Course along the anterior upper arm (**b**). Endpoint at the ipsilateral mastoid process (**c**). Pre-positioning for treatment in the area of the anterior shoulder (**d**). Change in the direction of triggerband treatment starting from the ipsilateral mastoid process (**e**). (© Anker 2022)

the trapezius muscle to the ipsilateral mastoid process.

- According to the direction of the body language, this triggerband can also be treated in the opposite direction (fig. 5.8e).
- In chronic cases, the body language may be ambiguous, even though the symptoms of painful movement restriction (e.g. in the context of chronic frozen shoulder) and pain-provoked palpation strongly suggest the presence of triggerbands. In these cases, treatment of a potential herniated triggerpoint at the shoulder should also be considered.

5.1.5.4 Triggerband Technique on the Back

Indications

- Restricted mobility or pulling-burning pain in the area of the back, hip, or knee (depending on the course)
- Possible mechanisms of injury: mechanical trauma (e.g. a strain of the back or a fall); chronic courses are common both in the area of the back and the thigh (e.g. in back pain with additional pulling pain in the leg)

- Typical body language: dynamic stroking with the fingers along the triggerband pathway

Course and treatment

- The typical pathway of triggerbands in the lower back extends in a first section from the thoracolumbar junction to the ipsilateral sacroiliac joint and in a second section along the sacrum to the coccyx. This section coincides with the course of the classic triggerbands on the outer or posterior thigh. They usually run from the coccyx, along the iliac crest over the buttocks to the knee. They are responsible for the typical triggerband symptomatology in the area of the hip or leg (fig. 5.2).
- Treatment of back triggerbands is performed with the patient standing and bent forward. Treatment in the lateral position is also possible, which may make palpation of the triggerband at depth easier in cases of high tissue tension.
- If the triggerband is treated starting from the coccyx, the starting point is usually found laterally at the transition to the sacrum. In the area of the back, the treatment pressure

should be directed so that the symptoms can be clearly provoked (fig. 5.9).

Practical tips

- Patients often describe triggerband complaints on both the right and left sides of the back. Consequently, both sides should be treated.
- If the pulling pain extends down the leg, treatment can also be performed with the patient standing. This treatment position offers the advantage of pre-stretching the triggerband. However, the disadvantage is that it is more difficult for the therapist to apply the necessary corrective force. Alternatively, for a course on the posterior thigh, pre-positioning in the prone position is suitable (possibly with one leg hanging laterally over the treatment table). For a course on the lateral thigh, treatment can be performed in the lateral position.
- According to Typaldos, the formation of triggerbands in the back can be the starting point for a variety of complaint patterns, which from an orthopedic perspective, are often associated with disc problems or spinal canal stenosis.

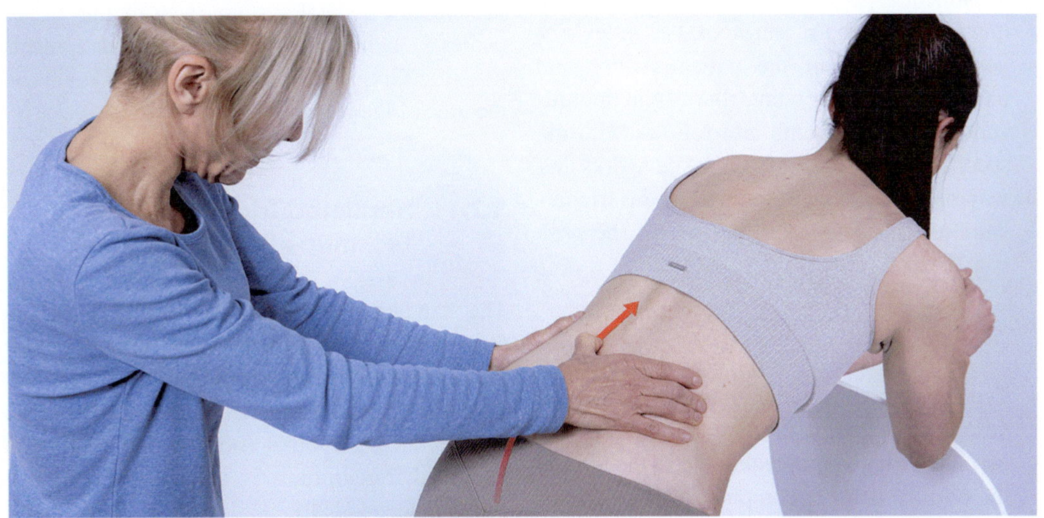

Fig. 5.9 Triggerband technique on the lower back. (© Anker 2022)

5.1.5.5 Adapted Triggerband Technique Above the Eye (Grain-of-salt Technique)

> **Background Information**
> The grain-of-salt technique is generally suitable for triggerbands in the area of the face, fingers, and toes. Based on experience, this variant is an option for the correction of triggerbands that are very close to the bone.

Indications

- Pulling-burning pain in the face or in the area of the eye; headache
- Possible mechanisms of injury: mechanical trauma (e.g. a fall onto the face); more frequently part of a facial or headache symptomatology
- Typical body language: dynamic stroking with the fingers along the triggerband pathway (e.g. in the area of the eyebrow)

Course and treatment

- The triggerband often runs from the temporomandibular joint to the root of the nose.
- Treatment is performed with the patient lying down. The therapist can hook her index finger at the root of the patient's nose and palpate the starting point. She begins mobilization with one thumb and follows with the second thumb. Step by step, she works her way through the entire course of the triggerband to the endpoint at the root of the nose (fig. 5.10).

Practical tips

- Typaldos recommends performing the above-described technique in combination with the herniated triggerpoint technique in the area of the orbit, if patients complain of pain behind the eyeball (see sect. 5.2.5.4).

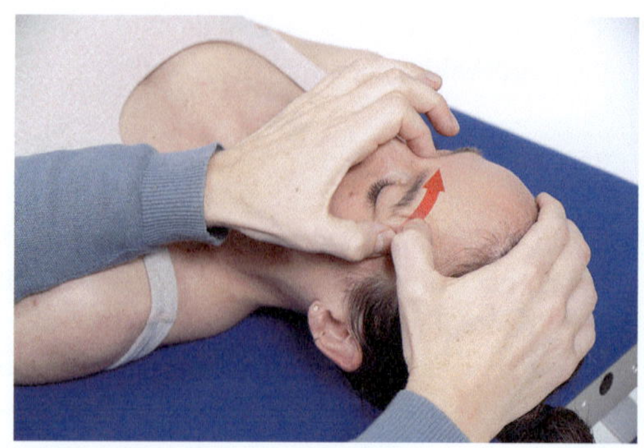

Fig. 5.10 Grain-of-salt triggerband technique on the face. (© Anker 2022)

5.2 Treatment of Herniated Triggerpoints

A herniated triggerpoint develops when tissue is pushed through and trapped by an adjacent fascial layer. This distortion subsequently causes a permanent blockage in the area of the smooth fascia, which is experienced by patients as a more or less painful restriction of movement (see 2.2).

The treatment of a herniated triggerpoint aims to return the protrusion back to the original fascial layer. This concept is also used in the correction of hernias as described in conventional medicine. However, it is rarely applied to the musculoskeletal system, even though orthopedics is familiar with hernia-like entrapments (e.g. the Grynfeltt hernia or the Petit hernia in the area of the back).

5.2.1 Herniated Triggerpoint Technique (HTP Technique)

The standard treatment of the Typaldos method for the correction of a herniated triggerpoint is the herniated triggerpoint technique, performed with the thumb. It can be used for both classic herniated triggerpoints (non-banded HTP) and herniated triggerpoints in the area of band-like fascia (banded HTP).

The correction is performed in three steps:

- Palpation of the herniated triggerpoint
- Reduction of the protrusion
- Complete repositioning

5.2.1.1 Palpation of the Herniated Triggerpoint

Typaldos describes typical locations on the body where herniated triggerpoints can occur (fig. 5.11a). In addition, specific body language can help localize the herniated triggerpoint and verify this by palpation (fig. 5.11b and c).

The palpatory quality of a herniated triggerpoint ranges from a spongy swelling in the tissue to a firm, nodular induration. This distortion is often located deep within the soft tissues, so the therapist's thumb must first skillfully penetrate this region. It is important to palpate gently so that the patient remains relaxed. If the palpation result is inconclusive, it may help to palpate bilaterally for comparison or to change the positioning of the region to be examined (and therefore its state of tissue tension) (fig. 5.12a and b).

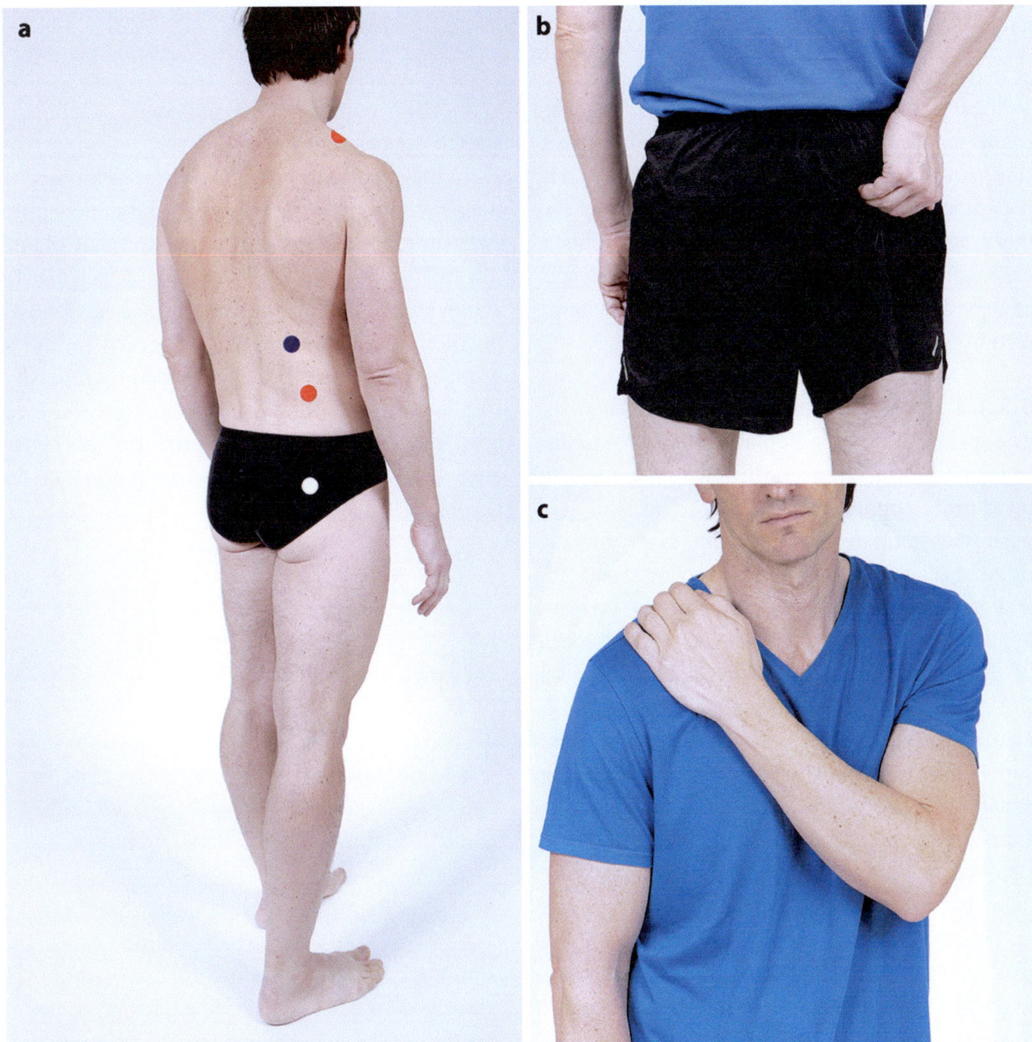

Fig. 5.11 Typical locations of herniated triggerpoints on the trunk. Bullseye HTP (white), belt HTP above the iliac crest (red), flank HTP in the area of the lower ribs (blue), shoulder HTP (red) (**a**). Body language in herniated triggerpoints at the gluteal region (**b**) and at the shoulder (**c**). (© Anker 2022)

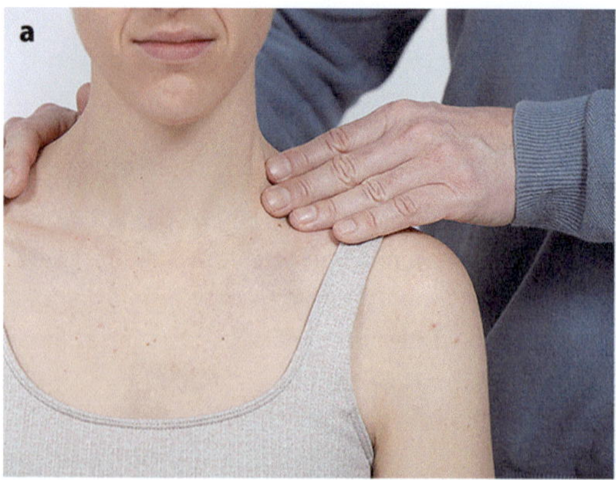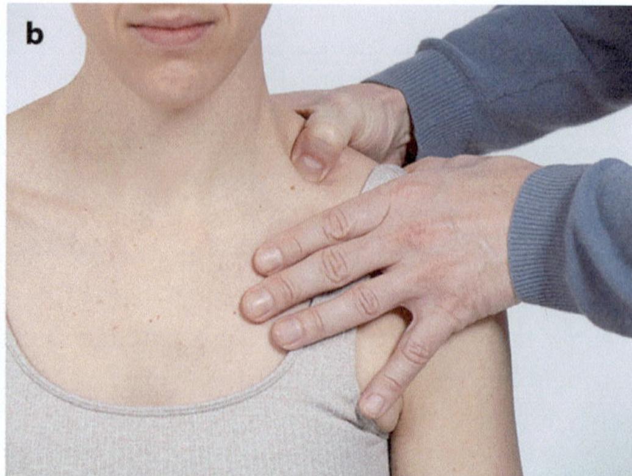

Fig. 5.12 Palpation of a herniated triggerpoint at the shoulder. It may be advantageous to first palpate broadly with several fingers (**a**) and in a second step to place the thumb precisely for repositioning (**b**). (© Anker 2022)

Ideally, the therapist both feels the herniated triggerpoint and, through palpation, elicits pressure pain or the patient's typical symptoms. The patient can assist during palpation by guiding the practitioner toward the protrusion. This is especially useful if the therapist has little experience with palpating the distortion or if the herniated triggerpoint is difficult to detect.

5.2.1.2 Reduction of the Protrusion

The pad of the thumb is placed on the pressure-sensitive protrusion according to palpation, and pressure is applied to the tissue. The goal is to push the herniated triggerpoint back into its original (usually deeper) fascial plane (fig. 5.13a and b). The amount and direction of pressure applied are adapted to the extent and direction of the protrusion. This means that just enough force is used to mobilize and reduce the herniated triggerpoint. The exact direction of pressure is determined by the shape of the protrusion canal through which the tissue has emerged from the deeper layers. Since this canal is not necessarily straight, the direction of pressure may also change during the course of treatment.

This maneuver, which is painful for the patient, can be facilitated by opening the passageway of the protrusion. This makes it easier to reduce the protrusion and shortens the duration of the uncomfortable treatment. For example, when treating a herniated triggerpoint in the shoulder girdle area, it may be advantageous to abduct the patient's arm and apply traction to stretch the passageway (fig. 5.14).

In the case of a distortion in the groin area, it may be helpful to reduce intra-abdominal pressure by manually pulling the abdominal organs toward the diaphragm. The same effect can be achieved by placing the patient in a head-down position, in which a herniated triggerpoint in the groin area can also be repositioned more easily. In general, the optimal positioning for the therapist can be verified, as this reduces the resistance that must be overcome to reposition the herniated triggerpoint.

Practical Tip

Depending on the location and type of tissue entrapment, considerable force may be required to reduce the protrusion. As a result, patients may experience more or less intense treatment pain. In addition, the technique can be very strenuous for the therapist.

It is therefore important that the therapist constantly seeks the optimal vector through which the protrusion can be mobilized as quickly as possible. In any case, prolonged static pressure on the protrusion should be avoided. If the herniated triggerpoint does not move, experience shows

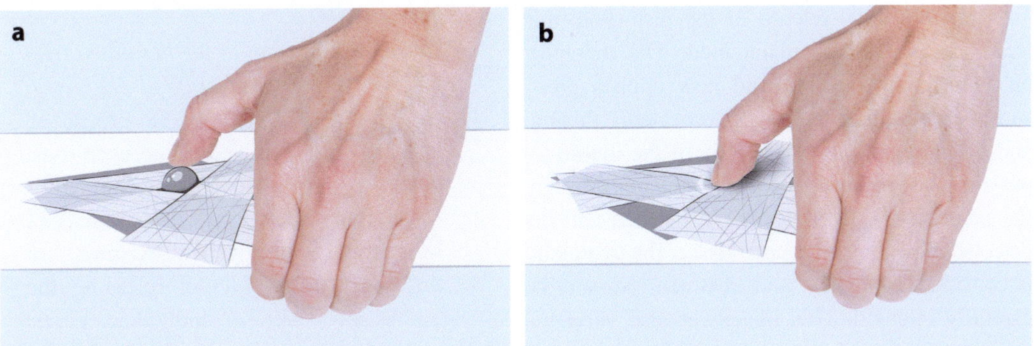

Fig. 5.13 Illustration of the herniated triggerpoint technique. Start repositioning with the pad of the thumb (**a**). Complete repositioning of the protrusion ("Milking the release") (**b**). (© Anker 2022)

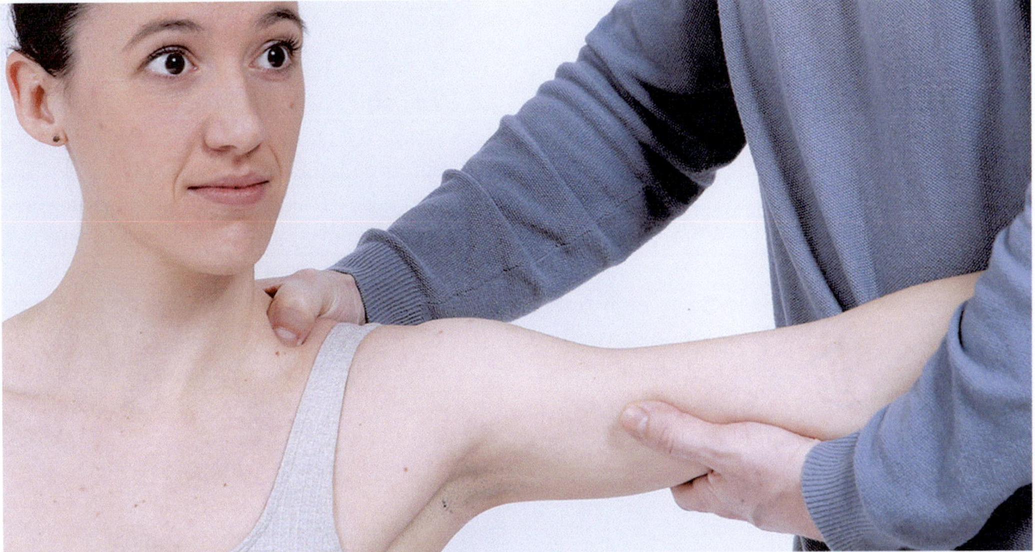

Fig. 5.14 Repositioning of a herniated triggerpoint at the shoulder with the arm abducted. (© Anker 2022)

that this is more likely due to the precision of the treatment than to a lack of force by the therapist.

The release marks the end of the second treatment step. The therapist perceives this tissue reaction as a progressive softening and reduction of the protrusion until it disappears. At the same time, patients describe a kind of relaxation in the affected region and a marked decrease in treatment pain despite continued treatment pressure.

5.2.1.3 Complete Repositioning ("Milking the Release")

The more completely the herniated triggerpoint is repositioned, the lower the risk of recurrence. The physiological protrusion canal remains anatomically present and is only closed by the functional repositioning of the tissue layers in this area. The more thoroughly the protrusion canal is cleared, the more effectively this closure occurs. For this reason, Typaldos recommends completing the herniated triggerpoint technique as follows:

After the initial release of the distortion, the treatment pressure is maintained. The therapist changes thumb position and now applies pressure with the tip of the thumb, repeatedly flexing and extending the distal phalanx of the thumb to push the last remnants of the protrusion through the passageway. If no further resistance can be detected indicating entrapped tissue, the treatment is considered complete and treatment pressure is carefully released. This maneuver also supports the repositioning of the overlapping layers, ensuring the functional closure of the hernial orifice.

Correction of a herniated triggerpoint should be performed with care. If the protrusion cannot be reduced, either the palpation must be checked or the technique or treatment position must be adjusted (e.g. by switching from a sitting to a lying down position when treating a herniated triggerpoint in the shoulder area).

Practical Tip

Compression of vessels, nerves, or other sensitive structures that must be passed on the way to the distortion should be avoided as much as possible. This makes the treatment less painful for the patient and allows them to relax more easily. As a result, less treatment pressure is often sufficient for repositioning.

In practice, complete repositioning of persistent herniated triggerpoints may extend over several treatment sessions. However, partial successes should be demonstrable after each therapy session, also because this confirms the FDM diagnosis.

Treatment of HTP Subtypes

In addition to the classic herniated triggerpoint, Typaldos describes two further subtypes (see sect. 2.2.1.1, fig. 2.9.) Their treatment requires partially adapted correction techniques:

- In the special form of the *herniated triggerpoint in the area of band-like fascia (Banded HTP)*, not only the protrusion but also the associated triggerband must be corrected. Typaldos recommends first repositioning the protrusion and immediately afterwards twisting out the triggerband, without releasing the thumb pressure. In individual cases, however, it may also be advantageous to first release adhesions in the area of the triggerband in order to facilitate repositioning of the herniated triggerpoint. After the protrusion has been corrected in a second step, the triggerband must eventually be completely re-sealed.

The order of treatment chosen depends primarily on the response of the entrapped tissue to the application of pressure. If the band-like herniated triggerpoint appears cemented in place by an adherent triggerband, repositioning is barely possible without first releasing adhesions. This particular correction is very physically demanding for the therapist and very painful for the patient. Therefore, after treatment, soft tissue pain may occur in the treated area, and rarely, bruising may also appear. For this reason, differentiated diagnostics in advance, precise palpation, and the avoidance of any roughness on the part of the therapist are an absolute priority.

- Treatment of the *pseudo-herniated triggerpoint* is performed using the triggerband technique instead of the herniated triggerpoint technique. In this case, there is no tissue protrusion, but rather an overlap of several chronic triggerbands, which appear as nodules on palpation. Treatment is performed with force to release the adherent nodule. This can cause severe pain for the patient, so the correction may need to be performed in stages.

5.2.2   Treatment Effects of the Herniated Triggerpoint Technique

Depending on the problem to be treated, the following therapeutic effects can be observed:

- If a herniated triggerpoint primarily impairs mobility, an immediate increase in the range of motion can be expected once the protrusion has been repositioned.
- Even in cases of pain-related movement restrictions, the extent of pain-free movement should be clearly increased immediately after correction.
- If the herniated triggerpoint is primarily associated with pain or tension, immediate resolution of symptoms is often not to be expected. Repeated treatment of the same herniated triggerpoint within the same therapy session is therefore not advisable, as patients need a therapy break to be able to assess the treatment effect.

The correction technique for the herniated triggerpoint can also be adapted according to the patient's problem:

- If the goal of treating a herniated triggerpoint is to improve movement, it is advisable to preposition the patient for correction in the direction of the movement limit. It may also be beneficial to passively move the affected joint into the restricted range during repositioning in order to enhance mobilization.
- In cases of pain or pain-related movement restrictions, it must be considered to what extent such forced mobilization is possible. Some patients tend to tense up during treatment, making repositioning more difficult. In this case, it is recommended to proceed gradually and to achieve an initial release through favorable positioning and/or involving the patient's breathing, which will then also be reflected in improved pain-free mobility.

5.2.3   Side Effects and Contraindications of the Herniated Triggerpoint Technique

As with the triggerband technique, open wounds, burns, or skin injuries in the area of the distortion are contraindications for the treatment of the herniated triggerpoint.

Apart from this, care must be taken during treatment of the herniated triggerpoint to ensure that *no unnecessary compression of vessels or nerves* occurs in the treatment area due to inaccurate positioning of the therapist's thumb. This may be indicated by increasing pain during treatment (even though the therapeutic pressure remains the same) or by tingling or numbness, e.g. in the patient's arm.

The herniated triggerpoint technique can cause muscle soreness-like symptoms after repositioning. These side effects can occur despite precise manual treatment and, once they have subsided, are not in themselves a contraindication for continuing treatment.

> **Background Information**
> Medically diagnosed hernias, such as inguinal hernias, can trigger symptoms of a herniated triggerpoint, such as movement restrictions, which can also be treated with the described correction technique. However, if severe pain in the abdominal and groin area occurs in addition, accompanied by nausea, vomiting, or cold sweats, caution is advised. There is a risk of necrosis of the entrapped tissue, so medical evaluation is urgently required.

5.2.4   Additional Measures for the Treatment of Herniated Triggerpoints

The positive effect of active movement on the reduction of a herniated triggerpoint is significantly less pronounced compared to triggerbands. Nevertheless, it is advisable to encourage patients, after successful manual correction, to move the treated area, as this supports the functional closure of the protrusion canal. In individual cases, it may also be helpful to prompt the patient to perform active movements during the application of the technique in order to mobilize the protrusion canal and thereby facilitate reduction.

In principle, *self-treatment* of a herniated triggerpoint is possible using appropriate aids (e.g. a triggerpoint stick). However, complete reduction is rarely achieved in this way, so symptoms often recur.

Complaints caused by herniated triggerpoints can only rarely be influenced by medication. Physical therapy approaches such as electrical stimulation or heat packs also have little lasting effect. Some patients may experience temporary symptom relief due to the loosening of tense smooth fascia and the resulting reduction in protrusion constriction. However, a mechanical reduction does not occur through such measures, so the deformation will persist and again cause symptoms.

Typaldos also considered surgical intervention for the correction of herniated triggerpoints. With surgical techniques already used for the reduction of hernias in conventional medicine, it would be conceivable to also correct herniated triggerpoints and to treat persistent entrapments surgically, for example in the back region. In clinical practice, however, this is only done in exceptional cases.

5.2.5 Treatment Examples

5.2.5.1 Shoulder HTP Technique— SCHTP Technique

> **Background Information**
> The treatment of the herniated triggerpoint at the shoulder (supraclavicular herniated triggerpoint—SCHTP) illustrates the change in perspective that the Fascial Distortion Model brings to the management of common clinical presentations:

> While classical treatment approaches for shoulder movement restrictions usually focus on joint structures, Typaldos emphasizes the importance of the herniated triggerpoint for mobilizing the shoulder.

Indications

- (Painful) restrictions in shoulder mobility, especially abduction and internal rotation; movement restrictions of the neck (especially rotation); tension in the shoulder girdle, tension headaches, or diffuse pain in the arm and fingers
- Possible mechanism of injury: mechanical trauma (e.g. a fall onto the shoulder or whiplash injury); often unknown cause
- Typical body language: pressing with several fingers of the opposite arm into the affected shoulder girdle area

Localization and Treatment

- Palpation of this herniated triggerpoint is performed in the region between the clavicle and the upper border of the scapula. Usually, the protrusion is located under the trapezius muscle, less commonly anteriorly directly above the clavicle or posteriorly above the scapula. Typaldos distinguishes herniated triggerpoints near the neck, which tend to restrict neck mobility, from those located more at the acromioclavicular joint, which have a greater impact on shoulder mobility.
- Reduction can be performed in a sitting or lying down position, either supine (fig. 5.15a) or prone, depending on the location of the herniated triggerpoint. The tightness of the surrounding tissue also plays a role, which can be reduced depending on the patient's position, thereby facilitating treatment.
- Reduction is performed using the herniated triggerpoint technique. Particular attention should be paid to opening the hernial orifice, for example by abducting and pulling on the patient's arm (fig. 5.14). Alternatively, the

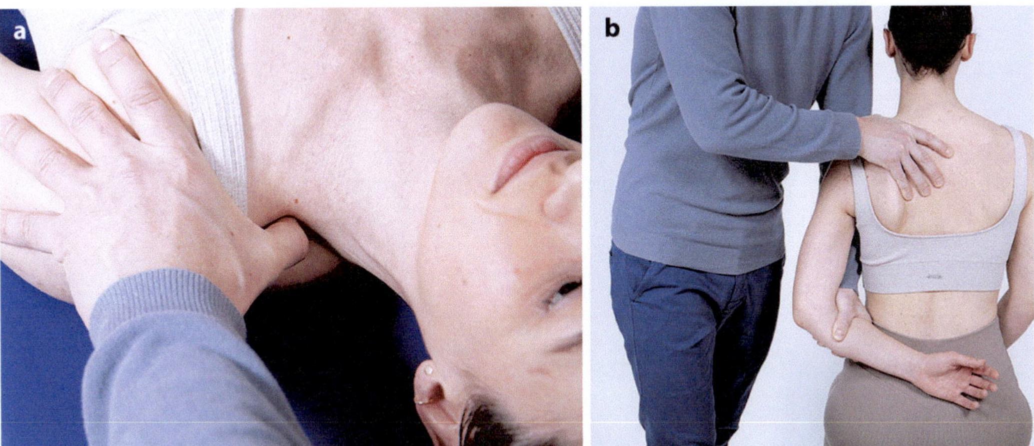

Fig. 5.15 Treatment of a herniated triggerpoint in the shoulder region. Technique in supine position (**a**). Technique for restriction of internal rotation of the shoulder in pre-positioning at the end of the range of motion with simultaneous passive mobilization (**b**). (© Anker 2022)

therapist can clamp the patient's arm between his thighs and extend his knees. This creates a strong traction force and also widens the protrusion canal. At the same time, both of the therapist's hands are free to press back the protrusion. The correction should not cause symptoms such as tingling or numbness in the arm or fingers.

Practical Tips

- If mobilization is the main focus, treatment should be performed at the end of the range of motion. In cases of chronic restriction, it may be advantageous to passively mobilize the shoulder at the same time as reducing the herniated triggerpoint (fig. 5.15b).
- If the protrusion is difficult to mobilize, changing the treatment position may help.

5.2.5.2 Herniated Triggerpoint Technique on the Groin

Indications

- (Painful) restriction of hip movement, especially flexion and external rotation; tension and pain in the groin or thigh

- Possible mechanism of injury: increased intra-abdominal pressure with simultaneous stretching of the groin area (e.g. due to heavy lifting), mechanical trauma (e.g. a strain), or in women during childbirth
- Typical body language: pressing several fingers into the hip crease

Localization and treatment

- Palpation starts at the thigh near the groin and proceeds towards the inguinal ligament in search of a nodular induration. This is tender to pressure and is clearly associated by the patient with her symptoms.
- The standard treatment position is the patient lying supine. Her leg rests over the therapist's flexed thigh to relax the groin area. Reduction is performed using the herniated triggerpoint technique and ends with a release of the herniated triggerpoint (fig. 5.16a).

Practical tips

- Treatment in the supine position can be facilitated if the patient pulls the deep tissues of the lower abdomen toward the diaphragma.

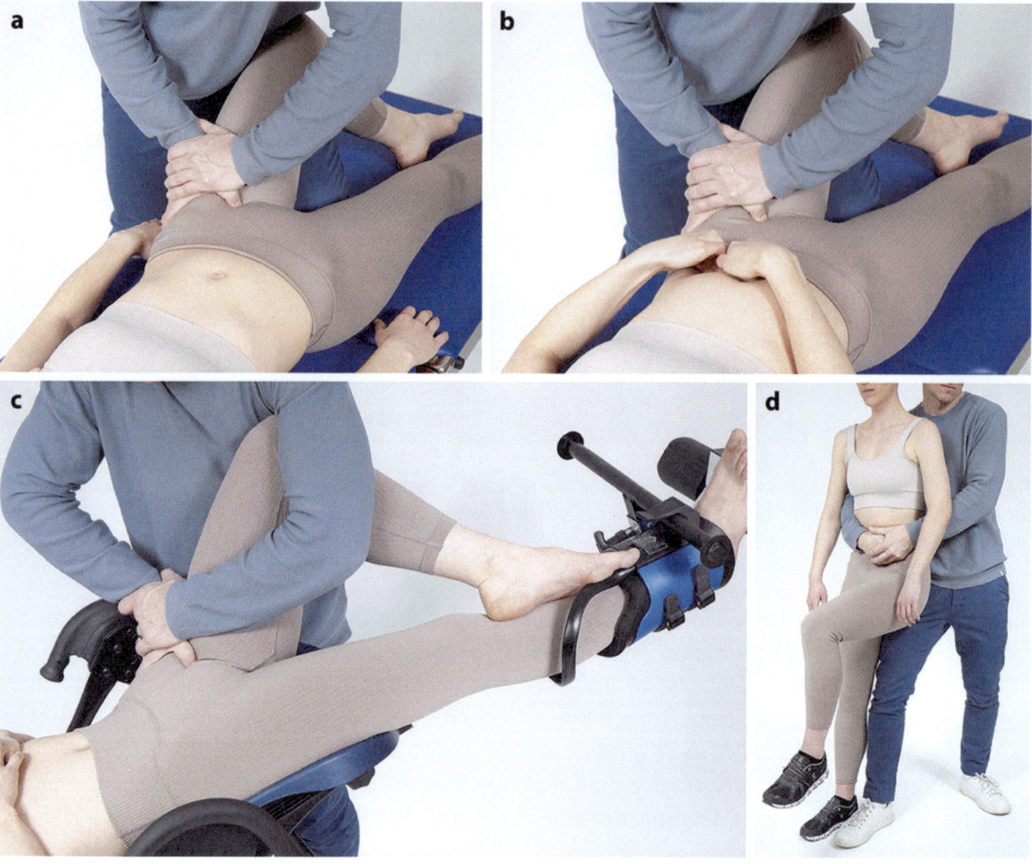

Fig. 5.16 Herniated triggerpoint technique at the groin. Standard positioning of the patient in the supine position (**a**). Supportive traction by the patient on the lower abdomen (**b**). Treatment in a slight head-down position using an inversion table (**c**). Alternative reduction technique with the patient standing (**d**). (© Anker 2022)

This reduces treatment pain and makes reduction easier (fig. 5.16b). The same effect can be achieved by performing the reduction in a slight head-down position (fig. 5.16c).

- Additionally or alternatively to the standard technique, a maneuver can be performed with the patient standing: she leans against the therapist while the therapist uses his hands to pull the deep tissues of the abdomen towards the chest. Under this traction, the patient performs a sweeping, circular external rotation movement to allow the entrapped protrusion to be released (fig. 5.16d).

5.2.5.3 Herniated Triggerpoint Technique on the Back

Indications

- Frequently painful restriction of back movement, especially extension or lateral flexion; sometimes extension-avoidance posture; persistent tension and pain in the back
- Possible mechanism of injury: increased intra-abdominal pressure with simultaneous stretching of the back, for example due to heavy lifting

- Typical body language: pressing several fingers or the thumb into the soft tissues of the back

Localization and treatment

- Typically, the herniated triggerpoint is located near the iliac crest (Belt HTP) or below the 12th rib (Flank HTP).
- If extension is restricted, the patient is treated while standing with arms supported (fig. 5.17). Alternatively, correction can also be performed in the lateral decubitus position or in a quadruped position. Reduction is performed using the herniated triggerpoint technique.

Practical tips

- If protective postures occur, treatment should aim for rapid realignment of the patient. The technique may need to be repeated several times for this purpose.
- The patient can be instructed to move actively during reduction (e.g. shifting the pelvis to the left or right) to ensure optimal widening of the protrusion canal.

5.2.5.4 Herniated Triggerpoint Technique on the Buttocks (Bullseye HTP)

Indications

- Pain and tension in the buttocks, back, or leg; often in association with existing back complaints; less commonly movement restrictions
- Possible mechanism of injury: fall onto the hip or back; significant weight loss or maximal exertion; often unknown trigger
- Typical body language: pressing several fingers, the thumb, or the knuckles into the buttocks

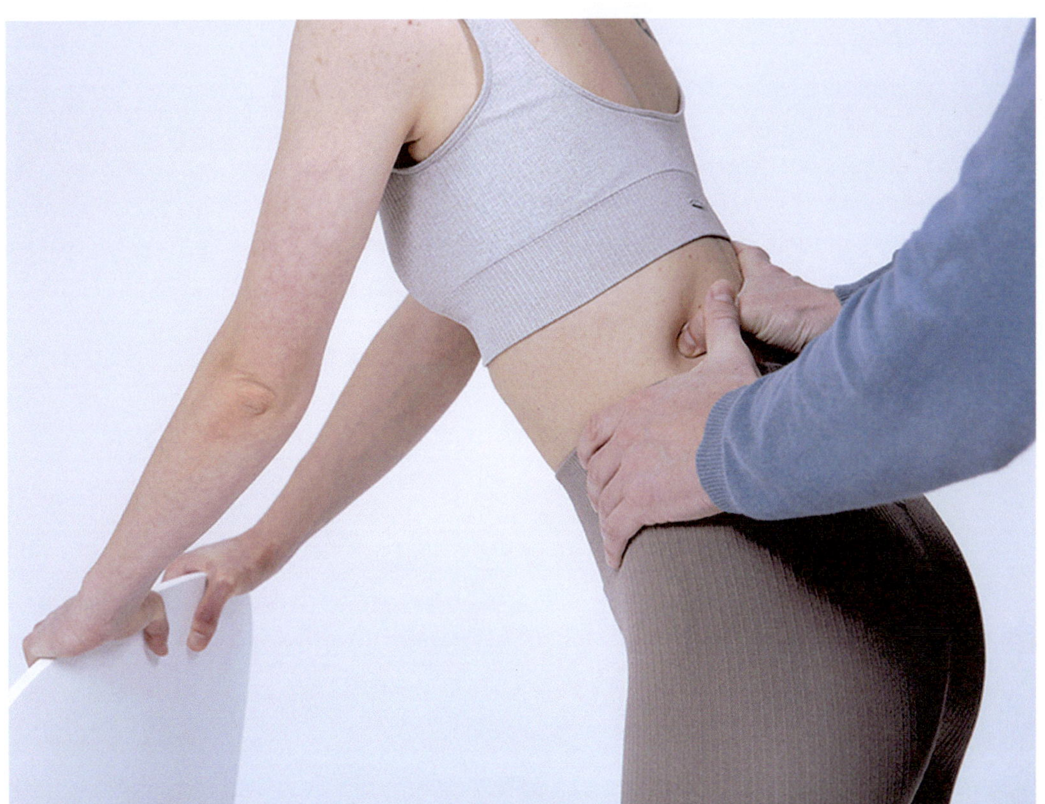

Fig. 5.17   Herniated triggerpoint technique in the flank area. (© Anker 2022)

Localization and treatment

- The protrusion is located centrally in the buttocks. This is the origin of its designation "Bullseye," the center of a target. Palpation and reduction often require considerable force. Supporting the treating thumb is recommended.
- Treatment is performed in the prone position or standing with arms supported. Reduction is performed using the herniated triggerpoint technique (fig. 5.18).

Practical tips

- If treated in the standing position, the patient can be instructed to move actively to ensure optimal widening of the protrusion canal (e.g. alternating flexion and extension of the knees).
- Typaldos describes a possible additional continuum distortion below the protrusion at the bone.

5.2.5.5 Herniated Triggerpoint Technique on the Orbit

Indications

- Pain in the area of the orbit or behind the eyeball
- Usually unknown mechanism of injury
- Typical body language: pressing with the thumb or fingers on the superior orbital rim

Localization and treatment

- The protrusion can be palpated in the area of the upper inner orbit at a small bony depression. A small, spongy, and pressure-sensitive induration can be felt with the tip of the thumb.
- Treatment is performed in the supine position, alternatively in a seated position. Reduction is achieved using an adapted herniated triggerpoint technique. The goal is a perceptible release (fig. 5.19).

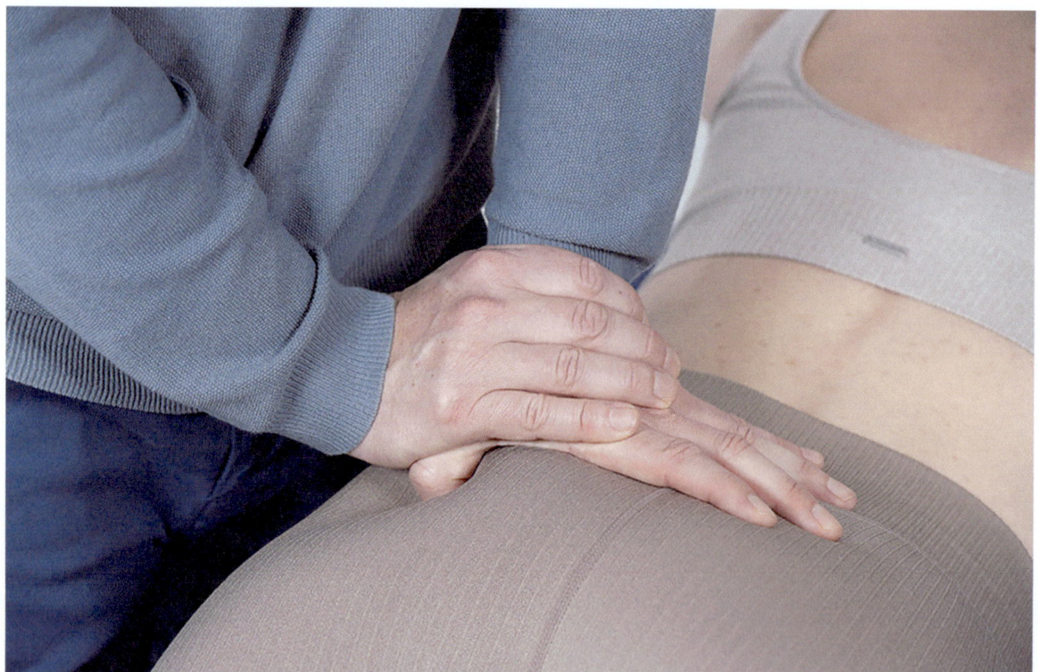

Fig. 5.18 Herniated triggerpoint technique at the buttocks. (© Anker 2022)

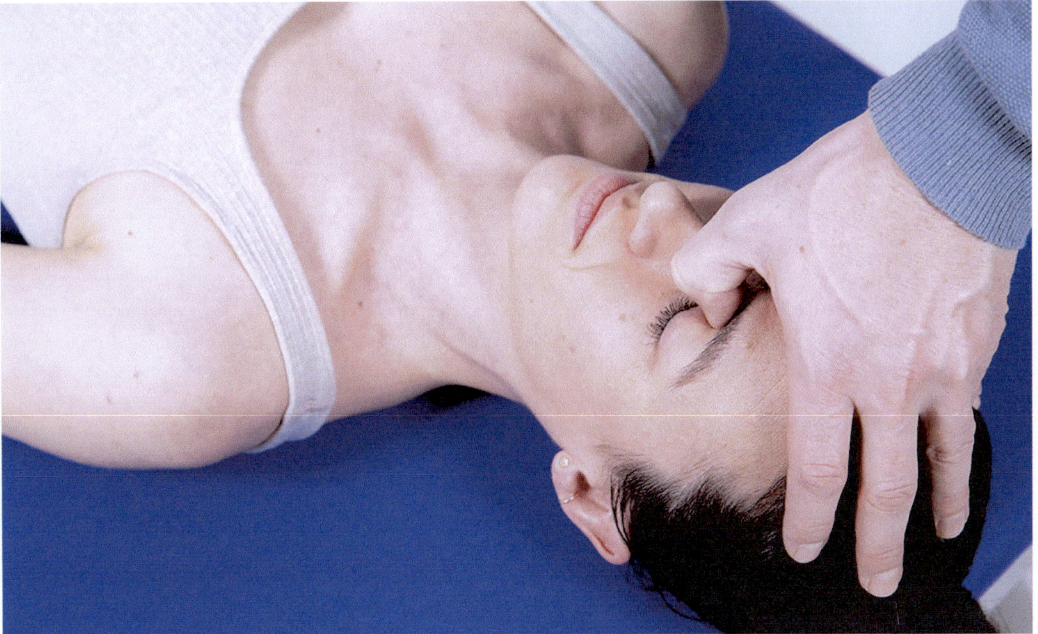

Fig. 5.19 Herniated triggerpoint technique in the area of the orbit. (© Anker 2022)

Practical tips

- If the therapist has a large thumb, the treatment can also be performed with the little finger.
- Typaldos additionally describes a triggerband from the temporomandibular joint, along the eyebrow to the root of the nose (see 5.1.5.5). In combination with the herniated triggerpoint, this is often responsible for pain behind the eyeball.

5.3 Treatment of Continuum Distortions

In continuum distortions, a part of a transition zone within the band-like fascia becomes stuck and forms a step-like deformation (see 2.3). The goal of any correction is to resolve this step, thereby allowing the transition zone to once again adapt as a whole to the forces acting upon it.

5.3.1 Continuum Technique

In the Typaldos method, a manual pressure technique performed with the tip of the thumb is used to correct the step formation of the transition zone. This continuum technique is the standard maneuver that can be applied to both everted and inverted continuum distortions. The procedure is as follows:

- Palpation of the continuum distortion
- Application of pressure until release

5.3.1.1 Palpation of the Continuum Distortion

An important clue to the localization of the continuum distortion is the typical body language (fig. 5.20). Precisely identifying the area for correction requires therapeutic skill, as these distortions are often located beneath a layer of soft tissue on the bone.

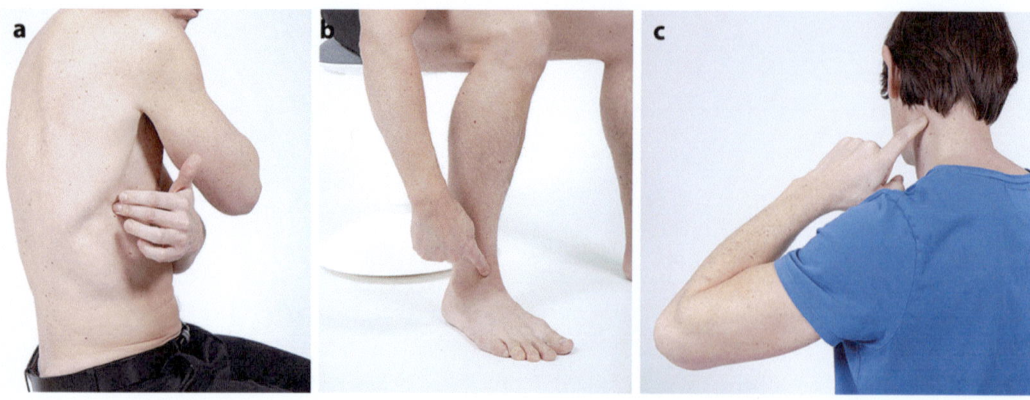

Fig. 5.20   **a** to **c**: Typical body language in a continuum distortion: pinpoint. (© Anker 2022)

The therapist's thumb tip penetrates the tissue without irritating the structures to be passed through. It is helpful to relax or appropriately position the affected area. Palpation is performed with millimeter precision in search of a tiny elevation, at most one to two millimeters in size (in everted continuum distortions), or a small depression (in inverted continuum distortions). Correct localization is confirmed when the typical pain can be elicited precisely and maximally, and the patient recognizes their symptoms.

Two points should be considered during palpation:

- The angle at which the therapist's thumb tip presses on the distortion plays a role. In continuum distortions, bony structures shift or become stuck along the course of the band-like fascia. Therefore, it is advisable to consider the anatomical alignment of the soft tissues in relation to the bone when applying pressure, and to align the thumb accordingly. This approach usually also leads to maximal provocation of pain, thereby confirming the accuracy of the corrective vector (fig. 5.21a and b).
- It may be advantageous to perform palpation (and subsequently treatment) of the continuum distortion in the position in which it originated. This provokes the symptoms and allows the patient to localize the pain point more precisely. In addition, it makes it easier for the therapist to find the correct corrective vector, which can, among other things, be derived from the mechanism of injury.

5.3.1.2 Application of Pressure Until Release

According to the optimal direction of pressure determined during palpation, the therapist uses the tip of their thumb to act directly on the distortion. With firm, targeted pressure, the step formation in the transition zone is reduced in this way. This applies to both everted and inverted continuum distortions (fig. 5.22a and b).

The applied force should lead to a reaction of the continuum distortion after 5 to 30 seconds, which Typaldos refers to as a "shift." Primarily, this means a marked decrease in pain within a short period of one to five seconds. The patient clearly perceives this release. Independently, the therapist may also perceive a change, as if the palpable irregularity on the bone is reduced or the area relaxes.

5.3.2 Treatment Effects of the Continuum Technique

Typaldos describes the response of a continuum distortion to the pressure technique with the "all-or-none principle": the step formation of the transition zone can either be completely corrected or does not respond to therapy at all,

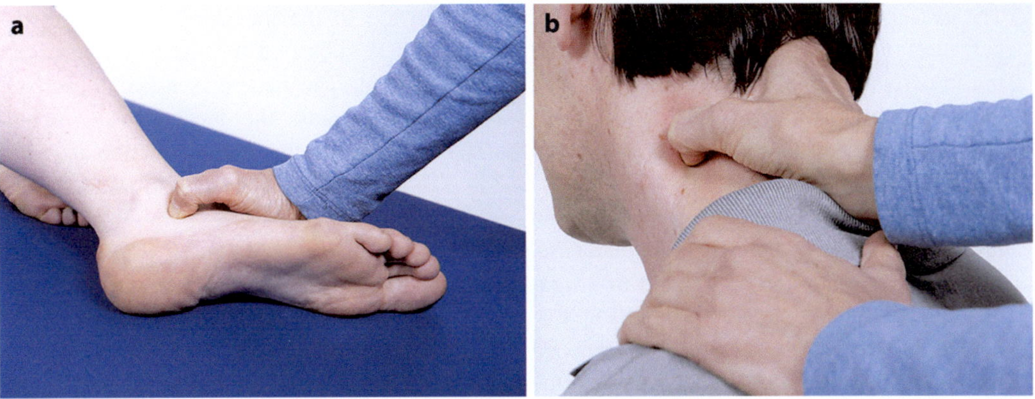

Fig. 5.21   Positioning of the thumb tip according to the anatomical alignment of the band-like fascia at the ankle (**a**) and at the neck (**b**). (© Anker 2022)

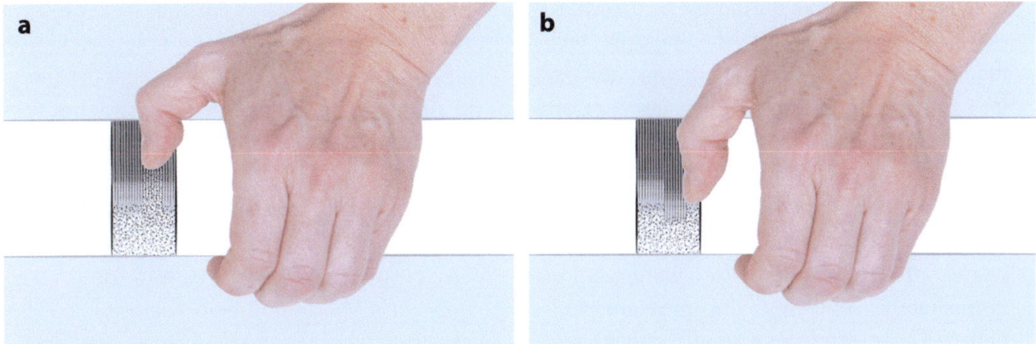

Fig. 5.22   Schematic representation of the continuum technique. Treatment of an everted continuum distortion: pressure directly on the bony fixed part of the transition zone (**a**). Treatment of an inverted continuum distortion: pressure on the edge of the distortion to reduce the step formation (**b**). (© Anker 2022)

similar to a light switch that only has an on or off position. Partial successes, as seen in the treatment of triggerbands or herniated triggerpoints, are not possible.

This is reflected in how the typical symptoms respond to the pressure technique:

- **The symptoms can be completely and sustainably resolved with the continuum technique**
  In this case, according to the all-or-none principle, a complete correction of the distortion can be assumed. Further treatment is not necessary.
- **The symptoms are only partially reduced**

The most likely explanation in this case is the presence of multiple continuum distortions, which must be resolved step by step until the maximum therapeutic effect is achieved. The presence of additional distortions, such as triggerbands, should also be considered.

- **The symptoms do not subside - no release occurs**
  After the diagnosis of a continuum distortion has been verified, there are usually two reasons for failure with the continuum distortion technique: either the direction or the amount of force must be adjusted to correct the transition zone.
- **The symptoms intensify during the course of treatment**

The cause of this reaction is often inaccurate palpation of the continuum distortion, resulting in compression of structures surrounding the continuum distortion.

- **The symptoms subside during correction but recur after treatment**

This can be interpreted as an indication of an inverted continuum distortion. In that case, part of the transition zone is fixed in a ligamentous configuration, and a type of step formation also develops. This can be reduced with the pressure technique by forcing the transition zone completely into its ligamentous configuration and creating a uniform level within the zone (fig. 5.22b). This provides the opportunity for the transition zone to readapt as a whole during the next configuration change. However, the pressure technique cannot transport stabilizing minerals into the transition zone, which are typically lacking in an inverted continuum distortion.

According to Typaldos, this deficiency explains the tendency for recurrence in this subtype. He therefore recommends the application of targeted *impulse manipulations* immediately following the pressure technique. These produce a unidirectional pull, drawing minerals from the bone into the transition zone. As clinical experience shows, this subsequently reduces the recurrence rate.

This approach is particularly suitable for continuum distortions in the area of joints. If the location of the continuum distortion does not permit such manual treatment, or if there are contraindications for thrust techniques, the following approach may be successful:

- Through *repeated application of the continuum technique*, the step formation is repeatedly corrected and fluid transport along the band-like fibers is increasingly improved. As a result, the supply of minerals to the transition zone normalizes over time, leading to resolution of the step formation.

- Another way to support mineralization of the transition zone is the use of *pinch techniques*. In this method, the tissue directly on top of the inverted continuum distortion is subjected to strong unidirectional traction. The patient is asked to actively move against the tensile force, or the therapist applies abrupt traction impulses to draw bony elements into the transition zone.

Background Information

Once the continuum distortion is corrected, from the perspective of the Fascial Distortion Model, there is no further need for protection. A particularly striking example in this context is the treatment of acute ankle trauma. Although conventional medicine assumes that immobilization, whether by bandage or offloading with crutches, is necessary to support the healing of strained ligamentous structures, treatment with the Typaldos method renders this approach obsolete if the patient's symptoms are due to continuum distortions. In such cases, successful treatment results in immediate and lasting improvement in mobility and load-bearing capacity, up to complete rehabilitation after just one therapy session.

5.3.3 Side Effects and Contraindications of the Continuum Technique

Side effects of the continuum technique can include *local pain or hematomas*, especially with inaccurate palpation. Such effects can be reduced by not exceeding the typical time span of 5 to 30 seconds until the shift occurs. Special attention should also be paid to palpation. Only the localized pain of the distortion described by the patient should be elicited, and no symptoms should occur in the area surrounding the deformation.

Contraindications are present if the patient's skin or tissue cannot withstand strong pressure (e.g. in the case of abrasions) or if the continuum distortion cannot be precisely palpated.

Practical Tip
If recurrences (apart from inverted continuum distortions) occur or if there is no positive treatment effect at all, caution is advised. In addition to reviewing the working hypothesis, a differential diagnostic evaluation of the involved structures may be necessary. This applies both in the context of a mechanism of injury due to physical trauma and in cases of localized bone pain that has occurred without any mechanical cause.

5.3.4 Additional Measures for the Treatment of Continuum Distortions

Apart from the continuum technique, *pharmacological interventions* or methods of physical medicine can also influence this type of distortion.

Similar to triggerbands, injections of steroidal anti-inflammatory medications can lead to a reduction in symptoms. Typaldos explains this by the potential of these substances to mobilize minerals within the tissue continuum and shift them into the transition zone. As a result, the zone completely shifts into the bony configuration, and the step formation is reduced. This provides the opportunity for the fixed area of the zone to move again during the next configuration change. However, in clinical practice, it is often observed that this therapeutic effect is not permanent.

Another alternative to manual treatment is the use of *shockwave therapy*. Its mechanical effect also reduces step formation and can thus resolve the symptoms of continuum distortions.

Background Information
A continuum distortion is not a wound, and therefore cannot heal. Nevertheless, this impression may arise because continuum distortions can disappear over time. This is not related to wound healing

mechanisms, but rather to the impaired, though usually not completely halted, fluid transport along the affected band-like fibers. The resulting reduced, but not completely blocked, mineral transport can slowly compensate for the step formation, causing the corresponding symptoms to resolve autonomously.

According to experience, this phenomenon is observed in connection with continuum distortions that cause pain. In persistent (low-pain) movement restrictions caused by this type of distortion, this form of autonomous correction occurs much less frequently.

5.3.5 Treatment Examples

5.3.5.1 Continuum Technique on the Anterior Ankle—AACD Technique

Background Information
This continuum distortion (anterior ankle continuum distortion) is, according to Typaldos, found in all patients after an ankle sprain. A typical symptom is inhibition of rolling over the ankle or foot.

Indications

- Restriction of movement during active dorsiflexion; localized pain at the joint or bone
- Possible mechanism of injury: typically occurs in the context of an acute ankle sprain; less commonly due to muscular weakness (e.g. as a result of a neurological disorder)
- Typical body language: pointing with individual fingers to a spot on the anterior ankle

Localization and treatment

- The patient's body language can help identify the distortion. However, in the absence of gestures, Typaldos recommends palpation at two typical sites: either in the joint space between the tibia and fibula, or in the ligament groove at the lateral malleolus.

- Treatment is performed using the continuum technique, which can be carried out with the patient sitting or lying down. First, the anterior ankle is relaxed by passive flexion. After palpating the distortion with the tip of the thumb, correction is performed with targeted pressure according to the orientation of the band-like fascia (fig. 5.23).

Practical tips

- The AACD technique is usually the first step in the treatment of an acute ankle sprain. The goal is to restore flexion mobility and improve the rolling mechanism. Subsequently, the distortions the patient notices while walking are then treated.
- A limitation of ankle dorsiflexion while standing (e.g. during stair climbs) can also be caused by triggerbands, tectonic fixations, or folding distortions of the ankle or the interosseous membrane of the lower leg.
- In clinical experience, complete restoration of ankle mobility after trauma is an important preventive measure to avoid recurrent ankle sprains.

5.3.5.2 Continuum Technique on the Sacroiliac Joint

Indications

- Localized pain at the joint or bone, often when walking or extending the back
- Possible mechanism of injury: acute strain in the pelvic area (e.g. after a fall); less commonly due to overuse
- Typical body language: pointing with individual fingers to a spot

Localization and treatment

- This often inverted continuum distortion is usually located deep in the joint space.

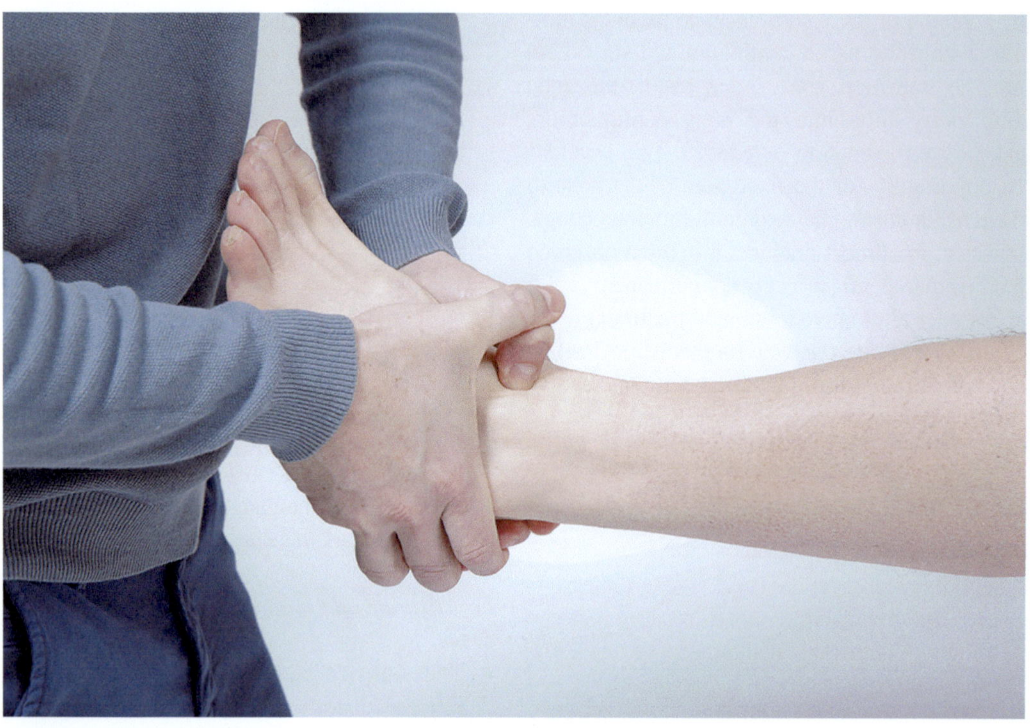

Fig. 5.23   Continuum treatment on the anterior ankle (AACD technique). (© Anker 2022)

- Correction is performed using the continuum technique until release is achieved (fig. 5.24a). Treatment is performed with the patient standing and arms supported. If this results in a satisfactory outcome, the treatment can be concluded. If symptoms recur (typical in inverted continuum distortions), the technique must be repeated and, in addition, an impulse manipulation technique (e.g. in the scissor position) should be applied.

Manual Impulse Treatment of the Pelvis in the Scissor Position

For this technique, the patient is positioned in a lateral decubitus position. The therapist stands astride behind the treatment table. She pulls the patient's lower hand or forearm close to his pelvis, thereby stabilizing the patient's trunk. Then she places the patient's upper leg over the edge of the treatment table and positions the impulse hand at the sacroiliac joint. She instructs the patient to turn his face toward the ceiling and rolls the patient slightly backwards towards herself. The impulse is generated by a sudden thrust of the hand at the pelvis forward while simultaneously stabilizing the patient's upper body (fig. 5.24b).

Practical tips

- The typical body language of pointing in this area can also be an indication of a tectonic

fixation or a folding distortion. In clinical experience, patients then describe a sensation of blockage or a deep-seated pain. In these cases, the impulse technique described above in the scissor position is also suitable.

5.3.5.3 Continuum Technique on the Knee

Indications

- Localized pain at the joint space or bone during movement or loading
- Possible mechanism of injury: acute dislocation or sprain of the knee; knee contusion; less commonly due to overuse
- Typical body language: pointing with individual fingers to a specific spot on the knee or patella

Localization and treatment

- According to the patient's description, the continuum distortion is palpated and treated in a position that provokes symptoms whenever possible.
- Correction is performed using the continuum technique and is repeated until the patient is symptom-free (fig. 5.25a). Treatment can be performed lying down, sitting, or standing with arms supported.

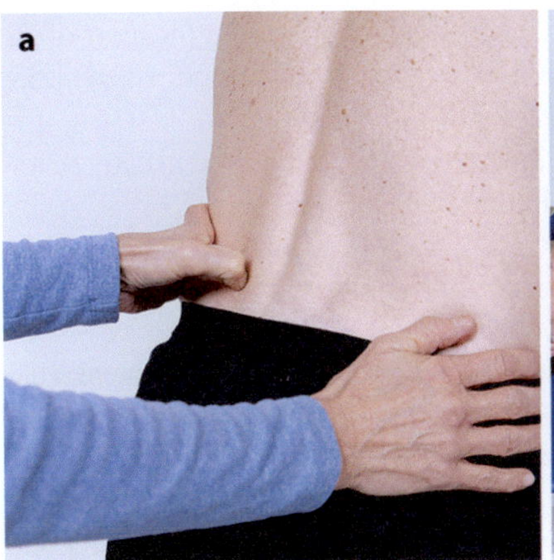
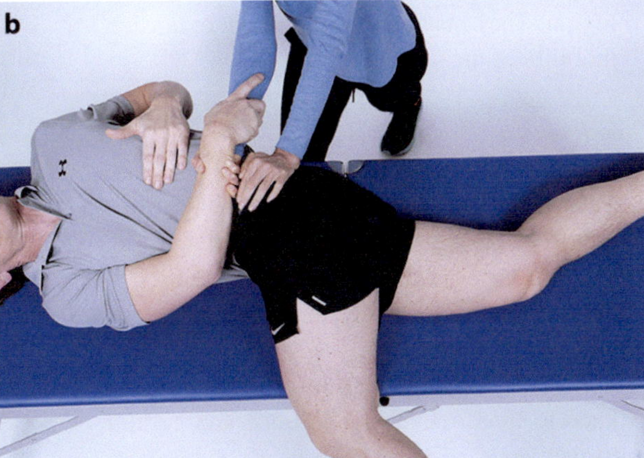

Fig. 5.24 Continuum treatment at the sacroiliac joint, continuum technique (**a**). Impulse-manual treatment in the scissor position for resolution of an inverted continuum distortion (**b**). (© Anker 2022)

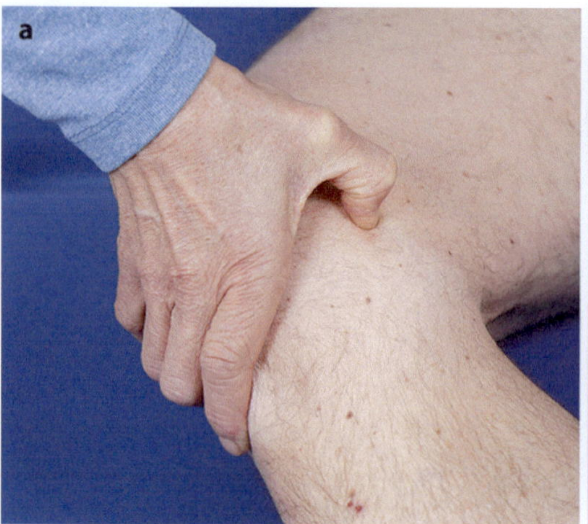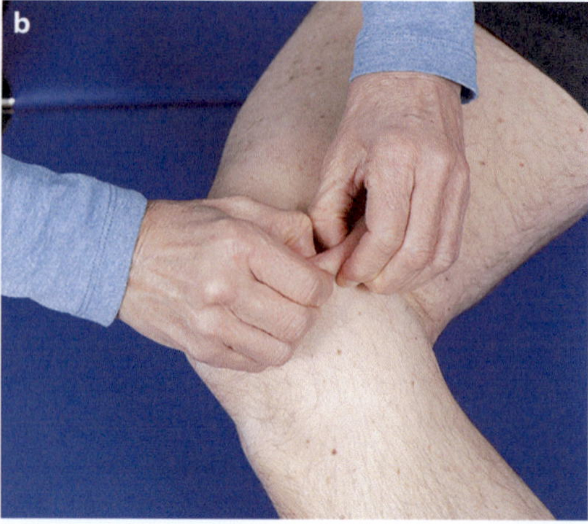

Fig. 5.25 Continuum treatment at the knee, continuum technique (**a**). Pinch technique for resolving an inverted continuum distortion (**b**). (© Anker 2022)

- In the context of contusions, inverted continuum distortions may occur, which are less effectively treated with the continuum technique. In such cases, impulse manipulation techniques can be applied. Another targeted option is the pinch technique (fig. 5.25b), which can be used to apply traction to the blocked transition zone. The skin fold overlying the distortion is grasped as close to the bone as possible and manipulated with a quick jerk. Alternatively, the patient can be asked to extend the knee against the therapist's resistance.
- *Continuum distortions in the popliteal fossa are another typical localization. These can be found at the posterior aspect of the femur, deep beneath the soft tissues of the popliteal region. They may restrict flexion or extension mobility of the knee.*

Practical tips

- The typical body language of pointing in this area may also indicate a folding distortion. In such cases, patients typically describe a deep-seated pain in the joint that cannot be palpated.
- The *pinch technique* can also be used at the knee to treat cylinder distortions and certain triggerbands.

5.3.5.4 Continuum Technique on the Ribs

Indications

- Localized pain at the bone after a rib contusion or rib fracture
- Typical body language: pointing with individual fingers to a specific spot on the ribs

Localization and treatment

- The patient knows the location and can guide the therapist to the distortion.
- Treatment is performed using the continuum technique in the pain-provoking position (fig. 5.26). Depending on the location of the distortion, treatment can be performed sitting or lying down.
- The initial goal is to reduce the usually severe respiration-dependent pain.

Practical tips

- Serial rib fractures or multi-fragment fractures should not be treated without medical monitoring.
- If the correction is too painful for the patient, the pain threshold can first be increased with

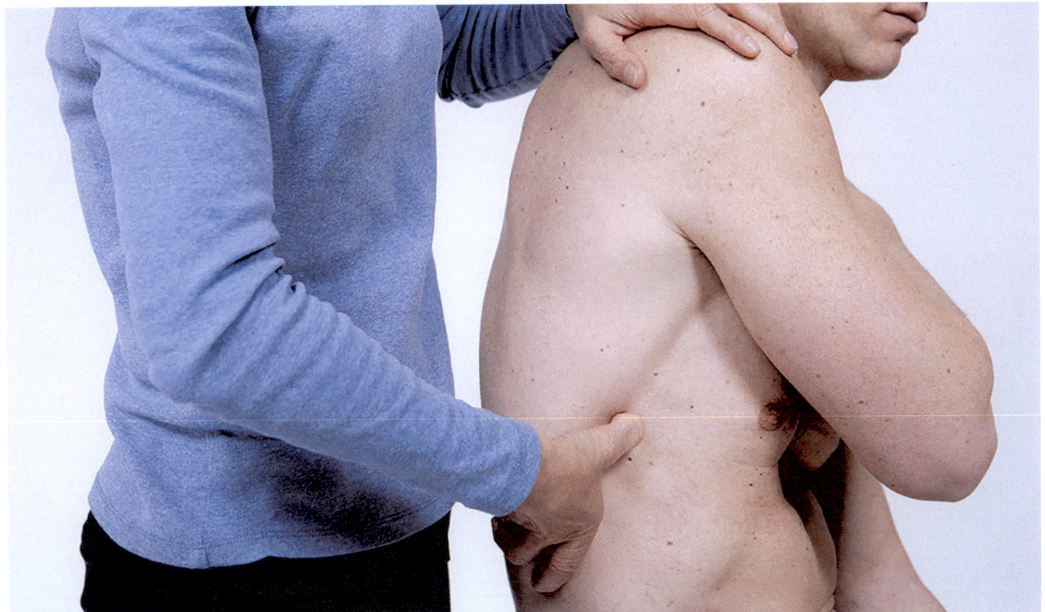

Fig. 5.26 Continuum technique at the ribs. (© Anker 2022)

ice or cold spray. Cold applications are also suitable immediately after treatment.

5.3.5.5 Continuum Technique on the Wrist—PWCD Technique

Continuum distortion at the lateral wrist (Posterior wrist continuum distortion—PWCD) frequently occurs in association with wrist sprains. According to Typaldos, it is one of the main causes of restricted extension mobility.

Indications

- Restriction of active wrist extension; localized pain at the carpal bones or at the transition to the forearm
- Possible mechanism of injury: traumatic cause; less commonly in the context of muscular weakness (e.g. due to a neurological disorder)
- Typical body language: pointing with the fingers to a specific spot on the lateral wrist

Localization and treatment

- The patient knows the location and can guide the therapist to the distortion.
- According to Typaldos, this everted continuum distortion is located on the thumb side, little finger side, or centrally on the dorsal wrist. Frequently, multiple continuum distortions can also be found.
- Treatment is performed using the continuum technique. It is recommended to apply traction to the wrist during correction (fig. 5.27).

Practical tips

- In the case of an acute wrist sprain, the primary goal is to restore pain-free wrist extension using the continuum technique.
- Folding distortions of the wrist or the interosseous membrane of the forearm are, according to Typaldos, other typical causes of restricted extension mobility.

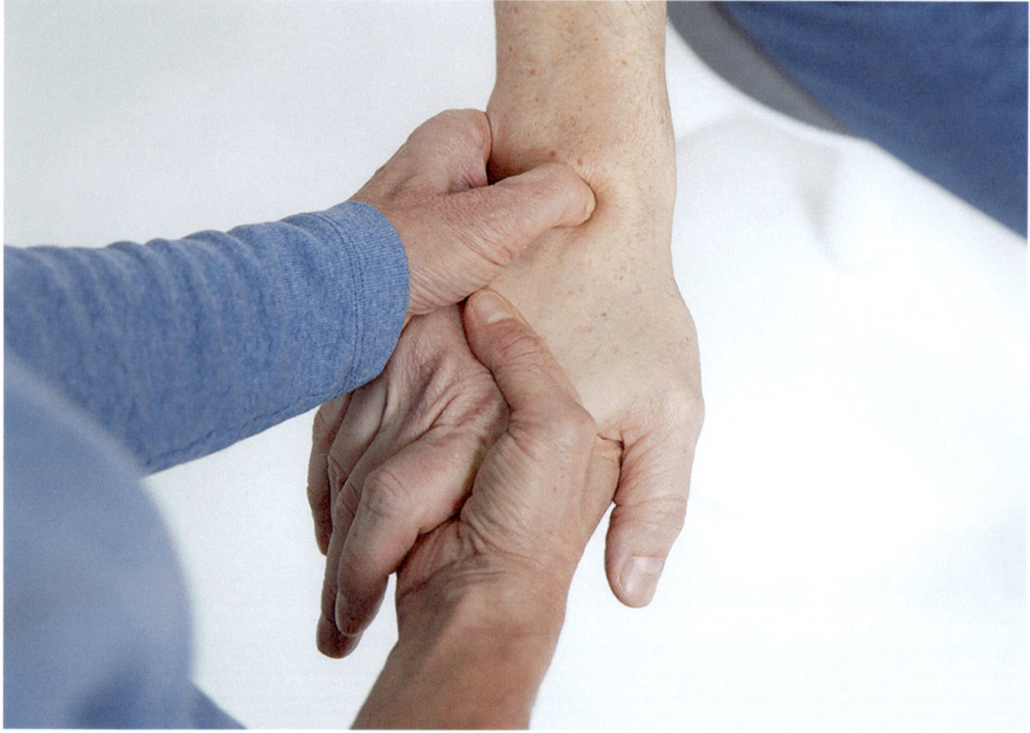

Fig. 5.27 Continuum treatment at the wrist (PWCD). (© Anker 2022)

5.4   Treatment of Folding Distortions

A folding distortion can be described as a dislocated or sprained folding fascia. Folding distortions impair the shock-absorbing function of this fascial type and cause movement- and load-related pain, swelling, or a feeling of instability in patients (fig. 5.30).

The goal of any treatment for a folding distortion is to restore the shock-absorbing function of the folding fascia. For the correction of folding distortions, especially in the area of the back as well as the joints of the arms and legs, the Typaldos method relies more on standardized procedures than on standardized techniques. The treatment is characterized by basic principles which can be implemented using various maneuvers, many of which are known from conventional manual therapy.

In contrast, the maneuvers for correcting folding distortions in the area of the interosseous membranes and muscle septa are more precisely defined. They are typical of the Typaldos method and follow established principles.

5.4.1   Principles of Treating Folding Distortions

In principle, a folding distortion can be resolved by reproducing or imitating the mechanism of injury. This means that an unfolding distortion, which arises through traction and twisting or shearing, can be resolved using the same vectors (fig. 5.28).

This relationship can be clearly illustrated using the example of shoulder dislocation. The dislocation occurs through a dislocation of the joint under traction. From the perspective of the Fascial Distortion Model, this leads to an unfolding distortion of the shoulder. The classic conventional medical therapy (known as the Hippocratic maneuver) again uses traction to reposition the joint. Thus, the repositioning of joints or bones, as is performed daily in orthopedics, can be considered the prototype of unfolding distortion treatment.

The treatment concept for refolding distortion is based on the same principle, and uses compressive forces to correct the folding fascia accordingly. For example, a sprained wrist with refolding distortion can be corrected using manipulation techniques under compression. Some therapists reject the use of compression in manual therapy, especially when it is primarily associated with applying pressure to individual anatomical structures. However, if we focus on the folding fascia, which is blocked in compression by the mechanism of injury in refolding distortion, this deformation cannot be resolved by applying traction, but rather requires the reapplication of a compressive force allowing the folds of the fascia to return to their original form (fig. 5.29).

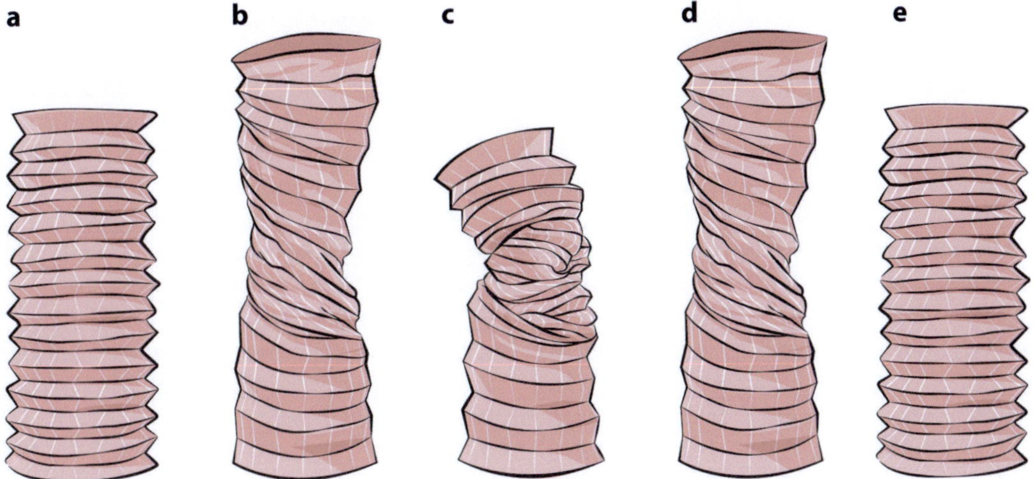

Fig. 5.28 a to e: Development and correction of an unfolding distortion. The intact folding fascia (**a**) is dislocated by traction and shearing movements (**b**). An unfolding distortion develops (**c**). To correct this distortion, traction and shearing movements are again applied (**d**), so that the folding fascia can finally return to its original form (**e**). (© Anker 2022)

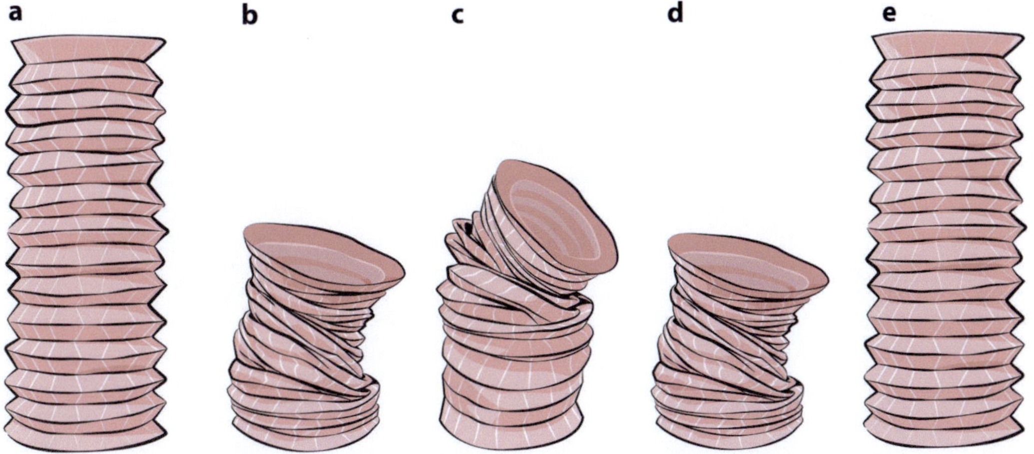

Fig. 5.29 Development and correction of an refolding distortion. The intact folding fascia (**a**) is sprained by compression and shearing movements (**b**). A refolding distortion develops (**c**). To correct this distortion, compression and shearing movements are again applied (**d**), so that the folding fascia can finally return to its original form (**e**). (© Anker 2022)

From these considerations, a two-step treatment process can be derived, which can be applied in particular to folding distortions of joints using mobilization or impulse-manipulation techniques:

- Determination of the correction vectors
- Manual treatment of the folding distortion

5.4.1.1 Determination of Correction Vectors

Unfolding and refolding distortions can be differentiated based on four criteria:

- *Mechanism of injury:* traction, hyperextension, and twisting of a joint are more likely to lead to unfolding distortions, whereas compression in an end-range joint position usually favors the development of refolding distortions.
- *Body language:* grasping a joint with the hand is a classic nonverbal indicator, which can be observed in both unfolding and refolding distortions (fig. 5.30a). For refolding distortions, the FDM recognizes another gesture, namely a dynamic horizontal stroking motion across the joint (fig. 5.30b). In contrast, there is no specific body language that exclusively indicates an unfolding distortion.
  In folding distortions involving the interosseous membranes or muscle septa, specific gestures can be observed, but these can barely be distinguished in terms of unfolding versus refolding distortion (fig. 5.30c).
- *Symptom dynamics over the course of the day:* unfolding distortions produce more symptoms during the day and with the increasing effect of gravity in the upright posture. In contrast, with refolding distortions, it is observed that more symptoms, such as pain or stiffness, are present in the morning and tend to resolve over the course of the day, or at least do not increase.
- *Manual testing:* if the therapist applies manual compression to a joint with an unfolding distortion, it will be uncomfortable for the patient, whereas applying traction will be relieving. Conversely, if the therapist compresses a joint with a refolding distortion, the patient will experience relaxation, while traction tends to provoke symptoms.

In addition to these four criteria, the following factors can influence the choice of correction vector:

- *Any treatment technique for folding distortions avoids reproducing the patient's typical symptoms (in contrast to the triggerband technique, the herniated triggerpoint technique, and the continuum technique, in which symptom provocation is a central element).*
  This means: If the correction vector is correct, the treatment—regardless of whether it is

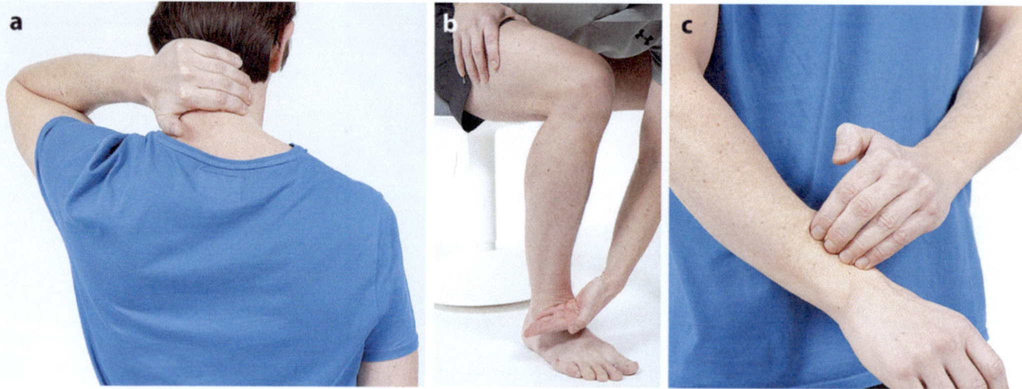

Fig. 5.30 Typical body language in folding distortions. Gestures at the neck (**a**). Gestures in refolding distortion at the ankle (**b**). Gestures in folding distortion of the interosseous membrane (**c**). (© Anker 2022)

performed with or without impulse—is painless and easily tolerated by the patient. This absence of symptom provocation also serves as a guide for the therapist when it is difficult to find the exact vector for correction.

- It can be advantageous to consider the dynamics of how the distortion developed. Folding distortions caused by a dynamic force (such as in a fall) often respond better to equally dynamic correction techniques with impulse than to treatments using sustained traction or compression without an acceleration component.
- However, it is not necessary to reproduce the magnitude of the force that caused the distortion. This means that a folding distortion caused, for example, by a traffic accident cannot be corrected more effectively by attempting to replicate the massive force of the accident. Regardless of the fact that such forces can hardly be applied by the therapist in the context of manual therapy, such an approach is potentially risky for the patient and can lead to injury. Furthermore, clinical experience shows that the dynamics of the force application are more decisive than its absolute magnitude.
- The body position in which the distortion occurred is often also suitable as the correction position. It may be that performing the folding distortion treatment in this position is particularly effective. In addition, resuming the injury position supports the patient's perception, making it easier to find the exact correction vector (see 3.1.4).

5.4.1.2 Manual Treatment of Folding Distortions

The main elements of the manual folding technique are traction for the unfolding distortion and compression for the refolding distortion. These are supplemented by additional movements such as rotation or shearing movements to release the deformed folding fascia.

The Typaldos method distinguishes between different forms of manual treatment. Whichever approach is chosen, the therapist corrects the folding distortion until its function is restored.

The following therapeutic approaches can be distinguished:

- Treatments with sustained traction or compression
- Impulse treatments with pre-loading in traction or compression
- Impulse treatments without pre-loading in traction or compression
- Treatment techniques for the interosseous membrane
- Treatment techniques for the muscle septa

5.4.2   Treatments with Sustained Traction or Compression

Non-thrust techniques can be used for uncomplicated folding distortions when constant traction or compression is sufficient to resolve the distortion, or when a thrust technique is contraindicated. The sustained traction or compression can be initiated either by the therapist or by the patient themselves.

In classical manual therapy, traction treatments play a major role. By applying a pulling force, joint surfaces aligned in parallel are separated and unloaded, and the surrounding structures are stretched. Unfolding techniques without thrust are performed in a similar manner, but their goal is to imitate the traction mechanism involved in the origin of the distortion. This allows the folds of the fascia to reposition themselves in an improved form after the traction is released. In this case, biomechanical considerations play a lesser role in selecting the appropriate vector for treatment. Rather, the extent and direction of traction are fundamentally adapted to the mechanism of injury.

With this form of unfolding technique, additional small movements can be introduced by the therapist while traction is applied. This can further support the resolution of the distortion. For example, in an acutely sprained ankle with unfolding distortion, gentle sustained traction combined with small mobilizing movements may be sufficient to correct the folding fascia.

The refolding treatment without thrust is performed in the opposite manner and utilizes sustained compression of the folding fascia to resolve the deformation. It is important to note that this does not focus on compressing joint surfaces; rather, the mechanism of injury of the distortion again determines the treatment vector. Additional passive movements or the introduction of shearing compression movements respect this principle. An example is a sprained ankle with refolding distortion, which can be corrected by therapeutic compression combined with passive mobilization.

For the treatment of such a refolding distortion, it is also possible for the patient themselves to apply compression to the folding fascia. For example, repetitive bouncing on a trampoline can be considered a form of compression treatment.

Folding distortion treatment without thrust is also an option for correcting persistent folding distortions, specifically as a preparation of the folding fascia for treatments with thrust.

(Contraindications such as cardiovascular diseases, increased intraocular pressure, neurological pre-existing conditions, etc., must be strictly observed during these maneuvers). In principle, the patient should be able to remain in the inverted position for at least 15 seconds to achieve a stretching effect on the folded fascia. Subsequently, mobilization techniques with thrust can be applied (fig. 5.31a).

A similar approach is used in the so-called *ball therapy*, which also works on the principle of sustained traction or compression. The patient lies in various positions over a large exercise ball to stretch or compress the fascia of the back. Additionally, the therapist can manually enhance the effect. This form of treatment is particularly well suited as a home exercise program for patients with persistent folding distortions (fig. 5.31b).

Inversion and Ball Therapy
A special form in this context is *inversion therapy*, which can be used for the treatment of the back and legs. In this technique, the patient is placed in an inverted position using various therapeutic devices, so that traction is generated by gravity.

5.4.3   Impulse Treatments with Pre-Loading in Traction or Compression

Impulse techniques have the advantage of reproducing the causative forces of folding distortions, including their dynamics. As is common

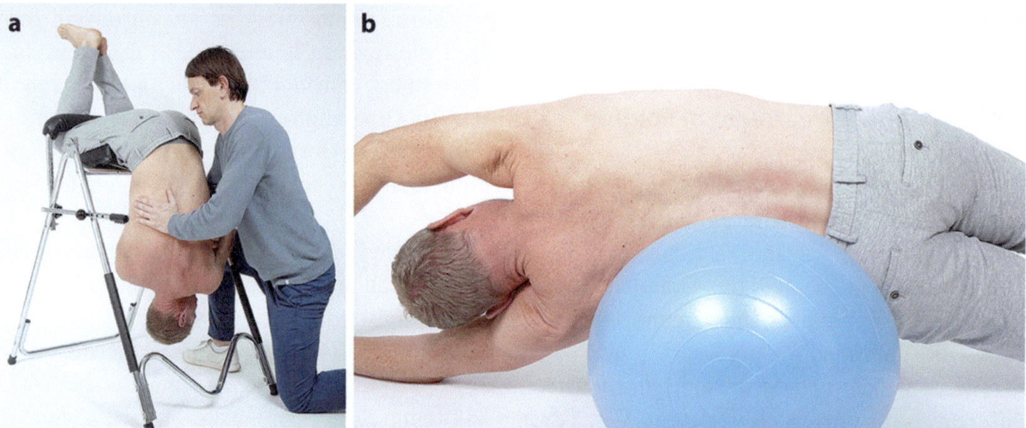

Fig. 5.31 Treatment of a folding distortion of the back with sustained traction or compression. Unfolding technique for the lower back on the inversion table (**a**). Ball therapy as unfolding treatment for the right side of the back, as infolding treatment for the left side of the back (**b**). (© Anker 2022)

in chiropractic manipulation maneuvers, the patient is positioned to take up the slack in the tissue. This pre-load is then intensified with a targeted impulse, so that the tension barrier is overcome and the distortion is resolved. When performed correctly, this technique is safe for and gentle on the patient, as well as time- and energy-saving for the therapist.

In manual therapy, pre-positioning is used to build up a *tension barrier.* To achieve this, various movement levers are combined. The goal is to focus the forces applied by the practitioner onto the area to be manipulated (e.g. a joint, a muscle septum, or an interosseous membrane). This allows the subsequent impulse to be delivered in a controlled and targeted manner.

In this context, the principle of finesse and force again plays a role. With impulse techniques, the primary concern is not the absolute magnitude of the applied force. Precise positioning of the patient, as well as focused and attentive work by the practitioner, are much more the key to success. This becomes even clearer when we recall that, in this type of distortion, the shock-absorbing folds of the fascia become stuck, and—unlike a chronic triggerband—no structural changes occur in the fascia.

> **Practical Tip**
> Impulse techniques transmit a sudden force from the practitioner to the patient. The thrust can range from a small jolt to relatively forceful application. To best adapt the impulse force to the needs of the patient, it is necessary to assume a controlled body position:
>
> - The feet are placed firmly on the ground. A slight step stance can be advantageous. Non-slip footwear is essential.
> - The knees are slightly bent.
> - The back is in a stable position, as neutral as possible.
> - If the impulse is delivered with the hands, it is advisable to slightly extend the wrists. It is also beneficial to keep the elbows close to the body. As a general rule, the alignment of the forearm corresponds to the direction of the impulse.
> - If the impulse is initiated via contact with the upper body, it is important to establish stable contact with the patient. A rolled towel positioned in front of your own sternum can be helpful (this is especially relevant for female therapists).
>
> The impulse is generated from the whole body and aims to break through the tension barrier (as if pushing open a swinging door).
>
> The patient's breathing can be taken into account, and the impulse can be delivered during the exhalation phase. Even more important, however, is to wait for the right moment for the impulse. Manual treatment is usually only successful when the patient is relaxed. To promote this relaxation, precise and pain-free handling of the entire technique is important.

In principle, all classic manipulation maneuvers of manual therapy can be used for the treatment of folding distortions with impulse, provided that the vectors created thereby correspond to the mechanism of injury of the folding distortion. For example, an unfolding distortion of the upper back can be very effectively corrected with the so-called *lift technique.* In this technique, the back of the seated or standing patient is suddenly pulled upward toward the ceiling by the therapist, creating traction in this area (see 5.4.5.5, fig. 5.39b).

In contrast, the classic *dog technique* generates significantly less traction. For this, the patient is positioned supine with arms crossed. The therapist places one hand under the patient's back to create a fixed point over which the vertebra to be treated is mobilized. The therapist then applies a more or less vertical impulse through the patient's elbows toward the treatment table. As a result, the unfolding effect is diminished compared to the lift technique described above, so the dog technique in its traditional form is not the first choice for correcting an unfolding distortion in the back region. (However, it is a suitable approach for correcting a tectonic fixation in this area; see sect. 5.6.5.2, fig. 5.66.)

If the use of standard treatment techniques does not yield a promising therapeutic approach, creativity on the part of the therapist will be required. Based on the principles for determining the correction vectors, the therapist can develop an individualized treatment maneuver for the patient.

Combined Folding Distortions

Unfolding and refolding distortions can occur in combination. This may be due to the mechanism of injury, for example, when, in the context of a knee injury, the joint is unfolded on the inside and folded on the outside. Combinations of folding distortions can also be caused by repeated traction or compression trauma. This can occur during a single trauma (e.g. in a bicycle accident with a somersault, where the body is compressed and stretched in various positions), but can also accumulate over time. Since they remain in the tissue as permanent deformations, refolding distortions from youth, for example, can cause problems in older age if an additional unfolding distortion occurs in the same region. In such cases, it is usually difficult for the therapist to clearly distinguish between the two subtypes based on the symptoms. However, it is clear that in such a situation, all folding distortions must be corrected in order to fully restore the shock-absorbing function.

Two treatment strategies are available for the management of combined folding distortions. Techniques can be used that simultaneously reproduce both traction and compression forces (e.g. manipulation techniques for the elbow or knee in a varus or valgus position, creating traction on one side of the joint and compression on the opposite side).

Alternatively, the components of a complex folding distortion can also be corrected step by step. The general strategy is to first treat the refolding distortion and then the unfolding distortion. It should be noted that any manual treatment of one subtype can provoke symptoms of the other. Sometimes, both the patient and the therapist must accept a reasonable compromise regarding symptom provocation during treatment.

5.4.4 Impulse Treatments without Pre-Loading in Traction or Compression; Acceleration Technique

If even more dynamics are required for the correction of a folding distortion, acceleration techniques without pre-loading can be advantageous. In this form of impulse manual treatment, the barrier position—where the impulse is ultimately to be delivered—is assumed and checked for painlessness. Then this position is released, the barrier is approached with momentum, and broken through with an impulse. For the success of the manual treatment, it is important that the patient can completely relax. This allows the therapist to treat the folding fascia with high acceleration but without excessive force. The acceleration technique at the knee is an example of this type of application (see sect. 5.4.5.3, fig. 5.35).

5.4.5 Treatment Examples

5.4.5.1 Folding Techniques on the Back in the Seated Position

Positioning the patient on a chair is suitable for both the manual treatment of folding distortions and for tectonic fixations of the back: the patient sits astride a chair and braces their knees—supported by cushions placed in between—against the wall. Their feet are hooked behind the chair legs, their arms are crossed, and their back is relaxed.

Indications

- Deep-seated, sometimes persistent back pain; often dependent on activity or time of day; feeling of instability or, less commonly, night pain

- Possible mechanism of injury: mechanical trauma (e.g. a sprain/strain of the back or a fall); onset may have occurred some time ago, as folding distortions permanently alter the fascial architecture
- Typical body language: placing the palm or back of the hand on the back (in both unfolding and refolding distortions); horizontal stroking over the vertebrae (especially in refolding distortions)

Unfolding Technique with Impulse

The therapist positions himself behind the patient in a deep squat. He rest his elbow on his thigh and places his hand next to the transverse processes on the patient's back, creating a traction lever on the patient's back. With the other arm, the therapist encircles the patient's torso under their crossed arms. Maintaining traction, the therapist rotates the patient up to the tension barrier (similar to the motion of a corkscrew). At the end, an impulse is applied in the direction of rotation (fig. 5.32a).

Unfolding Technique as Traction Mobilization

The therapist kneels on one knee behind the patient and places his elbow and hand as described above. Here too, his second hand passes under the patient's crossed arms. The therapist levers the patient's back into traction, rotates it, and rhythmically increases the pull. The patient is then rotated back to the neutral position and the traction is released (fig. 5.32b).

Refolding Technique with Impulse

The patient is positioned on the chair similar to the unfolding technique. The therapist stands behind the patient to the side. He stabilize the patient's back in an extended and slightly side-bent position. The therapist leans his axilla on the opposite shoulder girdle of the patient and encircles the patient's torso. The resulting compression is focused on the target area. The impulse intensifies this compression toward the patient's heel and adds a slight rotational movement (fig. 5.33a).

Refolding Technique as Compression Mobilization

The same technique can also be performed with rhythmic compression.

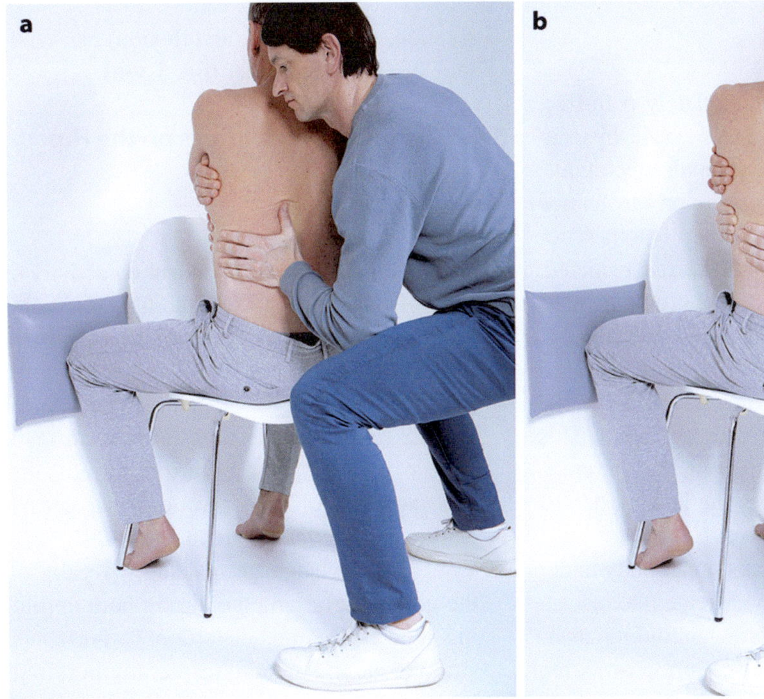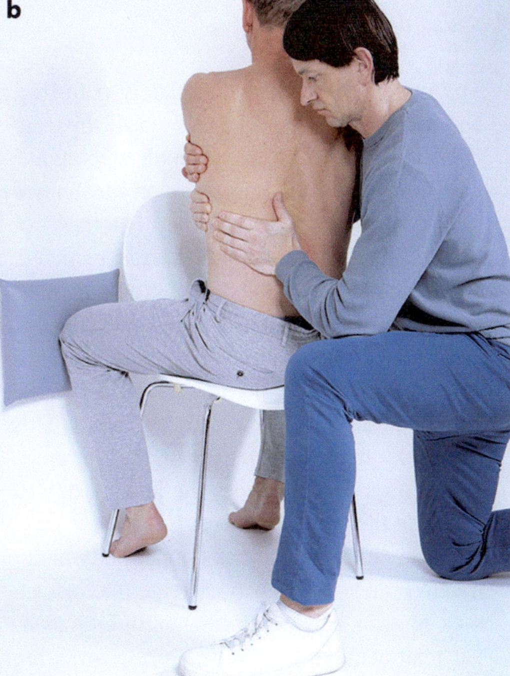

Fig. 5.32 Unfolding technique on the back in the seated position. unfolding technique with impulse (**a**). Unfolding technique as traction mobilization (**b**). (© Anker 2022)

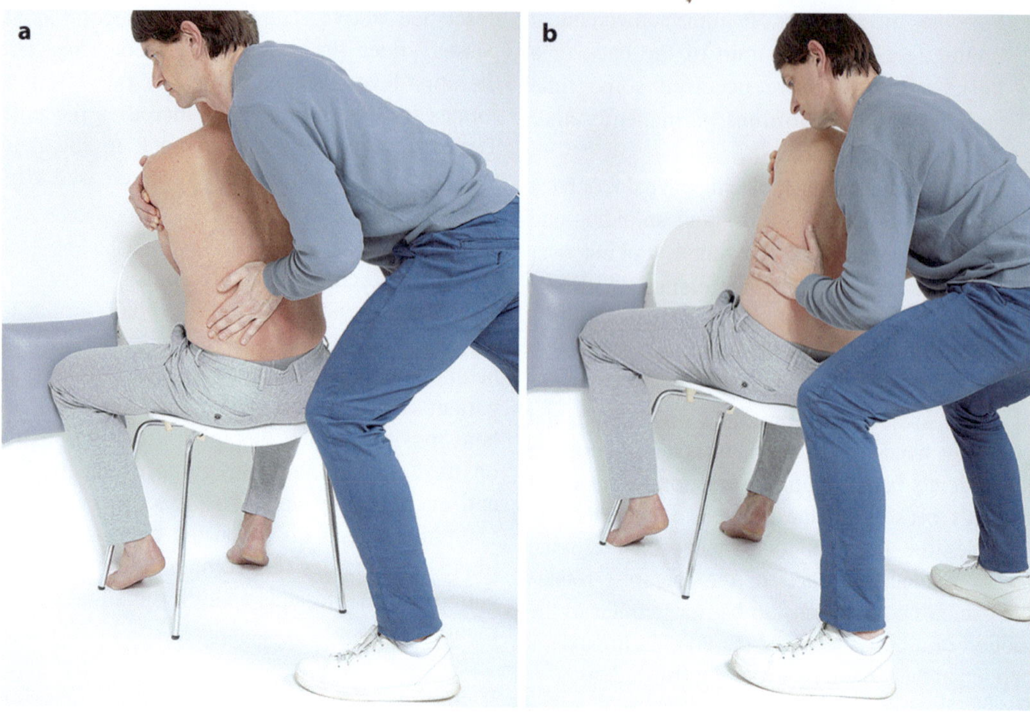

Fig. 5.33 Folding techniques on the back in the seated position. Refolding technique on the back (**a**). Variant of the unfolding technique: building the tension barrier by combining rotation, flexion, and side-bending (**b**). (© Anker 2022)

Practical tips

- The treatment must be completely pain-free, and the patient should be relaxed. If this cannot be guaranteed with an impulse technique, the corresponding mobilization technique should be used, or the working hypothesis or choice of technique should be reconsidered. For example, inversion therapy or ball therapy can be used as alternatives.
- These techniques can also be performed on a height-adjustable therapy table, with the patient sitting crosswise with legs apart. This can make treatment easier for the therapist, with a disadvantage being the lack of stabilization of the patient's knees.
- Solely rotating the patient's upper body under traction may not always create the necessary tension barrier for the unfolding manual treatment. In such cases, pre-positioning the patient with combined movements (e.g.

rotation, side-bending, and flexion) can facilitate building the barrier (fig. 5.33b).

5.4.5.2 Folding Techniques on the Hip

Indications

- Pain in the hip, often dependent on activity or time of day; feeling of instability; less commonly, significant restrictions in movement or nocturnal pain
- Possible mechanism of injury: mechanical trauma (e.g. a dislocation/sprain/fracture of the hip); onset may also have occurred some time ago, as folding distortions can permanently alter the fascial architecture
- Typical body language: placing the palm on the groin or grasping the hip (in both unfolding and refolding distortions); horizontal stroking along the groin (especially in refolding distortions)

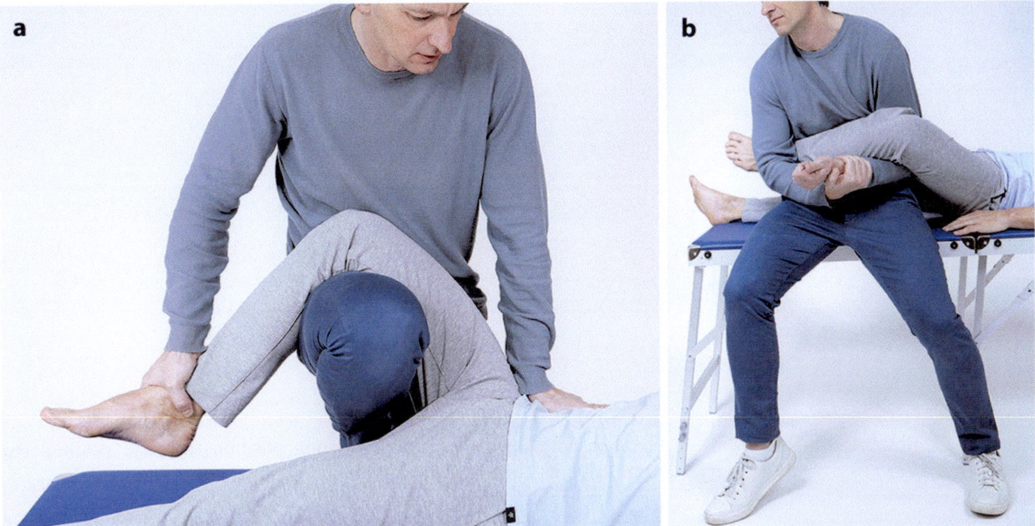

Fig. 5.34 Unfolding techniques at the hip. Unfolding technique with impulse in flexion (**a**). Unfolding technique with impulse in external rotation (**b**). (© Anker 2022)

Unfolding Technique with Impulse in Flexion Position The patient's leg rests relaxed over the therapist's thigh on the side away from the patient. The therapist stabilizes the patient's pelvis and lower leg by pressing with his hands towards the treatment table. The unfolding manual treatment is performed when the therapist simultaneously increases the pressure of his hands while abruptly rising onto his toes (fig. 5.34a).

Unfolding Technique with Impulse in External Rotation

The therapist sits at the edge of the treatment table and secures the patient's leg with his arms in front of his chest. When the therapist then leans forward and rotates away from the patient, traction and increased external rotation are applied to the hip. By abruptly intensifying the rotation of his upper body, the therapist initiates the unfolding impulse (fig. 5.34b).

Refolding Technique with Impulse in Flexion Position

This maneuver corresponds to the impulse technique in flexion position for a tectonic fixation of the hip (see sect. 5.6.5.3, fig. 5.68). Patients with refolding distortions also frequently complain of a feeling of stiffness, especially in the morning. In contrast to tectonic fixation, however, there is also pain in the joint.

Practical tips

- In cases of significant movement restrictions, the above-described maneuvers with impulse are difficult to perform and should be preceded by a mobilizing treatment technique (e.g. the tectonic pump technique) or by rhythmic traction or compression mobilizations.

5.4.5.3 Folding Techniques on the Knee

Indications

- Pain in the knee, often dependent on load or time of day; sensation of instability; joint swelling; less commonly, significant restrictions in movement
- Possible mechanism of injury: mechanical trauma (e.g. a strain/sprain of the knee); onset may also have occurred some time ago, as folding distortions permanently alter the fascial architecture

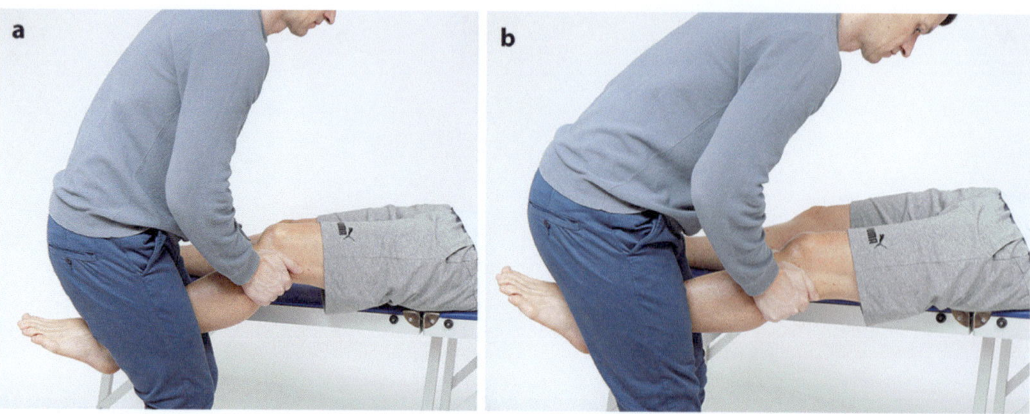

Fig. 5.35 Unfolding technique with acceleration impulse in extension. Starting position (**a**). End position (**b**). (© Anker 2022)

- Typical body language: grasping the knee with one or both hands (seen in both unfolding and refolding distortions); horizontal stroking across the knee (especially in refolding distortions); pulling and lifting the patella (in folding distortions in this area)

Unfolding Technique with Acceleration Impulse in Extension

The patient is lying down with the knee to be treated hanging over the edge of the treatment table. The patient's lower leg is held between the therapist's slightly flexed legs and the knee is grasped. The therapist moves the knee joint into a relaxed flexed position. The impulse is generated partly by a sudden pull of the hands towards the therapist's thigh, and partly by simultaneous extension of the therapist's knees (fig. 5.35a and b).

Refolding Technique with Impulse in Flexed Position

The patient is in the prone position and the therapist grasps the ankle of the flexed patient knee. Compression is applied along the patient's lower leg to the knee, and manipulation is performed with applying thrusts in various flexion and rotation angles (fig. 5.36).

Folding Technique with Impulse in the Frog-Leg Position

The patient is in the supine position and the therapist stands on the side to be treated. The patient's knee is flexed, the hip is externally rotated, and the leg is positioned as such in front of the therapist's torso. The therapist places one hand on the medial lower leg (with the fingers pointing toward their own abdomen). The second hand is placed on the lateral malleolus. The therapist rotates the patient's hip into maximal external rotation, pushes the ankle toward the patient's navel, and applies a thrust (fig. 5.37a).

Folding Technique with Impulse in the Reverse Frog-Leg Position

In the same starting position, the patient's knee is flexed and the hip is internally rotated. The therapist grasps the patient's medial malleolus with one hand and stabilizes the lower leg with the other hand close to the knee. (The patient's thigh remains abducted throughout.) The therapist pushes the lower leg outward with the hand on the medial malleolus, takes up the slack, and delivers an impulse (fig. 5.37b).

Practical tips

- The acceleration technique in extension is an adapted form of the "Whip technique" described by Typaldos. In this technique, the patient's leg is passively flexed at the hip and knee and lifted off the table. The therapist grasps the patient's lower leg near the ankle and pulls the leg abruptly toward the treatment table, where it lands in extension. This technique can generate significant

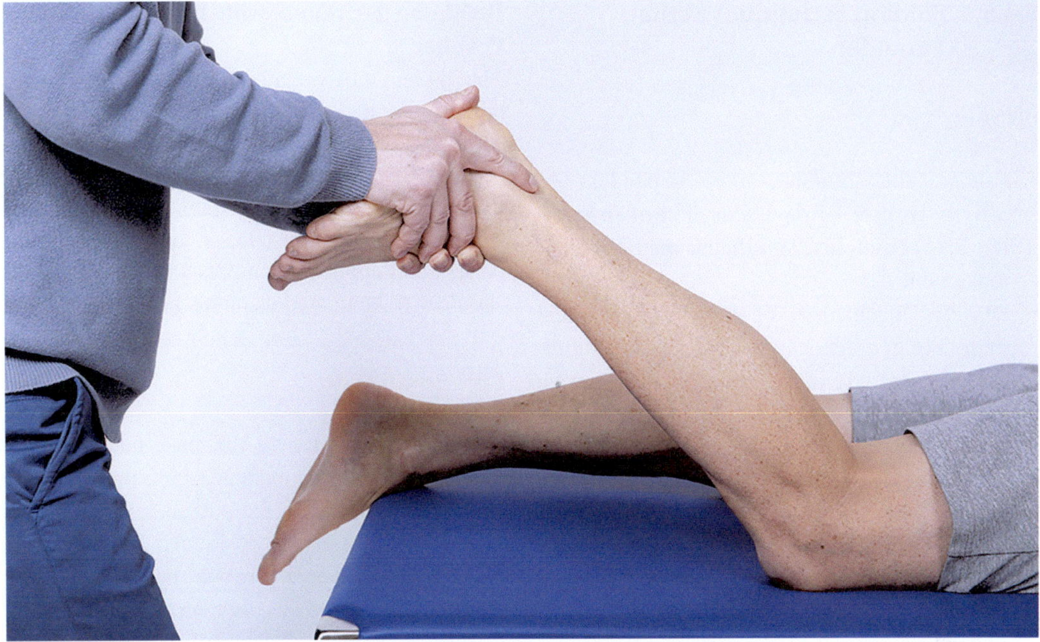

Fig. 5.36   Refolding technique with impulse in flexion. (© Anker 2022)

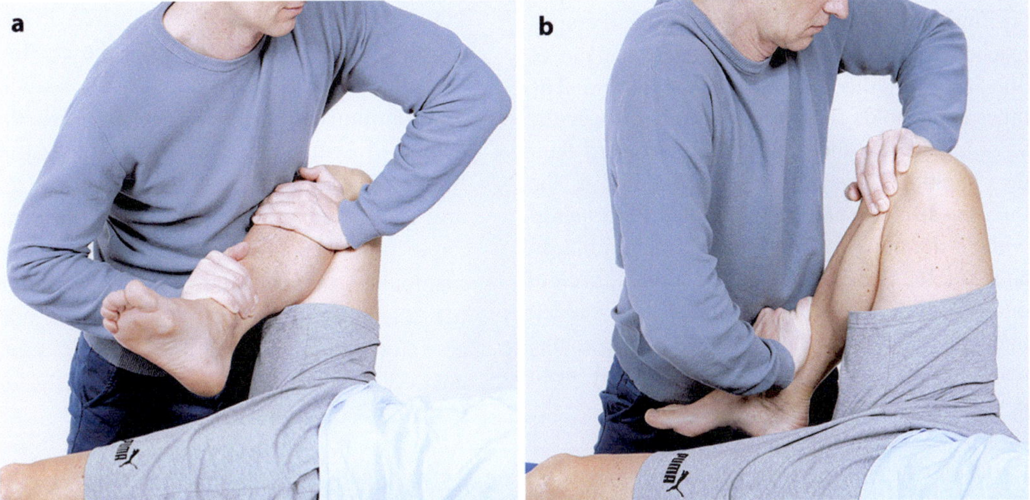

Fig. 5.37   Treatment of combined folding distortions at the knee. Folding technique with impulse in the frog-leg position (**a**). Folding technique with impulse in the reverse frog-leg position (**b**). (© Anker 2022)

traction at the knee, hip, and pelvic regions. However, it is more difficult to focus the force of manipulation.

- The refolding technique with impulse can be applied to both refolding distortions at the knee and at the ankle.

- For manual impulse treatment in the frog-leg position, good knee mobility is a prerequisite. Here, it is especially important to build up the tension barrier as effectively as possible, so that only a small, quick thrust is needed for the manual treatment.

5.4.5.4 Folding Techniques at the Shoulder

Indications

- Pain in the shoulder, often dependent on activity or time of day; sensation of instability; less commonly, significant restrictions in movement
- Possible mechanism of injury: mechanical trauma (e.g. a dislocation/sprain of the shoulder); onset may have occurred some time ago, as folding distortions permanently alter the fascial architecture
- Typical body language: grasping the shoulder with the hand (seen in both unfolding and refolding distortions); horizontal stroking over the shoulder (especially in refolding distortions)

Unfolding Technique with Impulse; Push-Out Technique

The patient sits or stands while the therapist positions himself closely behind. The therapist reaches across the opposite shoulder and places one hand on the patient's flexed elbow. The other hand holds the patient's forearm near the wrist and rotates the patient's palm toward their own shoulder. The barrier is established as the therapist lifts the patient's arm with both hands, without initiating flexion at the shoulder joint. In addition, the therapist pulls the patient's forearm outward. The impulse is generated by a sudden intensification of both movement components, resulting in a levering of the humeral head upward and outward (fig. 5.38a).

Refolding Technique with Impulse

The patient sits or stands while the therapist positions himself closely behind. The patient places the hand of the side to be treated on their opposite shoulder. The therapist embraces the torso and places both hands on the patient's flexed elbow. The therapist presses the shoulder against his own sternum and applies impulses at various angles of the shoulder (fig. 5.38b).

Refolding Technique with Impulse in Lateral Position

The patient lies on their side on the treatment table, with the shoulder to be treated on top. The therapist compresses the shoulder along the clavicle toward the patient's sternum to take up the slack. The other hand stabilizes the patient's sternum. The therapist leans his torso over the patient and applies a compression impulse to the shoulder to be treated using his body (fig. 5.38c).

Practical tips

- As an alternative to the push-out technique described above, manual techniques can also be performed with the patient lying down. In that case, the arm is positioned and traction is applied to the shoulder via the patient's forearm. It is possible to use constant traction until release, a rhythmic mobilization technique, or the application of impulses according to the position in which the distortion originated.
- Folding distortions in the shoulder region do not necessarily have to be localized in the shoulder joint itself. Frequently, the clavicle with its articular connections to the scapula and sternum, or the adjacent ribs, are the source of symptoms. This is especially true for complaints that occur when raising the arm above the horizontal. The push-out technique described above can also be used to manipulate the clavicular region. The refolding technique inthe lateral position is suitable for refolding distortions in the same area. Manipulation techniques for the ribs are explained in the following section.

5.4.5.5 Folding Techniques on the Ribs and Mid-Back

Indications

- Pain at the ribs or deep between the ribs; persistent symptoms; less commonly, significant restriction of movement; pain at the end of inhalation or exhalation

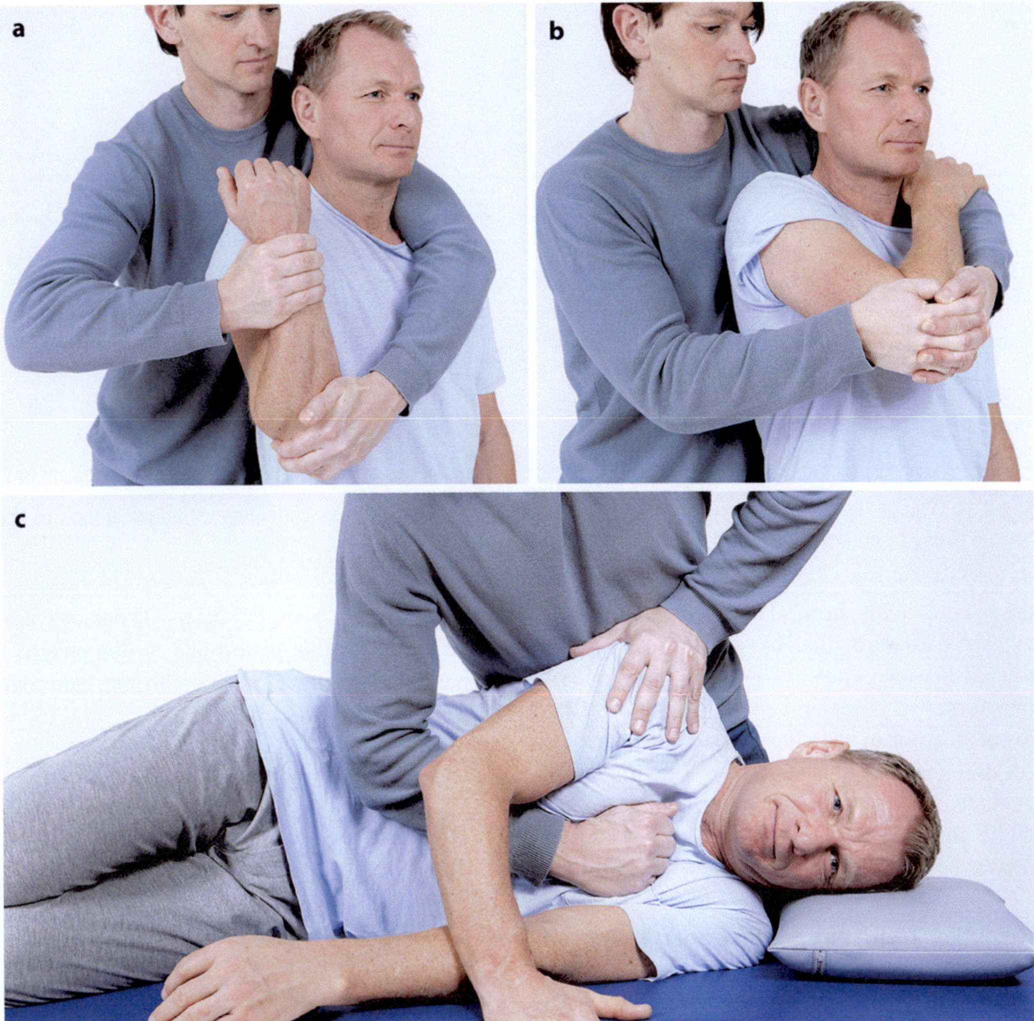

Fig. 5.38 Folding technique at the shoulder. Unfolding technique ("push-out technique") at the shoulder (**a**). Refolding technique with impulse in sitting position (**b**). Refolding technique with impulse in lateral position (**c**). (© Anker 2022)

- Possible mechanism of injury: mechanical trauma (e.g. a contusion or strain of the ribs); onset may have occurred some time ago, as folding distortions permanently alter the fascial architecture
- Typical body language: hooking the fingers onto the ribs or placing the hand on the back

Unfolding Technique on the Mid-Ribs; Star Folding Technique

This impulse technique is applied at the starting point of the star triggerband, hence its name.

For the manual treatment, the patient lies prone. The therapist stabilizes one rib near the costovertebral joint with one hand. The other hand is placed on the rib below. The therapist then pushes both hands apart and intensifies the traction with an impulse (fig. 5.39a).

Unfolding Technique on the Ribs and Back; Lift Technique

The patient sits and interlaces their fingers behind the neck. The therapist threads his hands through the patient's flexed arms and also places

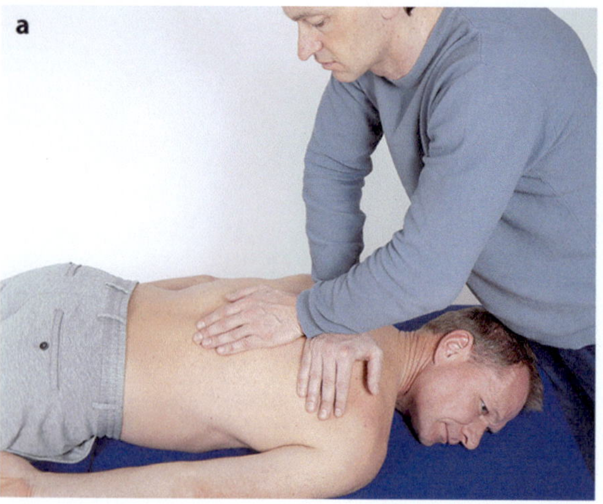
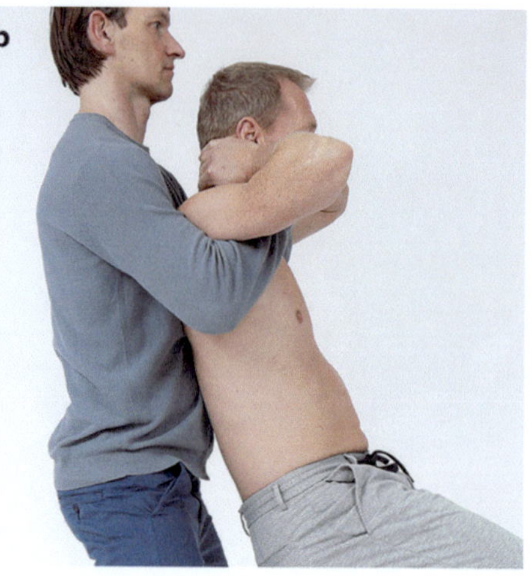

Fig. 5.39 Unfolding techniques at the ribs and back. Star folding technique (**a**). Unfolding technique at the ribs and back in sitting position (**b**). (© Anker 2022)

them behind the neck. The therapist pulls his elbows backward, thereby drawing the patient toward his own chest. (To focus the manipulation forces, it is recommended to place a rolled towel in front of the chest between the relevant rib and the patient's sternum). The impulse is generated by the therapist straightening his legs while simultaneously pressing his own sternum forward (fig. 5.39b).

Refolding Technique on the Upper Ribs in the Swimmer's Position

In the swimmer's position, the patient lies prone and supports their chin. The arm on the side to be treated rests, relaxed, in front of the head on the treatment table. For the impulse technique, the therapist places the thenar eminence on the area of the upper ribs and applies pressure toward the rib below. The other hand is placed on the patient's neck. The therapist tilts the patient's head away from the side to be treated, without the patient's chin slipping on the table. The impulse is delivered via the hand on the ribs. The hand on the neck stabilizes (fig. 5.40a and b).

Practical tips

- Unfolding distortions of the mid-ribs are often associated with triggerbands that run toward the neck (the so-called star

triggerband; see 5.1.5.1). Typaldos also describes folding distortions in this area as a possible starting point for chronic pain syndromes such as fibromyalgia.

5.4.5.6 Folding Techniques for the Neck

Background Information
Any manipulation or mobilization techniques in the neck region requires a review of possible contraindications (see 4.1).

Indications

- Pain or a feeling of instability in the neck; often dependent on the time of day; less frequently significant restriction of movement (in comparison to tectonic fixation, which primarily leads to a movement blockade but causes less pain)
- Possible mechanism of injury: mechanical trauma (e.g. whiplash or a neck sprain); onset may also have occurred some time ago, as folding distortions permanently alter the fascial architecture
- Typical body language: placing the palm on the neck (seen in both unfolding and

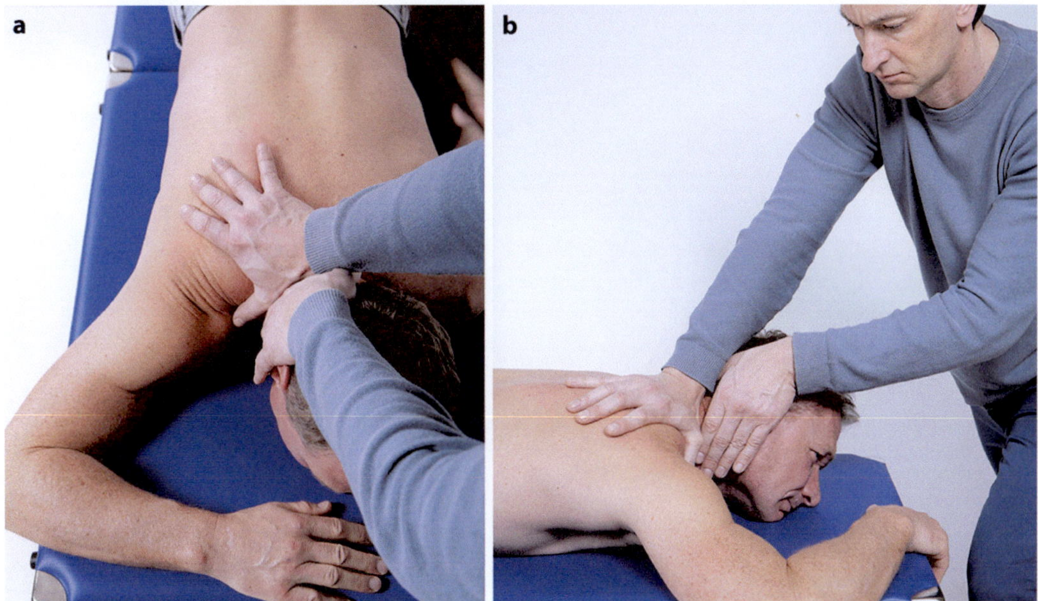

Fig. 5.40 Refolding technique at the upper ribs in the swimmer's position. Therapist's perspective (**a**). Positioning for the impulse (**b**). (© Anker 2022)

refolding distortions); horizontal stroking over the vertebrae (especially in refolding distortions)

Unfolding Technique as Traction Mobilization
Both thenar eminences of the therapist hook onto the right and left mastoid processes at the back of the supine patient's head. In this position, varying degrees of sustained traction or rhythmic mobilization in traction can be performed (fig. 5.41a).

Unfolding Technique with Thrust
The therapist stands at the side of the head end of the treatment table. He rolls the patient's head onto his forearm and place his index and middle fingers on the patient's chin. The base joint of the index finger of the therapist's other hand is placed behind the transverse process of the vertebra to be mobilized. The therapist tilts the patient's head toward this contact point and turns the face away and slightly upward. This positioning should create a tension barrier with slight traction on the opposite side of the neck, which can be overcome with a rotational thrust (fig. 5.41b).

Refolding Technique with Thrust
The therapist positions his hands behind the transverse processes of the relevant area of the patient's neck. He braces himself with his abdomen against the patient's head, without pressing it into flexion. Under the resulting compression, the therapist tilts the neck to one side and rotates it in the opposite direction to focus the forces on the respective vertebra. The thrust consists of an increase in compression and a simultaneous twisting movement of the therapist's hands toward the patient's sternum (fig. 5.41c).

Refolding Technique as a Mobilization Technique The same hand position can also be used for rhythmic mobilization.

Practical tips

- If a barrier cannot be established with the combination of lateral flexion and rotation of the patient's head, additional movements such as minimal translation (sliding) of the patient's head away from the therapist or increasing flexion or extension of the neck may help.

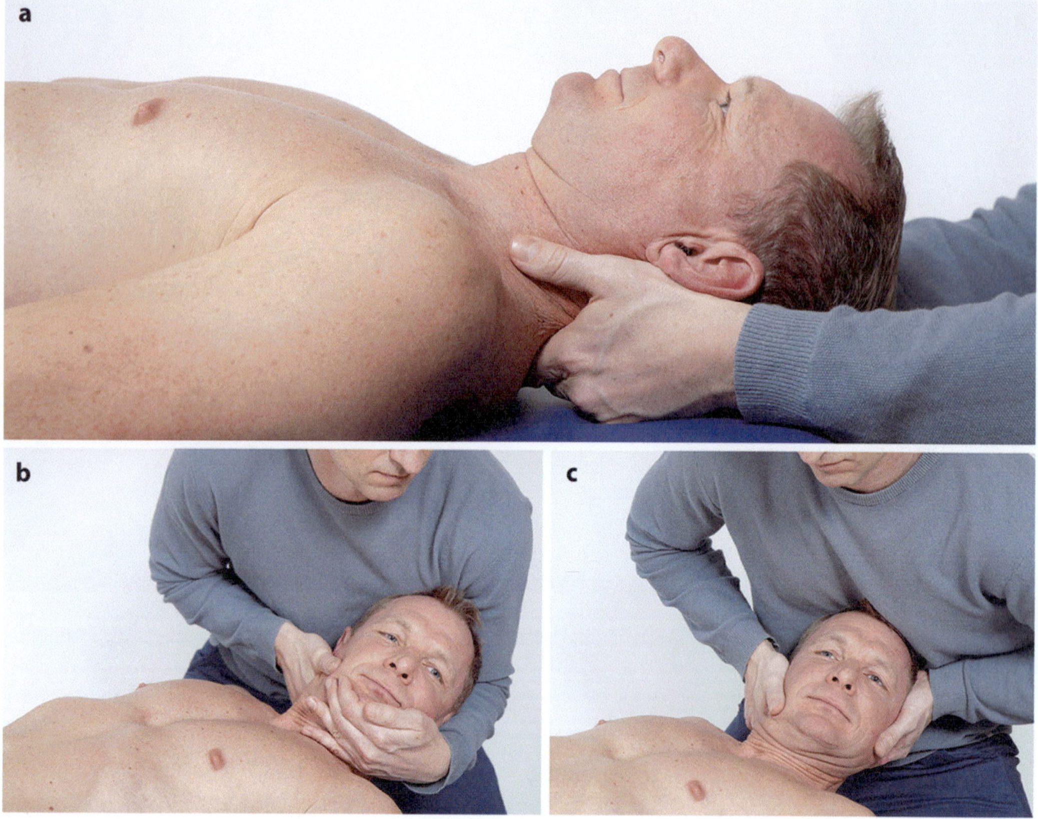

Fig. 5.41 Folding techniques for the neck. Unfolding technique as traction mobilization (**a**). Unfolding technique with thrust (**b**). Refolding technique with thrust or as mobilization (**c**). (© Anker 2022)

- The described thrust techniques are an adapted form of the original technique. In his books, Typaldos describes the thrust manual treatment of the neck with hand positions that primarily use rotation for establishment of the barrier, and for manual treatment. The techniques described above, however, use combined levers. This reduces the amount of pre-positioning in rotation, which is perceived as more comfortable by most patients, and facilitates the focusing of manipulation forces.
- These hand positions can also be used to treat tectonic fixations of the neck. If there is a global restriction of movement, the refolding technique as a mobilization technique is suitable. For local joint blockages, manipulations such as the unfolding technique with thrust are recommended. However, if a tectonic fixation is being treated, the traction or compression vectors (as in the corresponding folding techniques) do not need to be emphasized.

5.4.6   Treatment Techniques for the Interosseous Membrane

Folding distortions in the area of the interosseous membrane (IOM) lead to malpositioning of parallel-aligned bones relative to each other. This permanent deformation can result in persistent symptoms such as movement restrictions and load-dependent pain (fig. 5.42).

To correct the interosseous membrane, impulse manipulation techniques are suitable. Both unfolding and refolding distortions can be treated in this way. These techniques share the

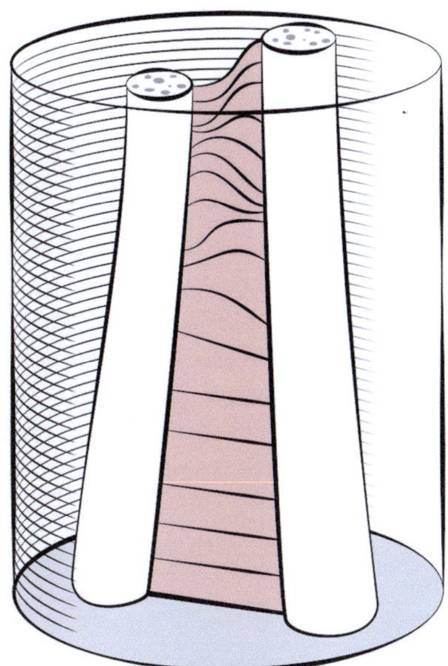

Fig. 5.42 Schematic representation of a folding distortion of the interosseous membrane. (© Anker 2022)

application of shearing impulses, which act on the membrane via the adjacent bones.

In general, the following sequence of techniques can be described:

- Pre-positioning of the membrane to be treated
- Manual treatment with shearing impulses

5.4.6.1 Pre-Positioning of the Membrane to be Treated

The membrane to be treated (e.g. in the area of the patient's forearm) is pre-loaded by separating the bones bordering the membrane, if an unfolding distortion of the membrane is being treated. If a refolding distortion is present, the bones are brought closer together.

Typaldos describes that pre-positioning is particularly effective if the *oblique orientation of the membrane* is taken into account, rather than pulling the bones apart or pressing them together at a right angle.

Practical tip

It is advisable to build up the tension barrier in the membrane step by step. This

means that the therapist first grasps the bone over which the main corrective impulse will be applied. Then, its bony counterpart is positioned so that the interosseous membrane limits this opposing movement. The tension created in this way is perceptible to both the patient and the therapist, but should not cause pain.

The contact with the bones should be as direct as possible, so that the surrounding soft tissues are compressed as little as possible. This ensures that the impulses applied during manual treatment act directly on the interosseous membrane, and that the technique is more easily tolerated by the patient.

5.4.6.2 Manual Treatment with Shearing Impulses

This treatment is generally performed using a *thrust* that exceeds the tension barrier created by the pre-positioning. After each impulse, the positioning is adjusted in order to address all parts of the membrane. This makes clear that a single manual impulse treatment is rarely sufficient to correct a folding distortion of the interosseous membrane. Rather, it is recommended to continuously adjust the direction and force of the impulse, as well as the degree of pre-loading, and to change the positioning of the hands on the patient.

The body position of the therapist also plays a role. As is generally the case with impulse techniques, the orientation of the therapist's forearms indicates the direction of the impulse force. In addition, manual treatment is easier to perform when the therapist's arms are extended, allowing the impulses to be initiated from the shoulders.

Practical Tip

Since the clinical distinction between unfolding and refolding distortion of the interosseous membrane is difficult and often not clear-cut, unfolding and refolding techniques are applied alternately. This approach leads to better results, especially in persistent distortions that cause movement restrictions. Additionally, the more impulses are applied to the membrane in different directions, the more likely a successful treatment outcome will be.

5.4.6.3 Folding Techniques on the Interosseous Membrane of the Forearm

Indications

- Restriction of movement of the forearm (especially pronation and supination), the wrist, or the elbow; deep pain in the forearm
- Possible mechanisms of origin: mechanical trauma (e.g. a fracture of the forearm or a sprain of the wrist); less commonly, overuse
- Typical body language: grasping the forearm with the hand; pressing with several fingers or deep rubbing between ulna and radius

Unfolding Technique with Impulse at the Radius

The therapist stands to the side of the seated patient and places his foot on the treatment table. The patient's forearm rests on the therapist's thigh. The therapist places the thenar of his hand behind the radius near the elbow and pushes it away from their own body. Hyperextension of the patient's elbow should be avoided. The second hand grasps the forearm at the wrist and pulls it toward himself. This opposing movement creates pre-loading in the membrane, which is reinforced with an impulse. The direction of the impulse is preferably oblique to the longitudinal axis of the forearm, directed toward the patient's elbow or wrist (fig. 5.43a).

Unfolding Technique with Impulse on Radius and Ulna

As in the technique described above, the patient's forearm rests on the therapist's thigh. The therapist again places the thenar of his hand behind the radius near the elbow and pushes it away from his own body. The second hand grasps the ulna from below and pulls it toward the patient's hand and toward himself. The resulting shearing creates pre-loading in the membrane. Subsequently, the impulse, which is directed almost parallel to the longitudinal axis of the bone, overcomes the barrier (fig. 5.43b).

Refolding Technique with Impulse on Radius and Ulna

The patient's forearm lies obliquely in front of the chest of the standing therapist. The therapist grasps the radius near the wrist with one hand and the ulna with the other. The therapist pulls and pushes the radius toward the patient's wrist while abruptly pushing the ulna in the opposite direction (fig. 5.43c).

Practical tips

- If the soft tissues of the forearm are very tense, it is advisable to loosen them before manual treatment, for example with the squeegee technique (see 5.5.1.3).
- The techniques described above are performed alternately and repeatedly. Unfolding and refolding distortions of the interosseous membrane cannot be distinguished diagnostically, at the same time, this can achieve a better mobilization effect.

5.4.6.4 Folding Techniques on the Interosseous Membrane of the Lower Leg

Indications

- Restriction of movement and stiffness of the ankle; load-dependent pain in the ankle, foot, or lower leg

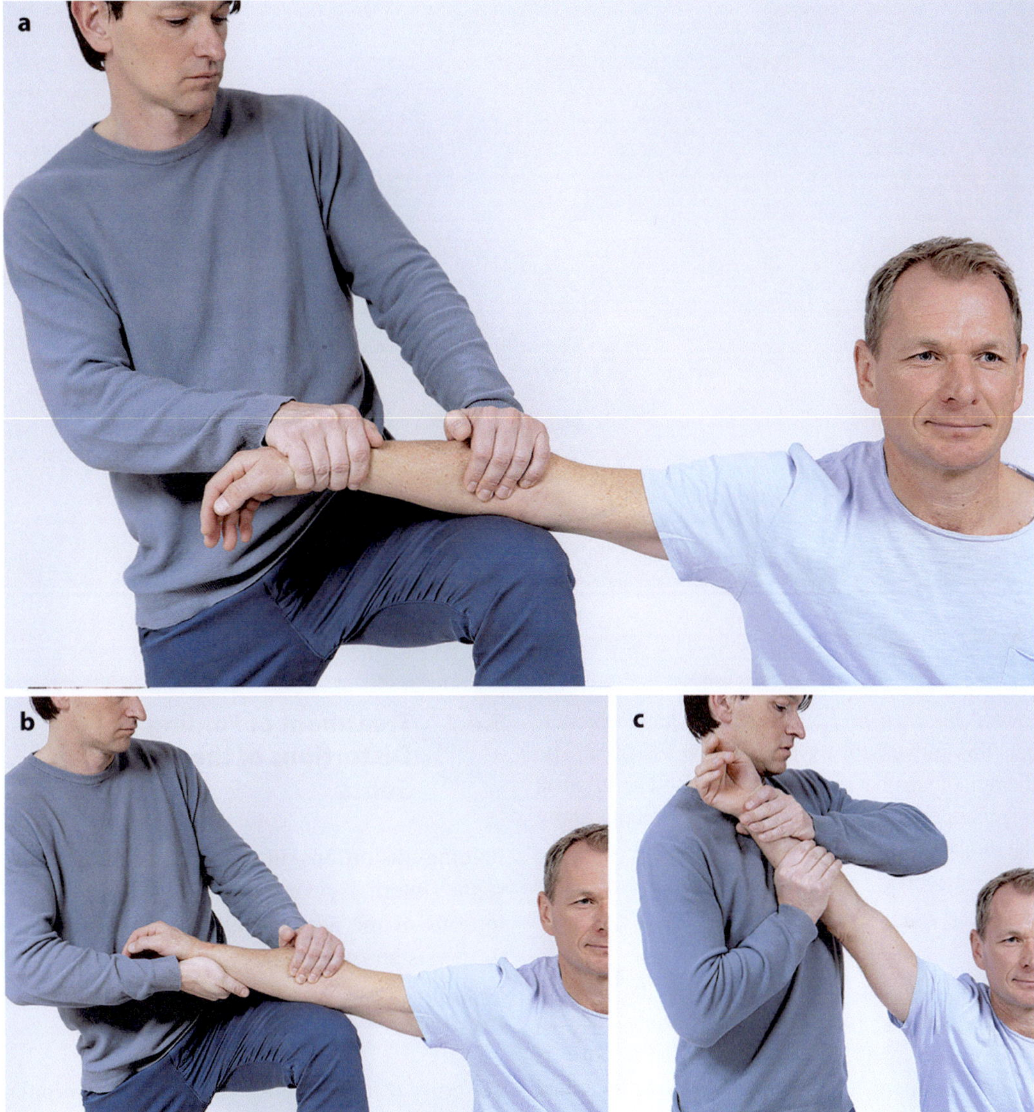

Fig. 5.43 Folding techniques on the interosseous membrane of the forearm. Unfolding technique with impulse at the radius (**a**). Unfolding technique with impulse at radius and ulna (**b**). Refolding technique with impulse at radius and ulna (**c**) (© Anker 2022)

- Possible mechanisms of origin: mechanical trauma (e.g. sprain or fracture of the ankle); less commonly, overuse
- Typical body language: grasping the lower leg near the ankle with the hand; pressing with several fingers between tibia and fibula; deep rubbing around the lateral malleolus

Refolding Technique on the Lower Leg with Impulse

The patient sits and places their lower leg on the therapist's thigh, who is seated at a right angle to the patient's leg. The therapist hooks the thenar of his hand just above the patient's lateral malleolus and pulls the fibula downward toward the foot and

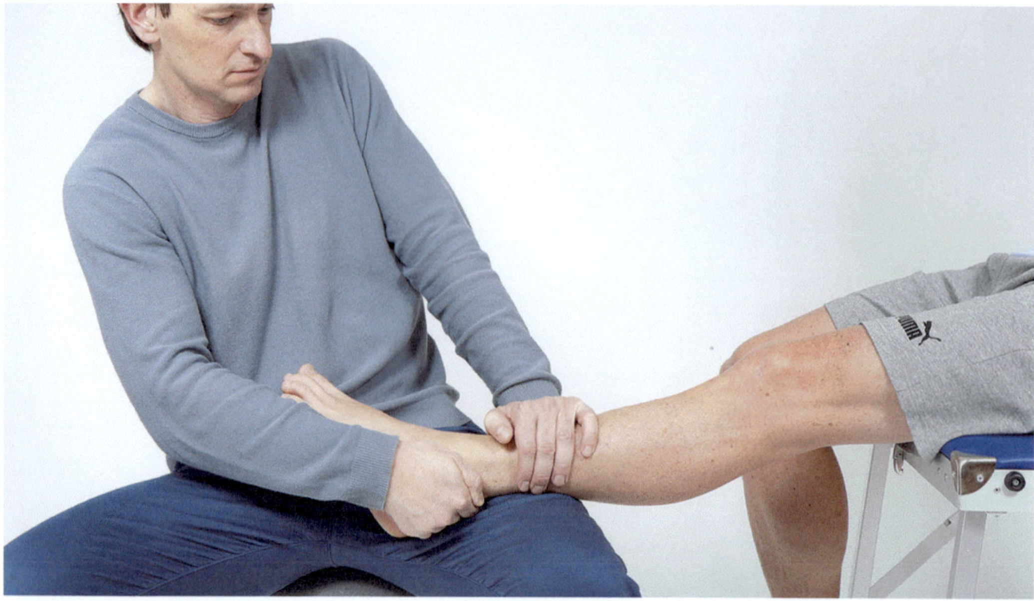

Fig. 5.44 Refolding technique on the interosseous membrane of the lower leg. (© Anker 2022)

toward his own body. The second hand counteracts this movement by pressing on the tibia. The therapist leans backward at an angle. The impulse is generated by abruptly pulling the fibula along the longitudinal axis of the bone (fig. 5.44).

Practical tips

- The technique described above is particularly suitable for treating complaints after an inversion injury of the ankle. If the impulse is directed more at a right angle to the longitudinal axis of the bone, the interosseous membrane can be treated up to the middle of the lower leg. This is often necessary in cases of lower leg fractures.
- After an inversion injury, it is often observed during examination—even when the soft tissue swelling has already subsided—that the ankle mortise appears visually wider. Based on experience, this can also be an indication of a possible folding distortion of the interosseous membrane.

5.4.7   Treatment of Folding Distortions of the Muscle Septa

Folding distortions in the area of the muscle septa (Intermuscular septum—IMS) cause distortions of the adjacent tissues. This can result in persistent symptoms, such as deep-seated pain in the soft tissues or movement restrictions (fig. 5.45).

To correct the folding distortion, manipulation techniques with impulse or techniques that require the active participation of the patient are suitable. The following basic elements characterize the techniques described by Typaldos:

- Pre-positioning of the muscle septum to be treated
- Manual treatment of the muscle septum with impulse or through active movement

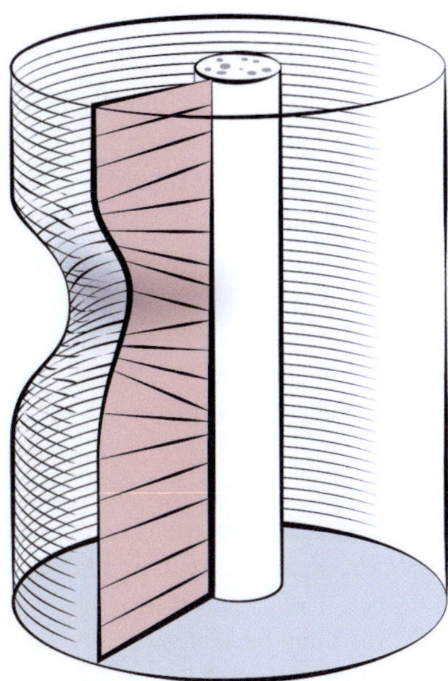

Fig. 5.45 Schematic representation of a folding distortion of a muscle septum. (© Anker 2022)

5.4.7.1 Pre-Positioning of the Muscle Septum

The goal of pre-positioning is to twist the muscle septum to be treated. This tensioning is achieved in two steps:

1. First, the therapist grasps the soft tissue area above which the impulse is to be applied, with a firm, broad grip. By additionally twisting this tissue (e.g. a muscle or muscle group), tension is transmitted to the corresponding muscle septum (the patient will feel this). If the therapist cannot hold the soft tissues firmly enough, a grip on the skin atop the relevant soft tissues is possible, as it is also anatomically connected to the muscle septum.
2. As a second step, the therapist twists the adjacent soft tissue area to pre-load the muscle septum in between. Alternatively, the therapist moves the bone to which the muscle septum is attached in the opposite direction, thereby creating a tension barrier.

Practical tip

Pre-positioning can cause pain in the patient. This may arise from the pre-loading itself or be caused by the grip or positioning. Such discomfort is acceptable up to a degree determined by the patient. However, joint pain or excessive painful pressure on soft tissues or bones should be avoided.

Ultimately, the treatment position of the patient can also play a role in building up tension. It may be advantageous to treat a folding distortion of a muscle septum in the calf with the patient standing, or to address a problem of the muscle septa in the upper arm using various shoulder positions.

5.4.7.2 Manual Treatment of the Muscle Septum with Impulse or through Active Movement

After positioning, correction of the septum can be approached using two different methods:

- **Manual treatment of the muscle septum with impulse**
  Along the longitudinal orientation of the muscle septum, or at a more or less oblique angle to it, repeated shearing impulses are applied. These should be varied in direction, intensity, and dynamics. The positioning of the body part to be treated in space, in relation to the therapist and the rest of the patient's body, can also influence effectiveness.
- **Manual treatment of the muscle septum through active movement by the patient**
  If the patient moves while the therapist manually pre-loads the muscle septum, a folding distortion can be resolved. Movements along the longitudinal axis of the septum, rotational movements, or combination movements are effective in this context, as they lead to

a dynamic increase in shear forces. These maneuvers reflect the mechanism of injury of the distortion, which is often associated with muscular activity or end-range active movement. Additionally, tensing the soft tissues (and therefore changing their volume) alters the vector acting on the septum.

Practical tip

As is usual in the treatment of folding distortions, therapy is continued until the expected improvement in function occurs. It should be noted that manual treatment can be perceived as very unpleasant by the patient, and the tissue fixed by the therapist's hand may become irritated. Therefore, breaks between individual applications may be necessary. Even more important, however, is to perform these techniques with the greatest possible care to avoid unnecessary irritation.

5.4.7.3 Folding Techniques for the Muscle Septa of the Arm and Shoulder

Indications

- Pain in the shoulder or upper arm; movement restriction (especially of internal or external rotation or arm elevation above the horizontal)
- Possible mechanism of injury: mechanical trauma (e.g. shoulder dislocation or bone fracture); overuse of the shoulder
- Typical body language: pressing between the muscles with several fingers; pulling on the soft tissues

Unfolding Technique with Impulse; Anchorage-Twist Technique

The therapist holds the flexor muscles with one hand and the extensor muscles of the upper arm with the other hand. He twists his hands in opposite directions, thereby creating pre-loading in the soft tissues. The patient is then asked to place their hand on their back against the therapist's resistance, which may already resolve the folding distortion. Additionally, the therapist can alternately manipulate the soft tissues abruptly in a diagonal-downward direction (fig. 5.46a and b).

Unfolding Technique with Impulse; Chicken-Wing Technique

The therapist stands behind the seated patient, whose arm rests, relaxed, over the therapist's thigh. As a first step, the therapist grasps the flexor muscles of the patient's upper arm and twists them to create pre-loading in the soft tissues. He then takes the patient's forearm, supinates it, and rotates the arm upward toward himself. This further takes up the slack. The impulse is mainly delivered with the hand

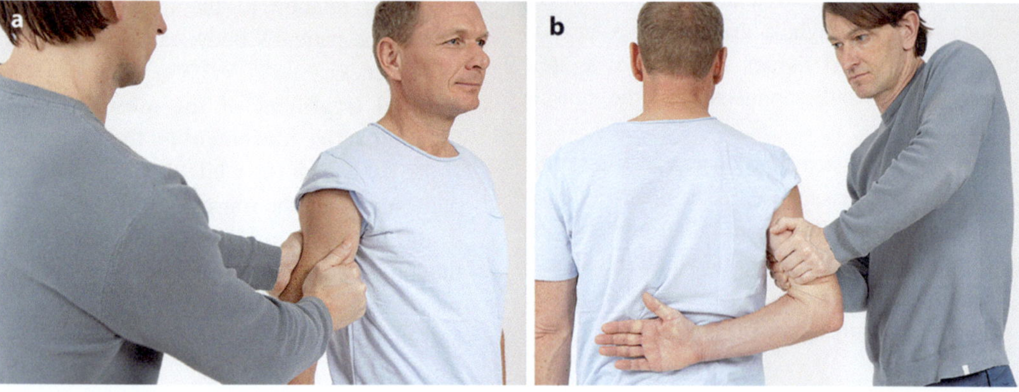

Fig. 5.46 Unfolding technique with impulse "Anchorage-twist technique": starting position (**a**). End position (**b**). (© Anker 2022)

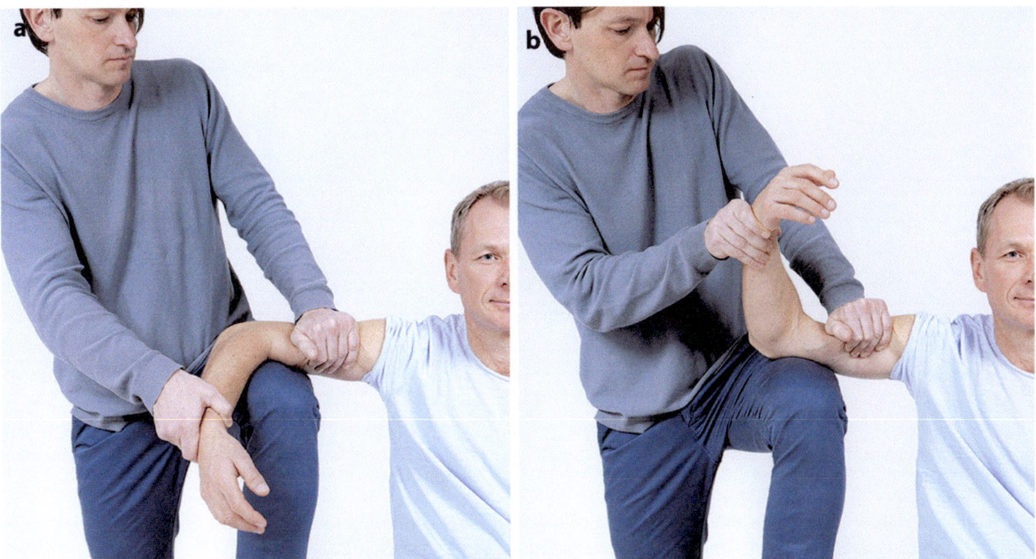

Fig. 5.47 Unfolding technique with impulse "Chicken-wing technique": starting position (**a**). End position (**b**). (© Anker 2022)

closest to the patient and is directed forward and toward the patient (fig. 5.47a and b).

Practical tips

Especially with the Chicken-wing technique, it can be difficult to grip the soft tissues to be treated securely enough, so that the hand does not slip during the impulse. It may therefore be advantageous to first perform rhythmic mobilization, and only proceed with impulses after the soft tissues have relaxed.

5.4.7.4 Folding Techniques for the Muscle Septa of the Lower Leg

Indications

- Pain in the calf; persistent complaints in the lower leg; cramps
- Possible mechanism of injury: mechanical trauma (e.g. calf strain or fracture of the lower leg); overuse

- Typical body language: pressing between the muscles with several fingers; pulling on the soft tissues

Unfolding Technique with Impulse in Supine Position
The patient lies on their back with the knee flexed. The therapist holds the inner part of the calf muscles with one hand and the outer part with the other hand. The therapist twists his hands in opposite directions to create pre-loading- in the muscle septum between the two soft tissue groups. Then, alternating, jerky impulses are applied diagonally downward (fig. 5.48a).

Unfolding Technique with Impulse in Prone Position
The therapist grasps the inner or outer part of the calf muscles and twists it toward the patient's thigh, thereby creating a tension barrier. With the other hand, the therapist holds the patient's flexed lower leg near the ankle and rotates it toward himself and in the opposite direction to the hand grip on the calf. The

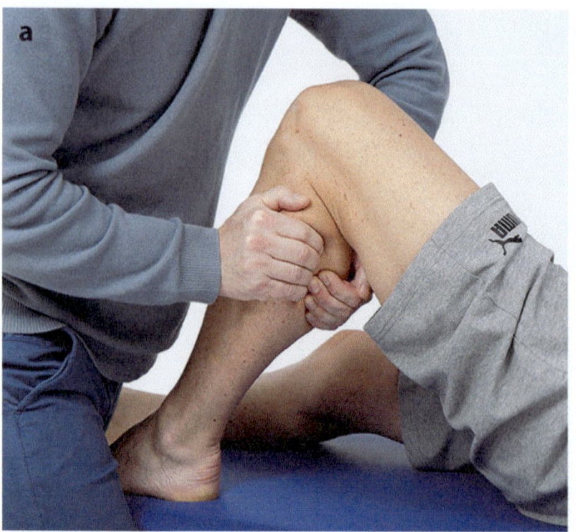
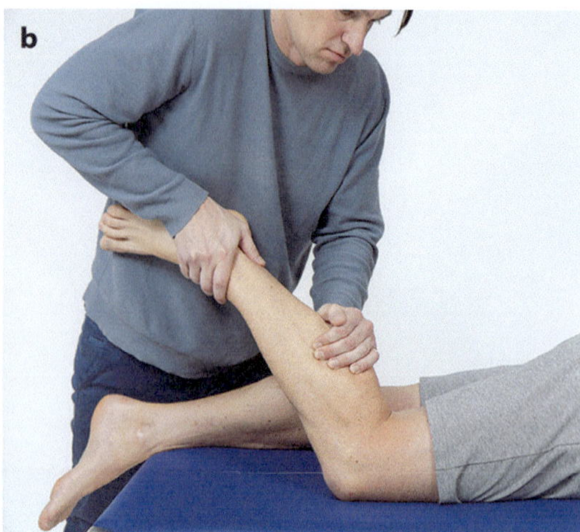

Fig. 5.48 Folding techniques of the muscle septa of the lower leg. Unfolding technique with impulse in supine position (**a**). Unfolding technique with impulse in prone position (**b**). (© Anker 2022)

impulse is mainly applied through the calf diagonally to the longitudinal axis of the lower leg (fig. 5.48b).

Practical tips

- Typaldos describes performing this technique in the prone position with the patient's legs crossed. The leg to be treated is placed over the other leg, with a cushion in between. This position allows for manual treatment on an extended leg, with the advantage of even more targeted tensioning. However, this position is difficult for many patients to assume.
- The technique in the prone position can also be used for the treatment of folding distortions of the thigh muscle septa.

5.4.8   Treatment Effects of Folding Techniques

According to Typaldos, when a folding distortion is successfully corrected, various *manipulation sounds* can be heard, regardless of the region being treated. The resolution of an unfolding distortion is accompanied by a popping sound, while a refolding distortion is usually associated with a kind of clicking sound. Interestingly, this clicking is often only heard

after the compression impulse has been applied, when the folding fascia relaxes again.

Such sounds indicate a successful treatment to both the therapist and the patient. At the very least, they can be interpreted as a signal to check the result of the treatment. However, the occurrence of these sounds should not be overemphasized, as they are sometimes difficult to perceive (especially in the area of the interosseous membrane or the muscle septa) and by no means always correlate with the desired functional improvement.

> **Practical Tip**
> Symptoms caused by folding distortions can gradually disappear with treatment. This means that a single successful manual treatment does not necessarily correct the entire functional impairment. This can be explained by the sometimes complex deformation of the fascial architecture, which requires several correction steps—possibly in a different starting position. At the same time, it is generally observed that pain caused by folding distortions often subsides immediately after correction, but only completely resolves after a certain period of time (hours to days).

After correction of a folding distortion, further rest is not necessary, as this is not a lesion but merely a malposition of the folding fascia. On the contrary, in the case of refolding distortions, the compression caused by gravity in everyday life (especially in the area of the legs and trunk) can even be therapeutically beneficial. There is a chance that the distortion will resolve on its own. For example, if a patient sprains their ankle due to a compression impulse, weight-bearing through walking or hopping is usually not only well tolerated but can also be used as therapy.

It follows that the prognosis for refolding distortions is generally better than for unfolding distortions, as unloading alone is not sufficient to correct the deformation.

5.4.9   Side Effects and Contraindications of Folding Techniques

Folding techniques are painless during application and do not inherently cause side effects. If complaints do occur after treatment, they are often related to improper application or misdiagnosis. For example, inadequate grip technique can cause *skin irritation*, especially if the manipulation is repeated. Another cause of side effects can be adhesions, which may be put under tension and partially torn by the jerky manual treatment during the procedure. Particularly in the treatment of chronic complaints, impulse techniques can therefore lead to painful reactions. For this reason, it is advisable to release adhesions before impulse manual treatment (for example, with the triggerband technique). As a result, mobilization of the folding distortion is easier.

Impulse techniques must be well tolerated by the patient, and the treated region must be able to withstand the load. The therapist must therefore consider in advance what forces will be generated by the respective technique. Under no circumstances should the application of an impulse worsen the symptoms, especially if alternative treatment options without impulse are available.

If there is a risk of side effects even with proper application of the technique, the therapist is obliged to discuss this with the patient in advance and obtain their consent.

5.4.10   Additional Measures for the Treatment of Folding Distortions

Typaldos describes a positive effect of *myofascial release techniques* on unfolding distortions. The area to be treated is gently placed under very light traction in order to wait for the tissue to relax.

Apart from manual treatment, Typaldos describes the effects of *non-steroidal anti-inflammatory drugs (NSAIDs)* on the symptoms of folding distortions. Although this group of drugs is primarily used in medicine for their anti-inflammatory properties, Typaldos emphasizes their mechanical effects. A folding distortion can cause swelling within the folding fascia, increasing its volume. As a result, the surrounding structures are sometimes painfully compressed, the flow of fascial fluids is blocked, and additional complaints arise. This roadblock effect is particularly pronounced in folding distortions. The positive effect of non-steroidal anti-inflammatory drugs is based on their ability to reduce the swelling caused by the folding distortion and thus interrupt the cascade of events described above.

In orthopedics and surgery, unfolding techniques, as mentioned above, have long been used. Fractures are reduced, artificial joints are inserted under traction, and dislocations are reduced using the Hippocratic maneuver. In all these cases, existing unfolding distortions are corrected, even without knowledge of the Fascial Distortion Model. However, FDM knowledge can expand the understanding of such treatment procedures and their significance, and help to optimally apply the corresponding techniques. Typaldos describes this using the example of a forearm fracture: if, before casting or surgical stabilization, not only the position of the bone but also the folding distortions of the interosseous membrane are corrected, clinical practice shows that the risk of developing post-traumatic movement restrictions or pain is reduced.

5.5   Treatment of Cylinder Distortions

Deformations of the cylinder fascia lead to a constriction of the structures they enclose, resulting in the typical symptoms of a cylinder distortion (see 2.5).

To correct the mechanical problem of this distortion, the mobile, adaptable architecture of the cylinder fascia must be restored. This requires disentangling the fascial coils and restoring their mobility. In the Typaldos method, techniques are used which place the cylinder fascia under traction or compression, thereby correcting it.

5.5.1   Manual Standard Techniques for the Treatment of Cylinder Distortions

Typaldos describes four different manual techniques which can be applied depending on the body region and type of the cylinder distortion. They form the basic repertoire of treatment techniques for cylinder distortions.

Three of the four techniques exist in both a traction and a compression variant, named after the main vector of the correction technique:

- double-thumb technique
- compression variant of the double-thumb technique
- squeegee technique
- compression variant of the squeegee technique
- indian burn technique
- compression variant of the indian burn technique
- pinch technique

Which of these techniques is used depends on the patient's symptoms and the observable body language (fig. 5.49a to c). The following correlations can be observed in clinical practice:

- Local symptoms of a cylinder distortion are treated with a locally acting correction technique, while regional complaints respond better to large-area treatments.
- The more a cylinder distortion causes constriction symptoms, the more promising are techniques that lift the cylinder fascia away from the underlying tissue.
- If cylinder distortions trigger jumping pain, these are treated locally one after the other until the symptoms disappear completely.

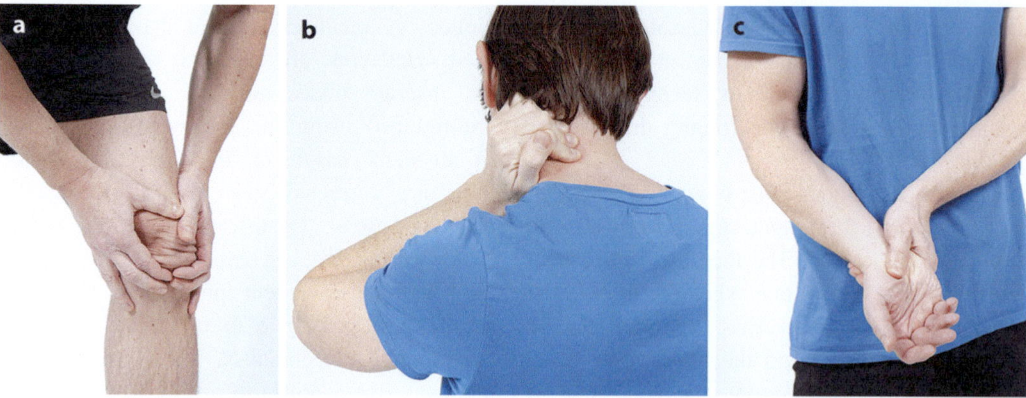

Fig. 5.49 Body language in cylinder distortions. Pinching gestures at the knee (**a**) or at the neck (**b**). Massaging gesture at the wrist (**c**). (© Anker 2022)

- Treating stuck cylinder distortions may trigger, as a result of the applied techniques, the phenomenon of jumping pain. This is considered a positive sign of the beginning mobilization of such stubborn cylinder distortions. Subsequently, the deformation is further treated locally until the symptoms disappear completely.
- Specific gestures indicate the particular effectiveness of certain correction techniques. These correlations are explained in the description of the individual techniques.

5.5.1.1 Double-Thumb Technique

The double-thumb technique is suitable for correcting small-area cylinder distortions, which are indicated by the patient with a similarly localized rubbing gesture. It can be applied anywhere on the body and produces no side effects. Therefore, it is also the technique of choice when the response to the treatment of a painful cylinder distortion cannot be predicted.

The therapist places both thumbs about 1 to 2 cm apart in the area of the cylinder distortion, and applies gentle pressure to make contact with the cylinder fascia beneath the skin. Then, the thumbs are pulled apart without sliding over the skin. The resulting stretch is clearly perceptible to the patient and is maintained until a relaxation of the tissue is felt. This release usually occurs after about 15 to 20 seconds.

Typaldos describes the structure of the cylinder fascia as similar to a lattice, with a deep and a superficial component. In the deeper layer, the cylinder coils are oriented parallel to the underlying bones, while on the surface, they are oriented at a right angle to them. This makes it necessary to perform the double-thumb technique in several directions in order to comprehensively correct deformations. If the deep layer is treated first, the thumbs are pulled away from the long axis of the bone (fig. 5.50a and c). For the more superficial area, the thumbs are rotated 90 degrees so that

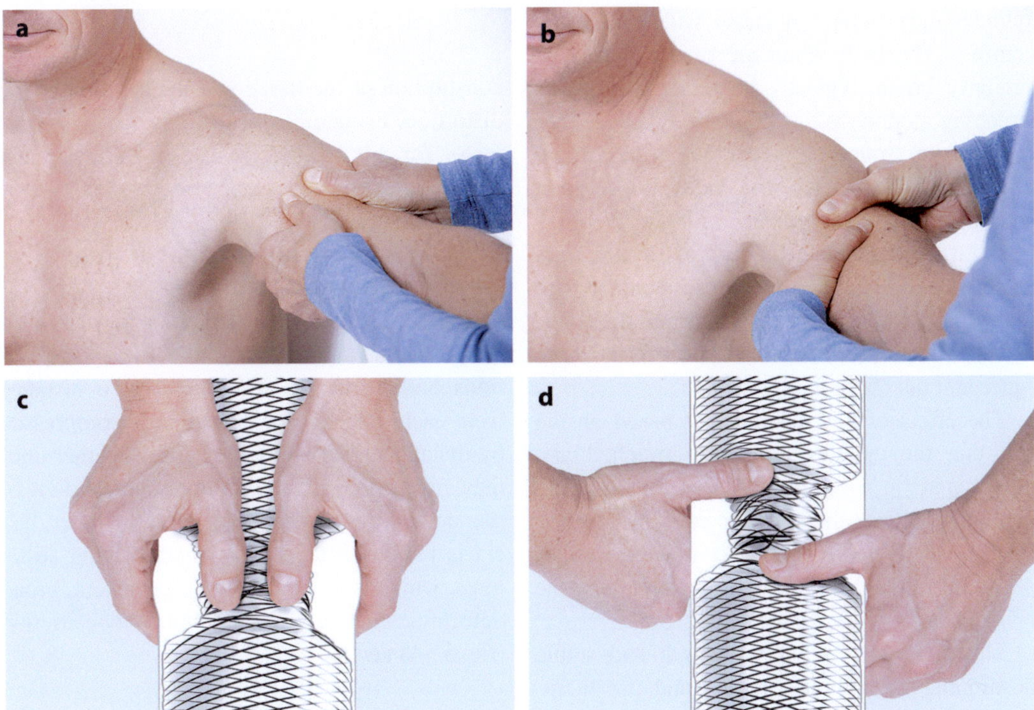

Fig. 5.50 Double-thumb technique. Treatment of the deep cylinder coils (**a**) and the superficial cylinder coils on the upper arm (**b**). Illustration of the technique for the deep (**c**) and for the superficial cylinder coils (**d**). (© Anker 2022)

traction can be applied along the long axis of the bone (fig. 5.50 b and d).

5.5.1.2 Compression Variant of the Double-Thumb Technique

Alternatively, the double-thumb technique can be applied in a compression variant (Compression Cylinder Variant—CCV). As with the traction variant, the thumbs first make contact with the cylinder fascia beneath the skin before being pushed together in this variant. The cylinder fascia is thereby compressed and slightly lifted until a noticeable release occurs (fig. 5.51a and b).

This technique is particularly advantageous in the treatment of persistent, localized distortions characterized by severe, pressing pain and a kind of gripping sensation. In such cases, a local pinching or tweaking body language is often observed.

5.5.1.3 Squeegee Technique

The squeegee technique is a vigorous manual maneuver, and is suitable for the treatment of cylinder distortions that cause widespread discomfort. The body language of the patient is similarly broad, typically involving a dynamic sweeping motion over an entire body area.

For the squeegee technique, the therapist spreads her thumb and index finger apart and forms a kind of clamp with the webbing between them. With this, she presses at a right angle into the soft tissue to make contact with the cylinder fascia and pushes through the tissue with this hand position, as if she were trying to squeeze it out (fig. 5.52a and b).

The effect of this technique is based on the fact that the cylinder coils are stretched and pulled apart in depth. In addition, the stripping motion mobilizes the cylinder coils by shifting fluid in the treated region. Like a wave, fluid is pressed through the tissue, thereby stretching the cylinder fascia from the inside (fig. 5.53).

This maneuver requires strength and stable positioning of both the patient and the therapist. Due to the friction generated on the skin, the technique can be painful for the patient and may cause skin redness. Depending on the

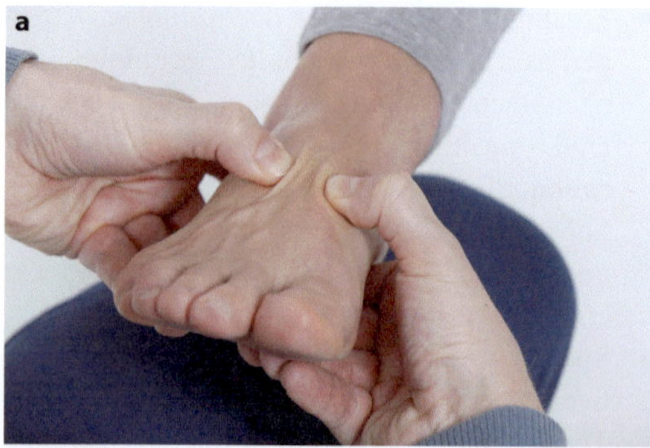
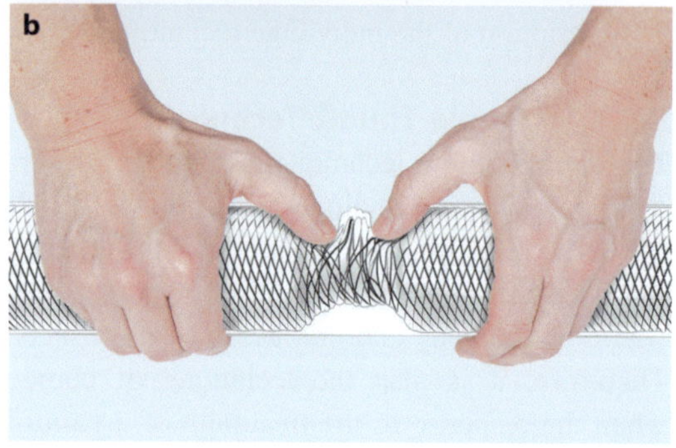

Fig. 5.51 Compression variant of the double-thumb technique. Treatment on the dorsum of the foot (a) and illustration of the technique (b). (© Anker 2022)

constitution of the tissue and the location of the distortion, hematomas occur only rarely. A risk factor for this can be the use of anticoagulant medication.

5.5.1.4 Compression Variant of the Squeegee Technique

The squeegee technique can also be used in a compression variant. First, the therapist positions both hands on the patient at a distance from each other. Then, the fascia is compressed by dynamically pushing the hands together until they meet. As with the compression variant of the double-thumb technique, the cylinder fascia is thereby lifted from the underlying structures, which is an advantage in persistent, broad deformities with a high potential for constriction (fig. 5.54a and b).

5.5.1.5 Indian Burn Technique

This technique is particularly suitable for the treatment of elongated body segments such as the

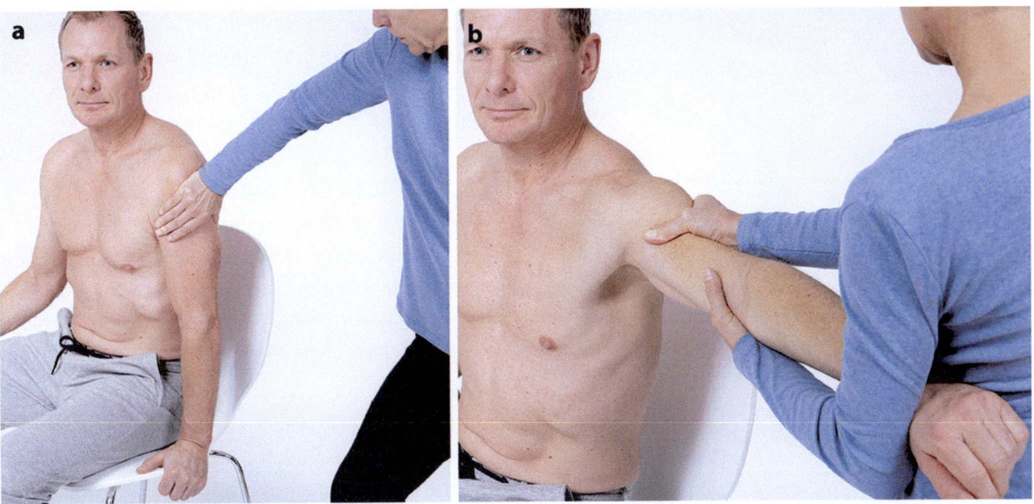

Fig. 5.52 Squeegee technique. Standard technique on the shoulder with the patient's arm supported (**a**). Variant with a push in the direction of the shoulder (**b**). (© Anker 2022)

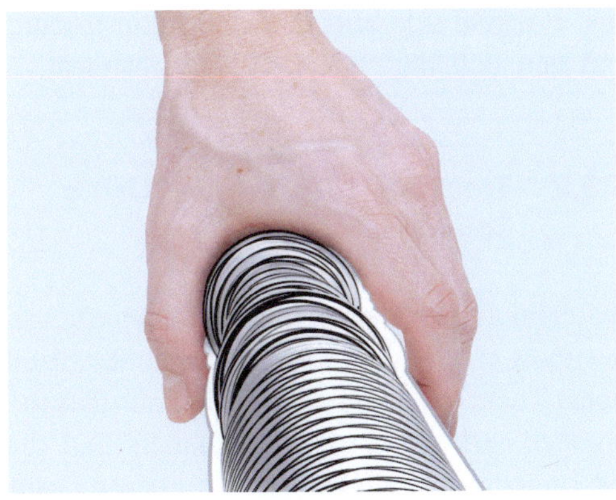

Fig. 5.53 Schematic representation of the squeegee technique. (© Anker 2022)

fingers, toes, lower legs, and forearms. Patients describe diffuse, deep-seated symptoms and present a pinching or kneading body language that wanders around the symptomatic area.

From childhood, we know this maneuver as a painful prank in which the forearm is firmly grasped with both hands and twisted in opposite directions, causing a burning pain. The Indian burn technique is performed similarly, but the cylinder fascia is first placed under traction before being twisted:

The therapist positions both hands (for example, on the patient's forearm) about a hand's width apart and encloses the soft tissue. In the first step, she pulls her hands apart to place the cylinder fascia under tension. In the second step, she twists the cylinder fascia in opposite directions and maintains the resulting stretch until the tissue tension noticeably decreases. If no release occurs, the technique can be repeated with the direction of rotation reversed (fig. 5.55a and b).

The technique is performed several times, and each time a release is achieved, the therapist moves her hands further along to gradually treat the entire painful region.

The maneuver is forceful and can cause pain in patients during treatment. If the treatment is difficult to tolerate, this is usually due to an insufficient traction component. The therapist must ensure the opposing pull is applied before twisting and is maintained throughout the entire maneuver.

Typaldos advises against using the Indian burn technique on the upper arm, ankle, and foot. In his experience, vigorous twisting can exacerbate existing cylinder distortions in these areas. He attributes this to a special and fragile architecture of the cylinder fascia in these regions.

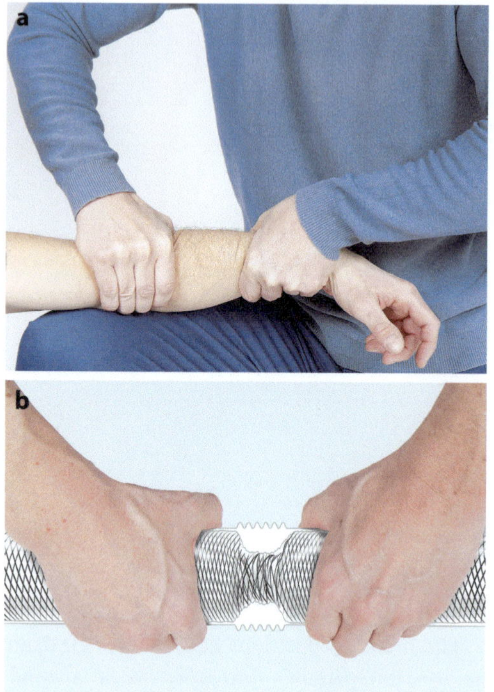

Fig. 5.54 Compression variant of the squeegee technique. Treatment on the forearm (**a**). Illustration of the manual grip (**b**). (© Anker 2022)

5.5.1.6 Compression Variant of the Indian Burn Technique

In the compression variant, the therapist first positions her hands at a distance in the region to be treated and pushes them together. Then, the compressed fascia is twisted in opposite directions and held until a release occurs. As with the

other technique variants under compression, this results in a more pronounced lifting of the cylinder fascia from the underlying structures (fig. 5.56a and b).

5.5.1.7 Pinch Technique

In the pinch technique, the therapist holds a skin fold (or the tissue beneath the skin) firmly and instructs the patient to actively move against the resistance of this fixation, until the tension resolves. This lifts the cylinder fascia away from the underlying structures, similar to the compression variants (fig. 5.57). The pinch technique is suitable for treating stuck cylinder distortions in combination with chronic triggerbands, as the intensive mobilization can also release adhesions.

However, this technique should be used with caution, especially in patients with sensitive tissue. Possible side effects include skin irritation and pain, both during and after the treatment.

5.5.2 Treatment Techniques Using Tools

In addition to these manual techniques, various tools can be used to correct cylinder distortions. Their advantage lies in the fact that they produce certain vectors for treatment that cannot be achieved with comparable intensity using the previously described manual grips. In addition, many of these tools can be used by patients

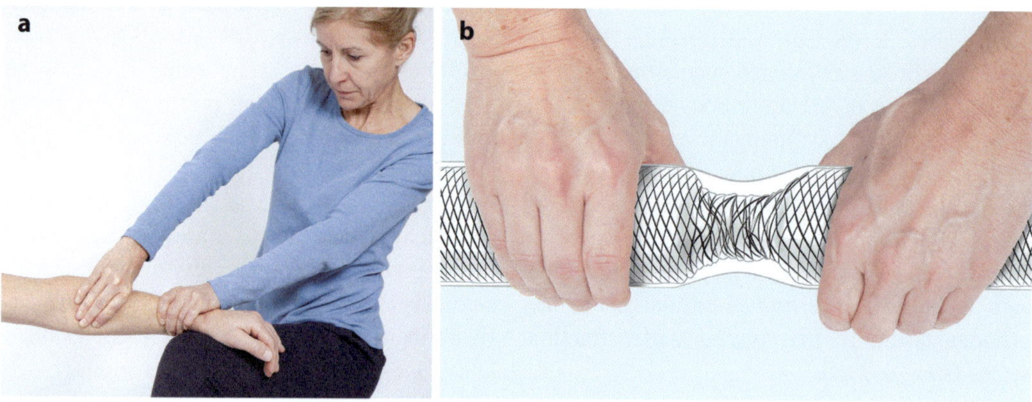

Fig. 5.55 Indian burn technique. Treatment on the forearm (**a**). Illustration of the manual grip (**b**). (© Anker 2022)

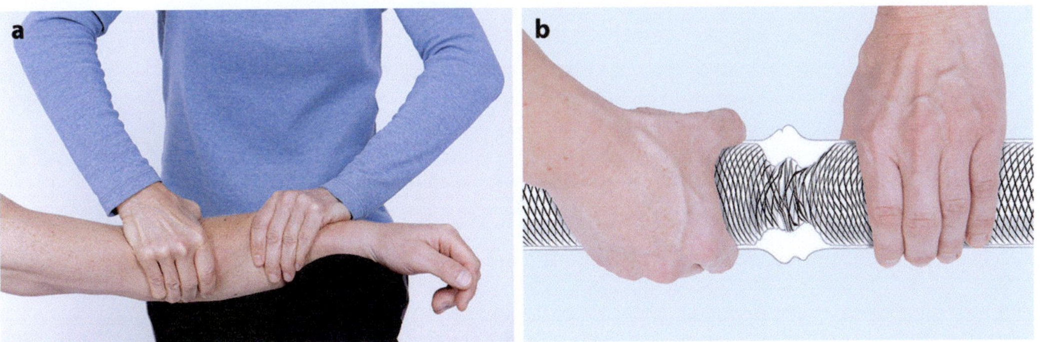

Fig. 5.56 Compression variant of the Indian burn technique. Treatment on the forearm (**a**). Schematic representation of the manual grip (**b**). (© Anker 2022)

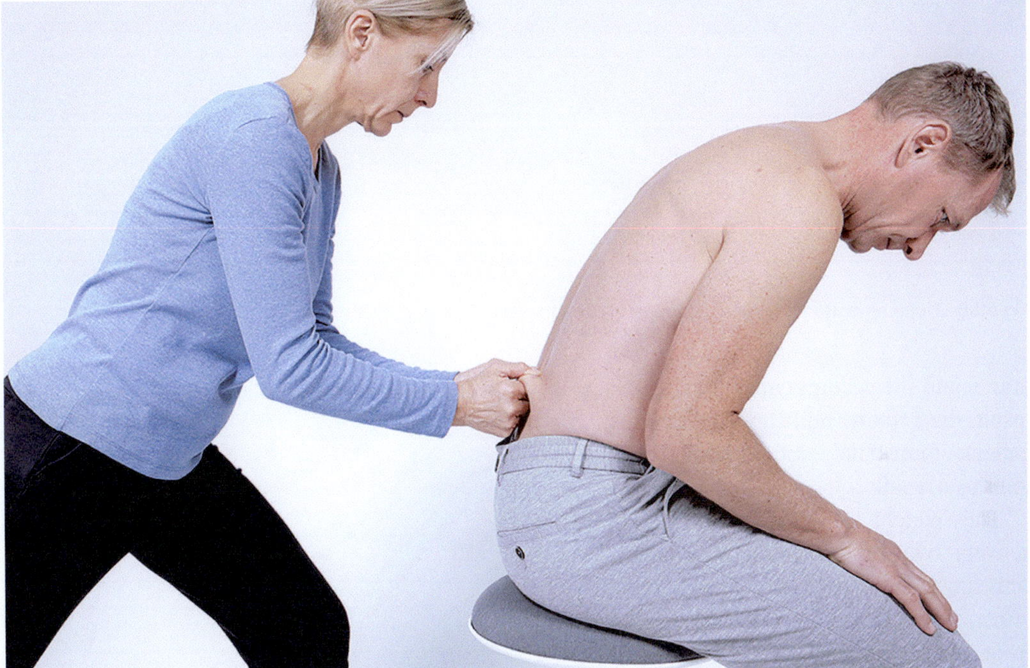

Fig. 5.57   Pinch technique. Manual grip at the lower back. (© Anker 2022)

themselves at home, allowing for autonomous continued treatment of cylinder distortions.

Typaldos experimented with devices that generate negative pressure (and therefore traction on the tissue) as well as with tools that induce tissue compression. Some of these approaches may appear unusual. However, in individual cases, they can be the key to a lasting resolution of the often troublesome symptoms of a cylinder distortion.

5.5.2.1 Cupping-with-Movement Technique

This technique is a standard treatment of cylinder distortions using a tool. It is particularly advantageous when cylinder distortions cause (painful) movement restrictions or when weakness or coordination disorders occur. One or more plastic or silicone suction cups are used, which are placed directly on or around the area of the cylinder distortion. The tissue is

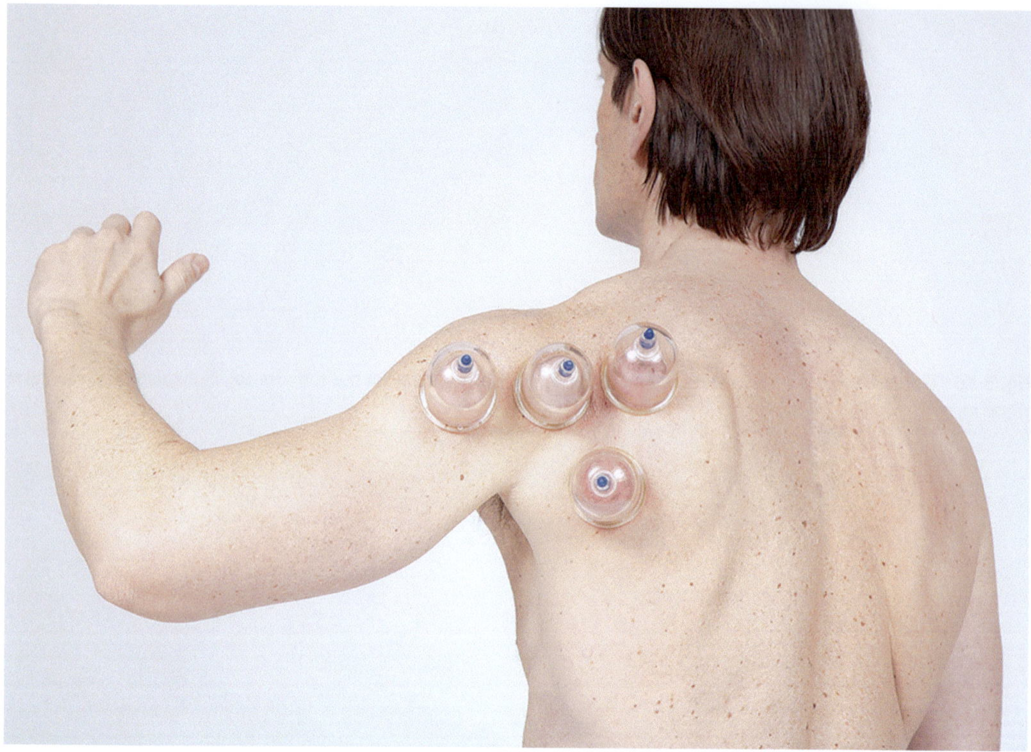

Fig 5.58   Cupping-with-movement technique at the shoulder. (© Anker 2022)

drawn into the suction cups, stretched, and, as a result, the cylinder coils are pulled apart. Often, patients immediately notice a reduction in symptoms as a result.

The patient is then instructed to move actively while the vacuum is applied. Muscle activation creates an additional mobilization effect, so that the cylinder coils are separated from each other (fig. 5.58).

When the pulling of the suction cups decreases, they can be reapplied in a slightly different position. The procedure is repeated until a stable improvement of symptoms is achieved. Typaldos recommends a maximum total treatment duration of 5 to 10 minutes (about one minute per application of the suction cups). It is important to inform patients that hematomas may occur as a result of the treatment.

5.5.2.2 KIWI© Technique

In addition to cupping with movement, there is another application utilizing the principle of stretching under vacuum. The KIWI© vacuum extractor is a suction cup commonly used in

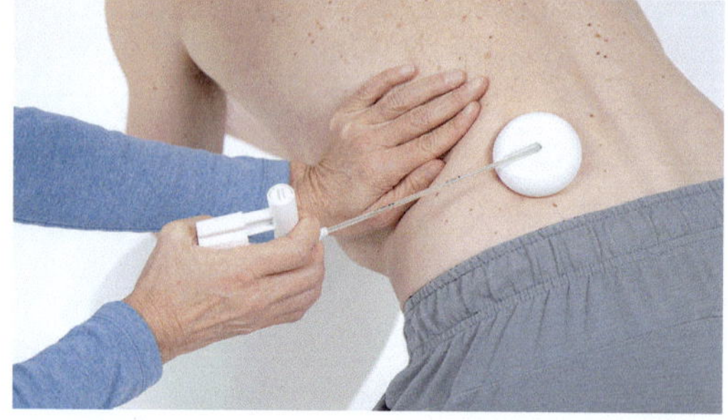

Fig. 5.59   Treatment of a cylinder distortion on the back with the KIWI© extractor. (© Anker 2022)

obstetrics. It can be applied to the area being treated, and pulled by the therapist in various directions over the underlying tissue. This process is repeated at different sites depending on the size of the cylinder distortion, in order to treat all parts of the affected cylinder fascia (fig. 5.59). This technique is particularly suitable for diffuse symptoms caused by cylinder distortions on the back or in the thigh area. For the treatment of deep-seated distortions, the mechanical effect of this device may be

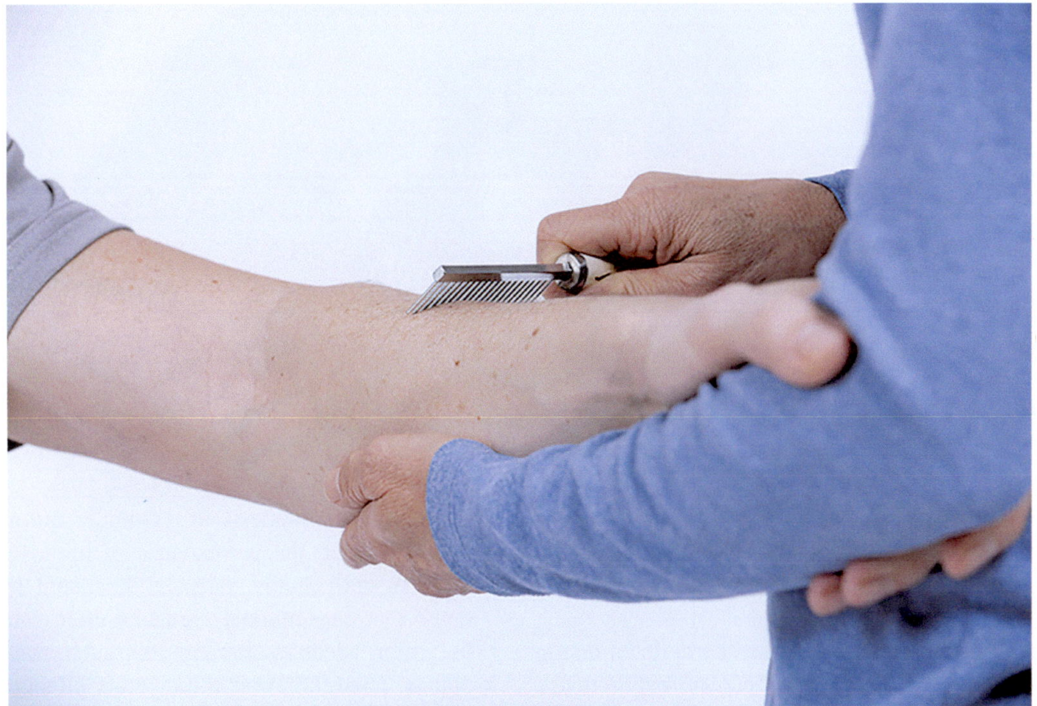

Fig 5.60   Comb technique on the forearm. (© Anker 2022)

insufficient. In such cases, cupping-with-movement or the pinch technique are often more suitable.

5.5.2.3 Comb Technique

The use of a steel comb has advantages in the treatment of cylinder distortions that occur together with chronic triggerbands. The comb technique releases both interlocked cylinder coils and adhesions of triggerbands. For this purpose, it is drawn over the skin in various directions with controlled pressure. This usually causes redness; pain due to excessive force should be avoided in any case (fig. 5.60).

5.5.2.4 Clamp Technique

Typaldos also experimented with compression tools for the treatment of cylinder distortions. Depending on the body region, he used different tools such as clamps or vices to pinch soft tissues or pin them against the underlying bone.

In these techniques, the patient is instructed to move against the resistance of the clamp or vice. Initially, this is very uncomfortable for the patient. After a few movement cycles, however, the movement should become visibly smoother and the resistance should noticeably decrease for the patient. The procedure can be repeated until the corresponding functional improvement is achieved (fig. 5.61a and b).

The effect of such clamping tools may be due to the fact that the cylinder coils are compressed and locally pinned. Active mobilization then generates shear forces in the tissue, which can resolve entanglements of the cylinder fascia. In clinical practice, it has been observed that this application has positive effects on existing folding distortions of the muscle septa and on chronic triggerbands as well. Therefore, this therapeutic approach is particularly suitable for complaints caused by a combination of these distortions.

5.5.3 Treatment Effects with Cylinder Techniques

As with the treatment of all other fascial distortions, we expect an immediate reduction of symptoms after the correction of cylinder distortions:

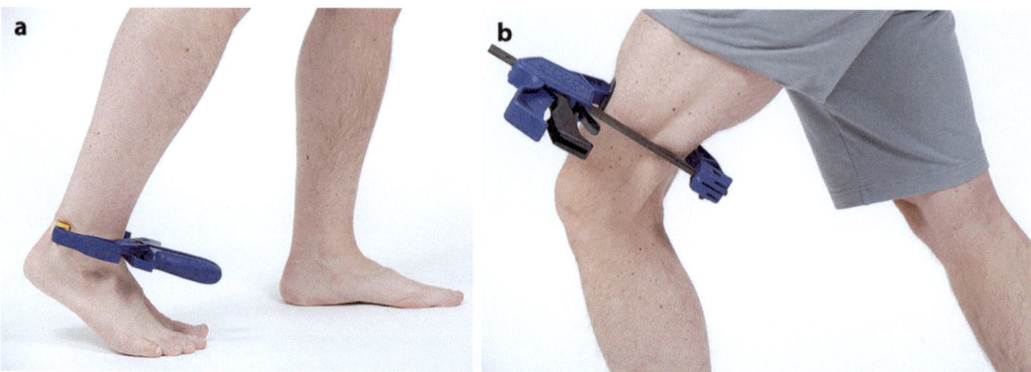

Fig. 5.61 Clamp and vice technique. Clamp treatment of the Achilles tendon (**a**). Vice treatment on the thigh (**b**). (© Anker 2022)

- Pain triggered by cylinder distortions often limits active mobility. Successful correction improves the patient's pain-free range of motion.
- If nocturnal pain is caused by cylinder distortions, significant relief can be expected the following night after appropriate treatment. The durability of these effects varies and, in line with the unpredictability of the cylinder distortion problem, may steadily improve or diminish again, making repeat treatments necessary.
- Typaldos describes a possible cause of muscle weakness as a mechanical disorder of the cylinder fascia. In particular, symptoms such as loss of strength, impaired inter- or intramuscular coordination, and muscular weakness in connection with immobilization or due to an acute neurological disorder (e.g. in the context of nerve root compression) can be positively influenced by correcting existing cylinder distortions. The effect is immediate, and ranges from a subjective feeling of strengthening to complete restoration of active mobility. Therefore, manual therapy lays the foundation for further active training. Through active contractions and the resulting change in volume, remaining tangled cylinder coils are pressed apart and released. This effect is also seen in the treatment of pain caused by cylinder distortions, which can be alleviated by active movement.
- Symptoms such as sensory disturbances, tremor, or cold sensations behave similarly to pain. An immediate treatment effect confirms the working hypothesis of a cylinder distortion. However, the permanence of improvement is individually variable. It should be noted that conventional medicine often cannot offer adequate therapy for such complaints. Therefore, even a temporary effect of the Typaldos method can bring a significant improvement in quality of life for patients.

5.5.4 Side Effects and Contraindications of Cylinder Techniques

The treatment techniques for cylinder distortions manipulate soft tissues and skin, sometimes vigorously. *If the treated tissues cannot withstand this mechanical stress (for example, in the case of skin abrasions), the techniques are contraindicated.*

In this context, it should be noted that not every technique produces the same mechanical stimulus. The double-thumb technique can be very well dosed and is the technique of choice when working on very sensitive tissue. Depending on the method used, *redness, soft tissue pain, or bruising* may occur as side effects. The latter, in particular, occurs regularly through cupping with movement or the KIWI© technique.

In clinical practice, it is evident that excessive treatment of cylinder distortions can have a detrimental effect on patients' symptoms. Especially when treating pain-inducing cylinder distortions, the treatment effect can become negative with repeated application of the correction technique after initial improvement. It is therefore advisable to limit the duration of manual treatment or to end it as soon as an obvious relief of symptoms is achieved. The correction can either be continued in a subsequent therapy session, or the patient can work independently on further resolving the cylinder distortion using appropriate tools.

5.5.5 Additional Measures for the Treatment of Cylinder Distortions

- Further positive effects in the treatment of cylinder distortions can be expected from *massage*. Patients often intuitively massage themselves, similar to the stroking, kneading body language seen with this distortion. As with the techniques of the Typaldos method, stroking and stretching the skin releases entanglements of the cylinder fascia.
- *Active movement* also helps reduce symptoms of cylinder distortions—at least temporarily. As previously mentioned, muscle contractions separate and push apart the entangled coils of the fascia from the muscle. This effect can also be observed with forms of electrotherapy that lead to muscle contractions.
- *Cryotherapy* can relieve pain caused by cylinder distortions. Additionally, it can be used to soothe irritation resulting from treatment. Ice rubs or cooling bandages are possible forms of application.
- In contrast, clinical practice shows a negative effect of direct heat application, especially in pain-inducing cylinder distortions. Irritation caused by manual treatment can also be exacerbated by heat. Although patients sometimes initially report a soothing effect, hot baths or similar measures can lead to a significant worsening of the problem after application.
- Unlike triggerbands, continuum distortions, or folding distortions, cylinder distortions are rarely significantly influenced by medication. It is more typical to observe that even high-dose pain medications cannot alleviate the sometimes dramatic symptoms, further increasing the suffering of patients with cylinder distortions.

5.6 Treatment of Tectonic Fixations

The FDM describes *primary and secondary tectonic fixations*. The former arise acutely and cause a local restriction of movement (e.g. a local blockade of a facet joint). The latter develop as a result of other fascial distortions. They are often associated with chronic complaints, and cause persistent, localized stiffness and limitation of movement.

The goal of treating a tectonic fixation is to restore the adaptability and gliding ability of the affected smooth fascia. This requires an improvement in the production and distribution of synovial fluid (or lubricating fluid), and the blocked joint or gliding surfaces must be mobilized.

Background Information
In his textbooks, Typaldos places the tectonic fixation of synovial joints at the center. However, in principle, all gliding planes of the body can be affected (e.g. the scapulothoracic gliding surface or gliding surfaces of internal organs). The measures for the treatment of synovial joints described in the following section can therefore also be applied in those areas.

5.6.1 Principles of Treating Tectonic Fixations

The concept of pain-free movement restrictions or blockades is a central element of osteopathy. Typaldos classically used osteopathic and chiropractic methods to resolve tectonic fixations. To resolve local joint blockades, i.e. primary tectonic fixations, impulse techniques proved particularly effective. These were less effective for the treatment of secondary tectonic fixations, which is why preparatory treatment steps were necessary.

For the correction of a tectonic fixation, Typaldos describes a multi-step treatment concept, which is used partially or completely, depending on the subtype of the distortion:

- Correction of all regional fascial distortions apart from the tectonic fixation
- Improvement of synovial fluid circulation
- Manual treatment of stuck fascial surfaces

5.6.1.1 Correction of all Regional Fascial Distortions Apart from Tectonic Fixations

This initial treatment step is particularly important for the correction of secondary tectonic fixations, which, according to Typaldos, are often caused by chronic triggerbands and folding distortions. The more completely these distortions are resolved beforehand, the easier it is to treat the tectonic fixation itself.

These causative distortions are not always immediately apparent to the therapist in FDM diagnosis, as patients with tectonic fixation primarily complain of restricted movement and stiffness. Therefore, the *analysis of the mechanism of injury underlying the symptoms* is of particular importance. For example, if a tectonic fixation of the shoulder develops following a dislocation fracture, there is a high probability of an additional folding distortion. If a sprained ankle becomes stiff after immobilization,

triggerbands, continuum distortions, or folding distortions, which developed during the injury, can trigger or maintain the tectonic fixation.

Provocation tests, such as active or passive end-range movement, are helpful in detecting these causative distortions. Triggerbands can be easily localized by the patient due to the pain they provoke. Continuum distortions, cylinder distortions, or folding distortions can also be revealed in this way. It is important for the therapist not to focus solely on the directly affected joint, but also to include adjacent articular and non-articular gliding surfaces in the treatment.

> **Background Information**
> The correction of fascial distortions, apart from the tectonic fixation, has a "door-opener function". Treating these distortions is expected to result in an initial improvement in mobility. As a result, synovial fluid is pumped more effectively through the affected joint, so that subsequent mobilization (as well as any other form of active movement) supports the resolution process of the tectonic fixation.

5.6.1.2 Improvement of Synovial Fluid Circulation

This treatment step aims to positively influence both the quantity and quality of synovial fluid in the affected joint (fig. 5.62a to c).

Typaldos describes various ways in which fluid circulation can be stimulated:

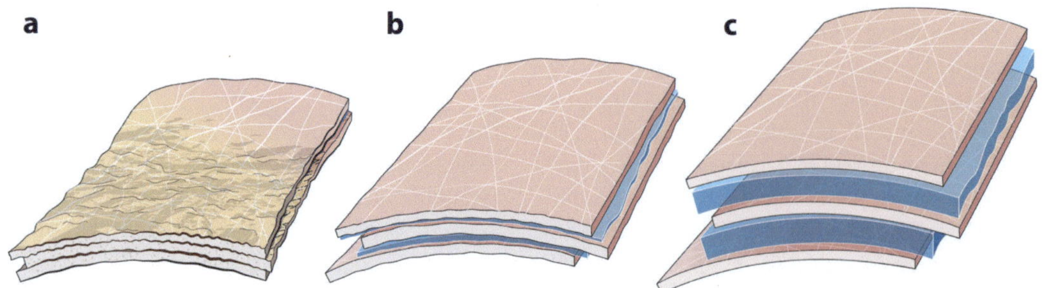

Fig. 5.62 **a** to **c**: step-by-step improvement of the circulation and production of (synovial) fluid in tectonic fixations, leading to reduced movement restriction. (© Anker 2022)

Hot packs, especially moist-warm compresses, have a positive effect on the suppleness of fascial structures. The application of heat relaxes the fascia and increases the viscosity of the synovial fluid. As a result, the stuck tissue can be mobilized more easily. However, it should be noted that in the presence of triggerbands or cylinder distortions, heat applications can intensify pain. Therefore, it must be decided on a case-by-case basis whether and at what point in the treatment hot packs should be used.

The *tectonic pump technique* is the core element of treatment, in which the therapist passively moves the tissue (and its fluids) to the end of its range of motion. Depending on the pattern of restriction, uniaxial movements, circumduction movements, or special combination movements are used, which are performed under (alternating) manual compression or traction of the joint.

In principle, the therapist first brings the restricted body part to its current movement limit, without provoking a hard end-feel. Mobilization then takes place in this position, with the therapist repetitively moving into and out of the area of stiffness. According to Typaldos, such a cycle should last three to five seconds, as the initial fascial response to therapy tends to be sluggish. Mobilization is continued until the resistance in the tissue noticeably decreases and the range of motion increases. Usually, it takes several minutes before the first improvements occur. In practice, many treatments of tectonic fixations fail because too little time is invested in the application of the tectonic pump technique.

This passive, end-range mobilization has multiple effects:

- It promotes fluid exchange in the smooth fascia through the constant alternation of compression and traction as well as stretching and relaxation.
- It stimulates the production of synovial fluid.
- It mobilizes the fixed tissue beyond the distortion-induced stop and thereby releases adhesions caused by triggerbands.

The tectonic pump technique can be painful for the patient, as mobilization is repeatedly performed at the end of the range of motion. The therapist is also physically challenged. Typaldos therefore recommends that the practitioner alternate with a colleague to generate sufficient intensity.

In the area of the joints of the arms and legs, the tectonic pump technique can also be performed in the *frog-leg position* or the *reversed frog-leg position.* In this technique, a shortened lever for mobilizing the stiff joint is created by flexing or extending the adjacent joints of the limb to their end range (which visually resembles a frog's leg). In this position, rhythmic mobilization at the end of the range of motion can be performed.

Background Information

Typaldos describes even impulse manipulations being performed in the frog-leg position. However, in clinical practice, this does rather not improve fluid circulation, but may be advantageous for improving the fascial gliding.

Regardless, the frog-leg position can also be used for the correction of folding distortions at the limb joints, especially for combinations of unfolding and refolding distortions at the elbow and knee.

In certain body regions—such as the back or shoulder—the *plunger technique* can be used in addition to the tectonic pump technique. For this, a suction cup is affixed to the area to be treated, and a pumping mobilization is performed by repeatedly pulling and pressing. The intense traction possible with the plunger technique is perceived by patients as particularly relieving. Technically, fluid is pumped between the adhering gliding surfaces, and the tissue is mobilized at the same time; an effect that also positively influences existing adhesions.

5.6.1.3 Manual Treatment of Fixed Fascial Gliding Surfaces

In the treatment of secondary tectonic fixations, blocked gliding surfaces are released in a third step after the tectonic pump technique. For the correction of primary, local fixations such as joint blockages, these manipulations can usually be started directly.

In this treatment step, various *manual techniques with and without impulse* are used, which *mobilize parallel gliding surfaces by applying force or speed.*

In the areas of the neck and back, classic chiropractic manipulation maneuvers can be used. They correct joint blockages by means of a forced gliding impulse. However, for pain that is perceived by the patient as deeply localized (as is typical with folding distortions), they are not optimal. In these cases, techniques that primarily apply traction or compression to the folding fascia are necessary.

If impulse techniques are not possible or are contraindicated, rhythmic mobilization techniques can be used, which also produce gliding movements parallel to the joint surface. These manual therapy techniques are applied forcefully in the Typaldos method to release both the gliding surfaces of the joint and to achieve a mobilizing effect on the surrounding soft tissue envelope.

5.6.2 Treatment Effects of Techniques for Tectonic Fixations

In primary tectonic fixations, following successful mobilization, an immediate improvement in symptoms can be expected. A blockage can occur abruptly and can be resolved just as quickly through targeted manual impulse treatment.

However, if tectonic fixations arise in connection with other, usually pain-inducing fascial distortions, greater therapeutic effort is required to reduce the often persistent movement restrictions. At this point, perseverance and determination are needed, as success often only occurs when a certain treatment intensity is achieved. This also requires the patient's commitment to consistently follow the therapy and to immediately integrate the achieved improvements in movement into daily life or to maintain them through targeted exercise programs.

5.6.3 Side Effects and Contraindications in the Treatment of Tectonic Fixations

Every maneuver must be applied with consideration—depending on the patient, their goals, and the type of injury. In particular, vigorous mobilization during the tectonic pump technique can be painful and may lead to side effects after treatment, such as *soft tissue pain or fatigue.* It is important to inform the patient in advance of the treatment, and to convey that pausing during mobilization is possible at any time.

When using impulse manipulations or leverage techniques, any contraindications must be observed, as already explained in the section on manual treatment for folding distortions.

Reduced bony stability, whether due to an incompletely healed fracture or decreased bone density, is a prime example here. Rejection of this form of therapy by the patient or her lack of understanding of the treatment's intent can also prevent the use of such interventions.

5.6.4 Additional Measures for the Treatment of Tectonic Fixations

- Through *regular active movement*, patients can support the treatment. Similar to the tectonic pump technique, the focus is on rhythmic, repeated mobilization of the maximum possible range of motion, and it may be advantageous to avoid excessive force.

Depending on the problem, starting positions can be chosen that reduce the influence of gravity (e.g. moving a shoulder while lying on the back). Aids (e.g. elastic bands) can also be used to reduce muscular effort during movement execution. This enables repeated performance of mobilizing movements over a certain period of time. In addition, this can reduce the partially negative effect of strong muscle contractions on the mechanics of a joint with restricted movement.

- *Joint infiltrations* can have a certain effect by increasing the fluid volume. According to Typaldos, it does not seem to be crucial which substance is administered (e.g. saline solution, cortisone, or artificial joint lubricant). What is more important is that the tectonic pump technique is applied following the infiltration. This supports the diffusion of the fluid between the joint partners and reduces their "magnetic" attraction.
- Tectonic fixation is the only fascial distortion that benefits from *direct heat applications*. As already described in the treatment process, heat increases the viscosity of the synovial fluid and improves the elasticity of the tissue. A hot shower before an active mobilization program or movement in warm water takes advantage of this effect.
- Finally, the *importance of prevention* in connection with secondary tectonic fixations should be mentioned again. After physical trauma, the goal is to prevent a tectonic fixation as much as possible by prescribing immobilization only as long as absolutely necessary, and by treating associated fascial distortions as soon as possible.

In conventional medicine, the *side effects of immobilization* with regard to mobility and physical function are often underestimated. Especially in older patients, after injuries with significant bleeding into the tissue, and in patients with a high proportion of band-like fascia, adhesions and subsequently tectonic fixations may develop rapidly, which can only be treated with considerable therapeutic effort.

5.6.5   Treatment Examples

5.6.5.1   Treatment of Tectonic Fixations of the Shoulder

Indications

- Restriction of movement of the shoulder or shoulder girdle; pain is not the primary symptom
- Possible mechanisms of origin: primarily as a result of mechanical trauma; secondarily as a result of injury, surgery, or chronification (e.g. chronic frozen shoulder)
- Typical body language: self-mobilization; characteristic movement restriction (compensation of limited arm abduction by increased forward elevation of the arm or backward bending of the trunk; see sect. 2.6.4, fig. 2.26)

Tectonic Pump Technique in the Supine Position
The patient lies at the edge of the treatment table. The therapist grasps the forearm near the wrist and moves the shoulder into maximal possible extension and then into flexion. The mobilization is repeated slowly and rhythmically until the resistance to movement decreases and a greater range of motion is possible (fig. 5.63a and b).

Tectonic Pump Technique in the Frog-Leg Position
The therapist flexes the patient's shoulder and elbow. With one hand, he grasps the elbow and applies gentle compression to the shoulder. The second hand holds the forearm and wrist. The therapist mobilizes the shoulder with a rotational movement by rotating the elbow toward the patient's face and pulling the wrist outward (fig. 5.63c).

Tectonic Pump Technique in the Reverse Frog-Leg Position
The therapist flexes the patient's shoulder and elbow. With one hand, he grasps the elbow and

applies gentle compression to the shoulder. The second hand holds the forearm and the flexed wrist. The therapist mobilizes the shoulder with a rotational movement by rotating the elbow inward and pulling the wrist outward (fig. 5.63d).

Manual impulse treatment in the scissor-position

The patient lies in a lateral position with the affected shoulder on top. The therapist stands behind the treatment table. One hand is placed flat on the shoulder, while the other hand holds the patient's lower arm and stabilizes the upper body. The therapist creates a manipulation barrier by gently compressing the shoulder and pushing it forward. The impulse is delivered by increasing the gliding movement forward or downward (fig. 5.64).

Practical tips

- Typaldos describes the possibility of manual impulse treatment in the frog-leg position. However, the required range of motion is only present in exceptional cases (e.g. in primary tectonic fixations of the shoulder).
- Particularly in secondary fixations, the focus is on the tectonic pump technique. In this context, fixations should be considered and treated not only in the shoulder joint, but also in the shoulder girdle, neck, and thorax.
- Gliding mobilization techniques, as used in classical manual therapy, are equally suitable for promoting movement. In the Typaldos method, they are generally applied more forcefully.

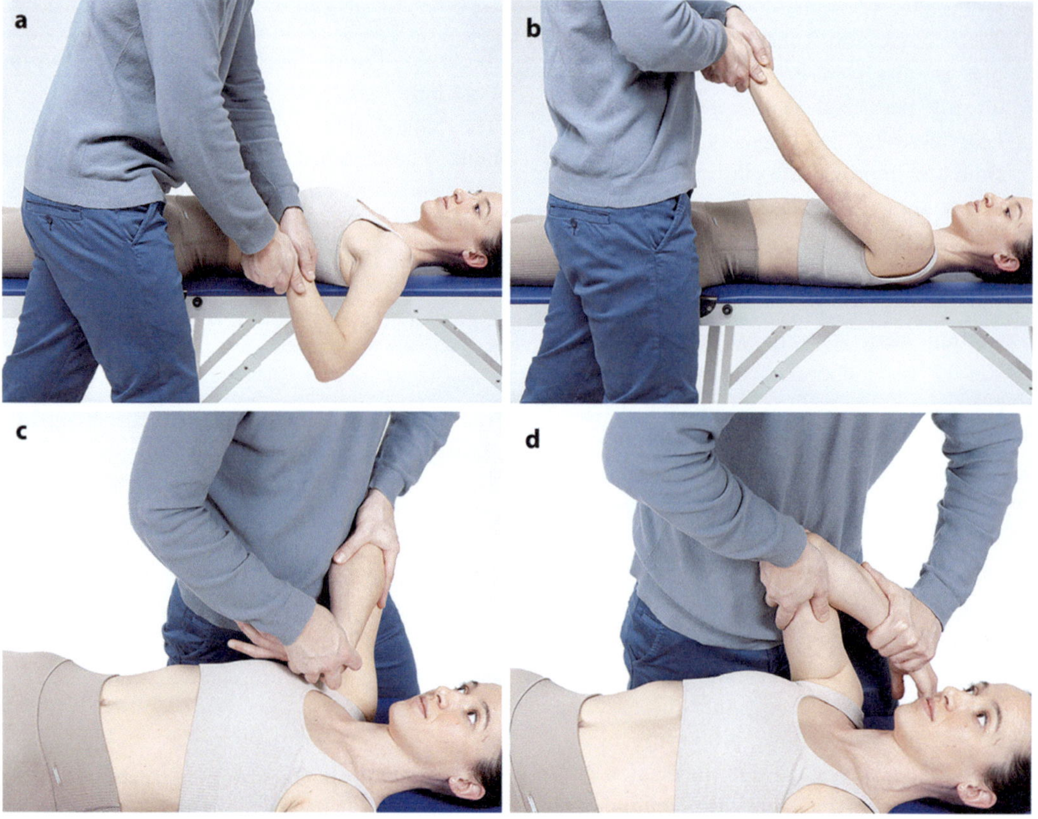

Fig. 5.63 Tectonic pump techniques at the shoulder. Mobilization in extension (**a**). Mobilization in flexion (**b**). Mobilization in the frog-leg position (**c**). Mobilization in the reverse frog-leg position (**d**). (© Anker 2022)

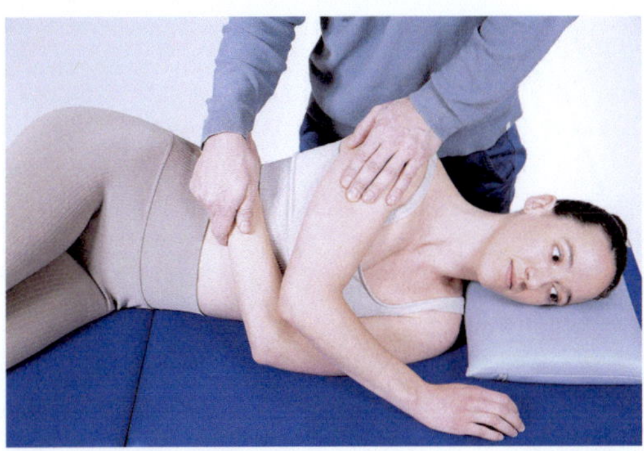

Fig. 5.64 Impulse-manual treatment of the shoulder in the scissor-position. (© Anker 2022)

5.6.5.2 Treatment of Tectonic Fixations of the Back

Indications

- Restricted mobility of the back; sensation of blockage; less commonly, pain
- Possible mechanisms of origin: primarily as a result of mechanical trauma; secondarily following injury, surgery, or in the context of chronic complaints
- Typical body language: pressing both hands into the back; placing fingers on the stuck area; self-mobilization

Pumping Technique with a Plunger
The patient lies in the prone position, and the suction cup is applied to the area to be treated. Mobilization is performed by rhythmically lifting and releasing (fig. 5.65a).

Impulse Technique in the Chair Position
The patient sits astride a chair and braces their knees against a wall on a cushion. She hooks her feet behind the chair legs, crosses her arms, and relaxes her back. The therapist stands in a deep squat position behind the patient. He supports his elbow on his thigh and his hand on the side of the patient's back. The therapist grasps the patient's upper body and rotates them to the tension barrier. The impulse is delivered in the direction of rotation. (fig. 5.65b).

Impulse Technique in the Supine Position; Dog Technique
The patient is positioned supine with their arms crossed in parallel (fig. 5.66a). The therapist stands at the side of the treatment table and rolls the patient toward himself. He places his hand under their back so that the thenar and hypothenar eminences are in contact with the corresponding transverse process (fig. 5.66b). By moving the patient's elbows, he focuses the manipulation forces and then applies a more or less vertical impulse toward the treatment table (fig. 5.66c).

The dog technique can also be performed in a flexed back position. For this, the therapist places one hand on the upper back and positions the patient's head in flexion. The therapist lifts the patient's upper body and delivers the impulse as it is lowered back onto the treatment table (fig. 5.66d).

Practical tips

- In tectonic fixations, pain is not the predominant symptom. As an exception, Typaldos describes fixations of the lower back that can cause centrally localized deep pain.
- If, during the impulse technique on the back in rotation, it is not possible to establish an appropriate barrier, introducing additional movements such as side bending toward the fixation or increasing flexion or extension of the back may help.
- Alternatively, the *manual impulse treatment of the back in the scissor-position* can also be used. This technique corresponds to the impulse technique for the pelvis in the scissor- position (see sect. 5.3.5.2, fig. 5.24). This manual treatment not only produces traction in the area of the sacroiliac joint (for correction of inverted continuum distortions and unfolding distortions), but also a rotational movement in the lower back. Therefore, it is suitable for the treatment of both primary and secondary tectonic fixations.
- The impulse technique on the back in rotation is suitable for treating tectonic fixations of

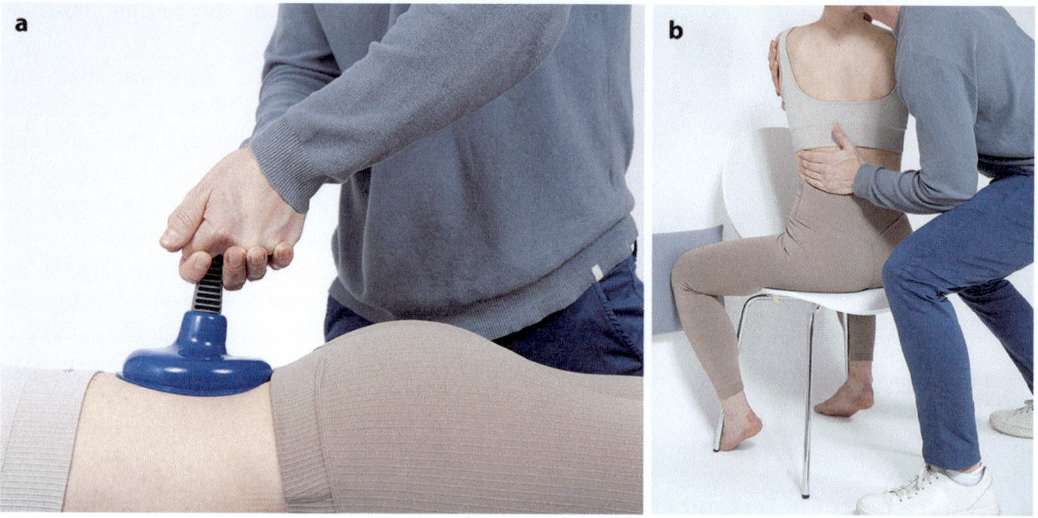

Fig. 5.65 Tectonic mobilization techniques. Pumping technique with a plunger (**a**). Impulse technique in rotation (**b**). (© Anker 2022)

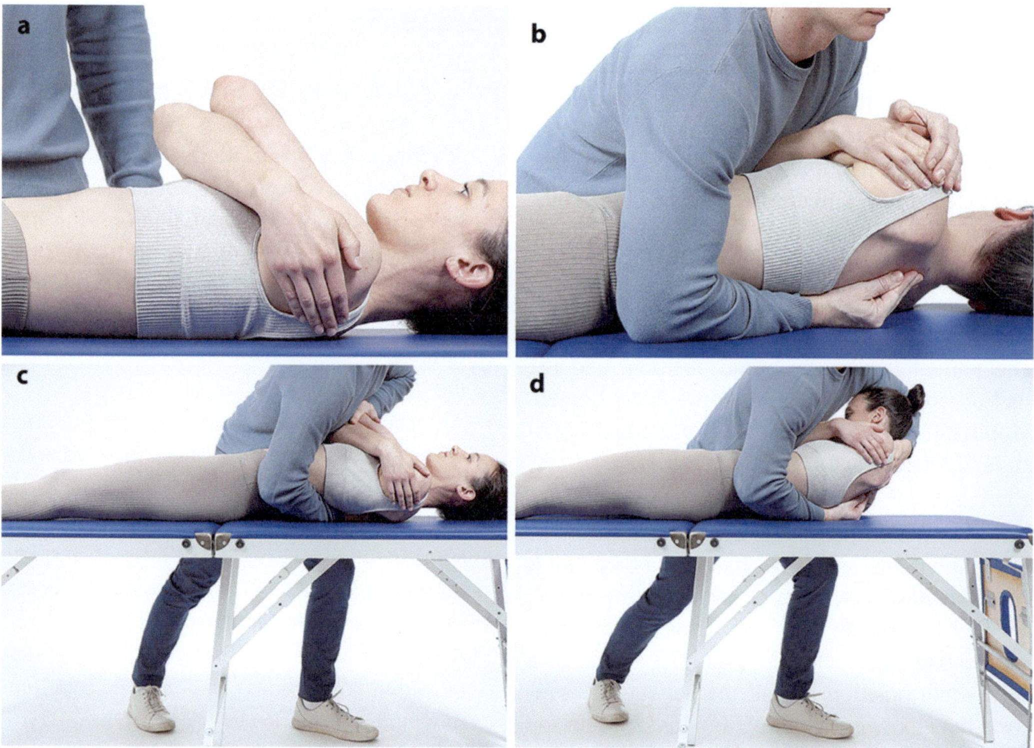

Fig. 5.66 a to d: Impulse technique on the back "Dog technique." Positioning of the patient (**a**). Possible positioning of the therapist's hand under the back (**b**). Barrier setup and impulse with the back extended (**c**). Variant in flexed back position (**d**). (© Anker 2022)

the lower or middle ribs as well. The plunger technique can also be used for scapula tectonic mobilization.

5.6.5.3 Treatment of Tectonic Fixations of the Hip and Pelvis

Indications

- Restricted mobility of the hip, pelvis, or lower back; sensation of blockage; less commonly, pain
- Possible mechanisms of origin: primarily as a result of mechanical trauma; secondarily following injury or surgery
- Typical body language: supporting the pelvis with both hands; self-mobilization

Tectonic Pump Technique in the Frog-Leg Position

The therapist grasps the patient's flexed knee with one hand. The second hand is placed on the lower leg near the ankle. The therapist flexes the hip and rotates it outward. The joint is rhythmically compressed and mobilized by simultaneously pressing the patient's knee outward and toward the floor, while moving the ankle toward the patient's abdomen. The higher the chosen flexion position, the more this maneuver mobilizes the pelvis and lower back (fig. 5.67a).

Tectonic Pump Technique in the Reverse Frog-Leg Position

The therapist grasps the patient's flexed knee with one hand. The second hand is placed on the patient's medial malleolus or inner thigh. The therapist flexes the hip and rotates it inward, while the hip remains abducted. The joint is rhythmically compressed and mobilized by rotating the patient's knee inward and simultaneously pressing the lower leg outward and upward. The higher the chosen flexion position, the more this maneuver mobilizes the pelvis and lower back (fig. 5.67b).

Impulse Technique in Flexion Position

The therapist grasps the patient's knee and flexes the hip. He positions himself next to the treatment table, facing the patient's feet. The second hand is placed, palm up, deep in the patient's groin to apply compression to the hip. Then, the therapist abruptly compresses the patient's hip by pressing on the knee while simultaneously pushing the hand in the groin away from himself (fig. 5.68).

Practical tips

- Especially in cases of secondary fixations, the use of inversion therapy has proven effective as preparation for the tectonic pump technique (see sect. 5.4.2)

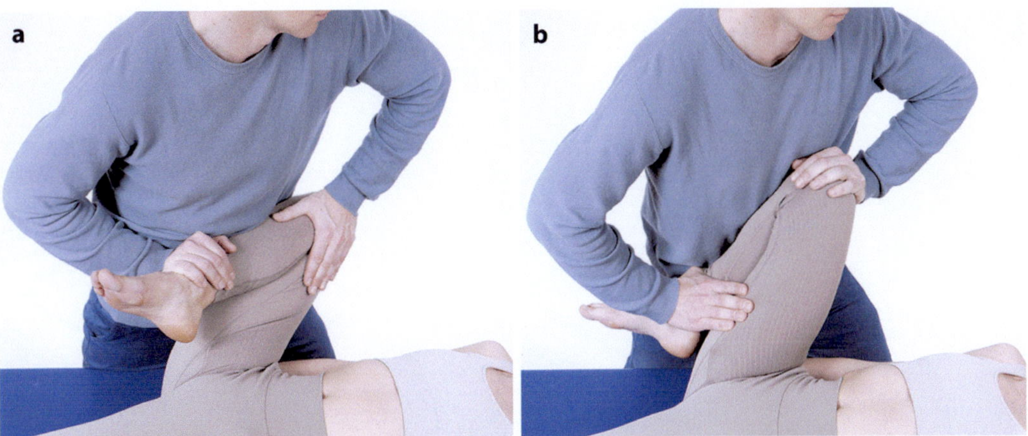

Fig. 5.67 Tectonic pump techniques of the hip and pelvis. Mobilization in the frog-leg position (**a**). Mobilization in the reverse frog-leg position (**b**). (© Anker 2022)

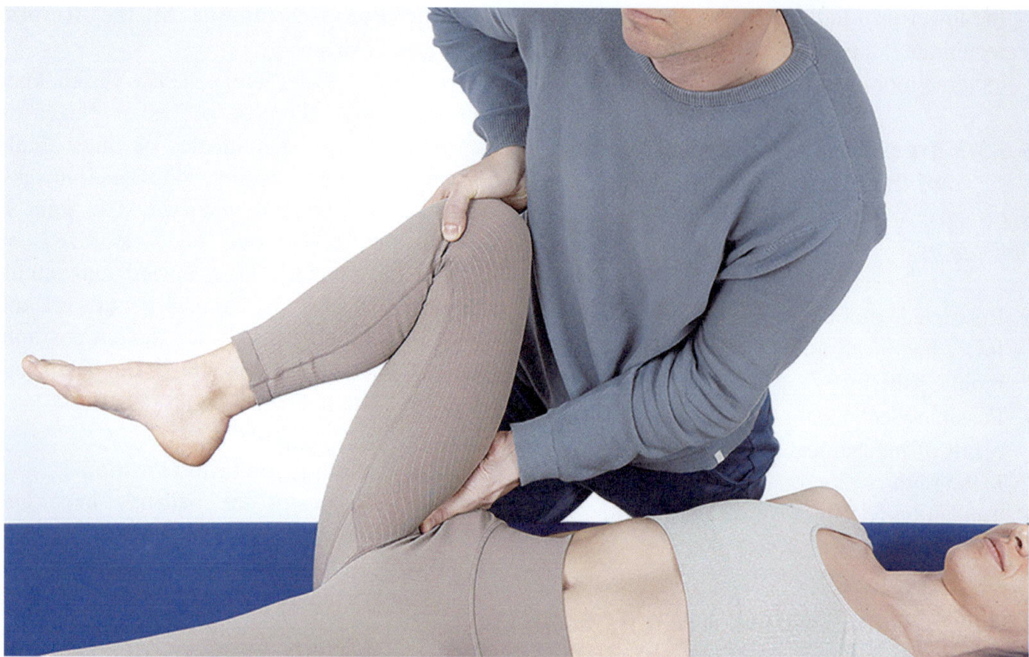

Fig. 5.68 Impulse technique in flexion for tectonic fixation of the hip. (© Anker 2022)

- Typaldos describes the possibility of a manual impulse treatment in the frog-leg position. However, the necessary range of motion is only present in exceptional cases.
- The impulse technique can be used as a stand-alone treatment for primary tectonic fixations of the hip or pelvis (in the sense of a blockage). For secondary fixations, manual impulse treatment is recommended following the tectonic pump technique.

6

Appendix

6.1 Flowcharts for the Treatment of Shoulder Complaints

For certain specific patterns of complaints, Typaldos outlines sequences of simple tests and resulting treatment steps in flowcharts in his textbooks (see sect. 4.2). These instructions are intended to make his method easily applicable in medical practice, especially for therapists with little experience in clinical application. For example, Typaldos provides a step-by-step guide for the treatment of ankle sprains (see sect. 4.2, fig. 4.2) or for correcting restrictions of shoulder movement (fig. 6.1 and 6.2). These treatment sequences have proven effective in clinical practice. Nevertheless, they should not be misunderstood as dogma. With increasing experience and a solid understanding of the Typaldos method, therapists should be able to deviate from the established sequence in individual cases, with appropriate justification.

6.2 Distortion Matrix

This overview (fig. 6.3) presents the six fascial distortions in comparison. The most important elements of FDM diagnosis and treatment are listed.

6.3 European Fascial Distortion Model Association (EFDMA) and its International Partner Organizations

The EFDMA was founded in Vienna/Austria in 2006 as a non-profit association. Its goal is to sustainably promote the Fascial Distortion Model (FDM) and the Typaldos method throughout Europe, thereby enabling all patients in Europe to receive qualified treatment according to the Fascial Distortion Model (FDM) according to Typaldos.

The association's main activities focus on

- regulating and promoting high-quality training for medical professionals,
- disseminating the Fascial Distortion Model developed by Stephen Typaldos, D.O., through public relations,
- promoting scientific studies on FDM and the Typaldos method, and
- the international exchange of experience in close cooperation with other international FDM associations.

The EFDMA certifies instructors who teach the Fascial Distortion Model and the Typaldos method according to a Europe-wide curriculum. Graduates of this medical training can become full members of the EFDMA.

© The Author(s), under exclusive license to Springer-Verlag GmbH, DE, part of Springer Nature 2026
S. Anker, *Fascial Distortion Model in Clinical Practice*, https://doi.org/10.1007/978-3-662-72081-3_6

FLOWCHART FOR ACUTE SHOULDER PAIN

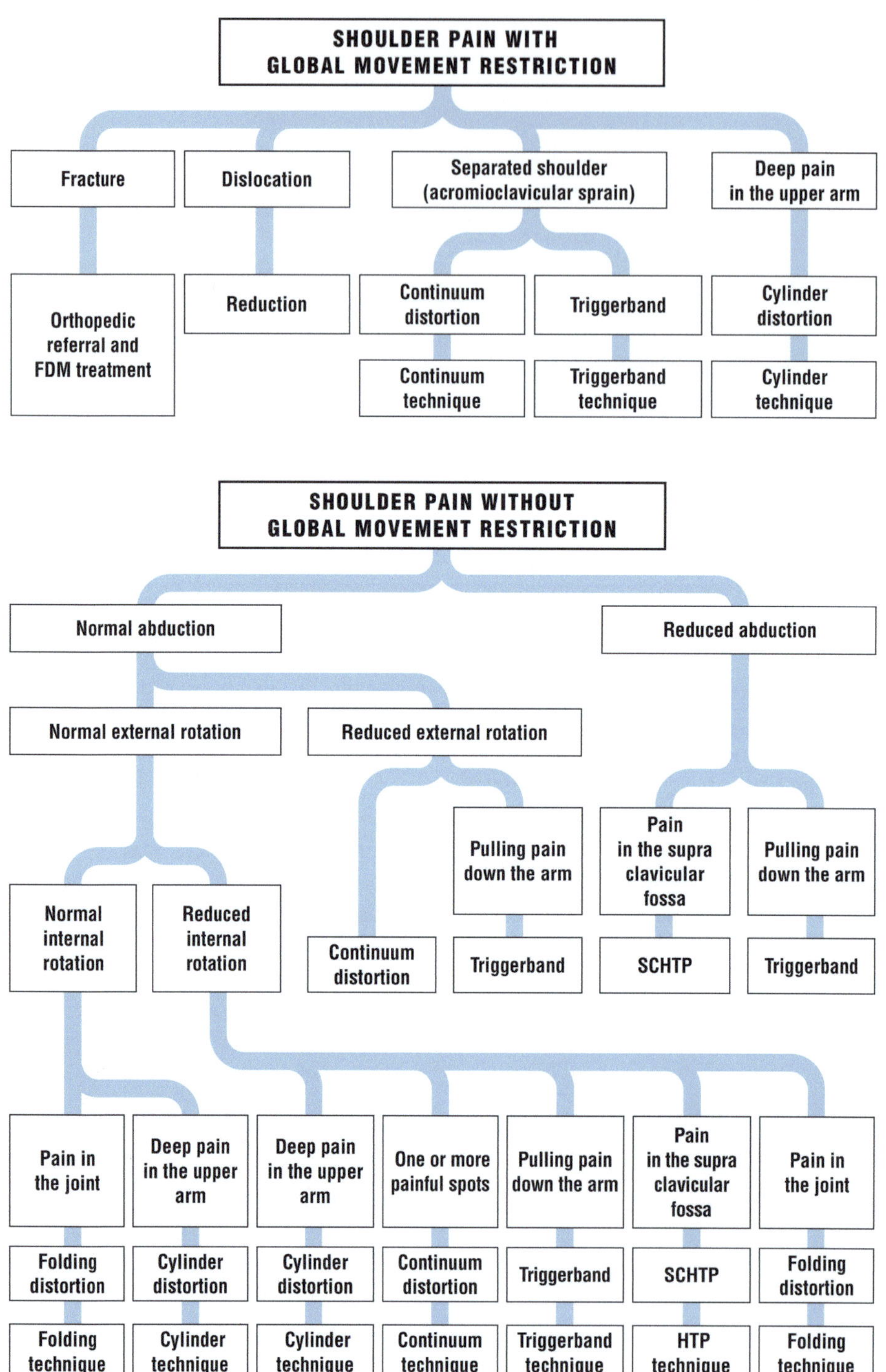

Fig. 6.1 Flowchart for the treatment of acute shoulder pain [1]

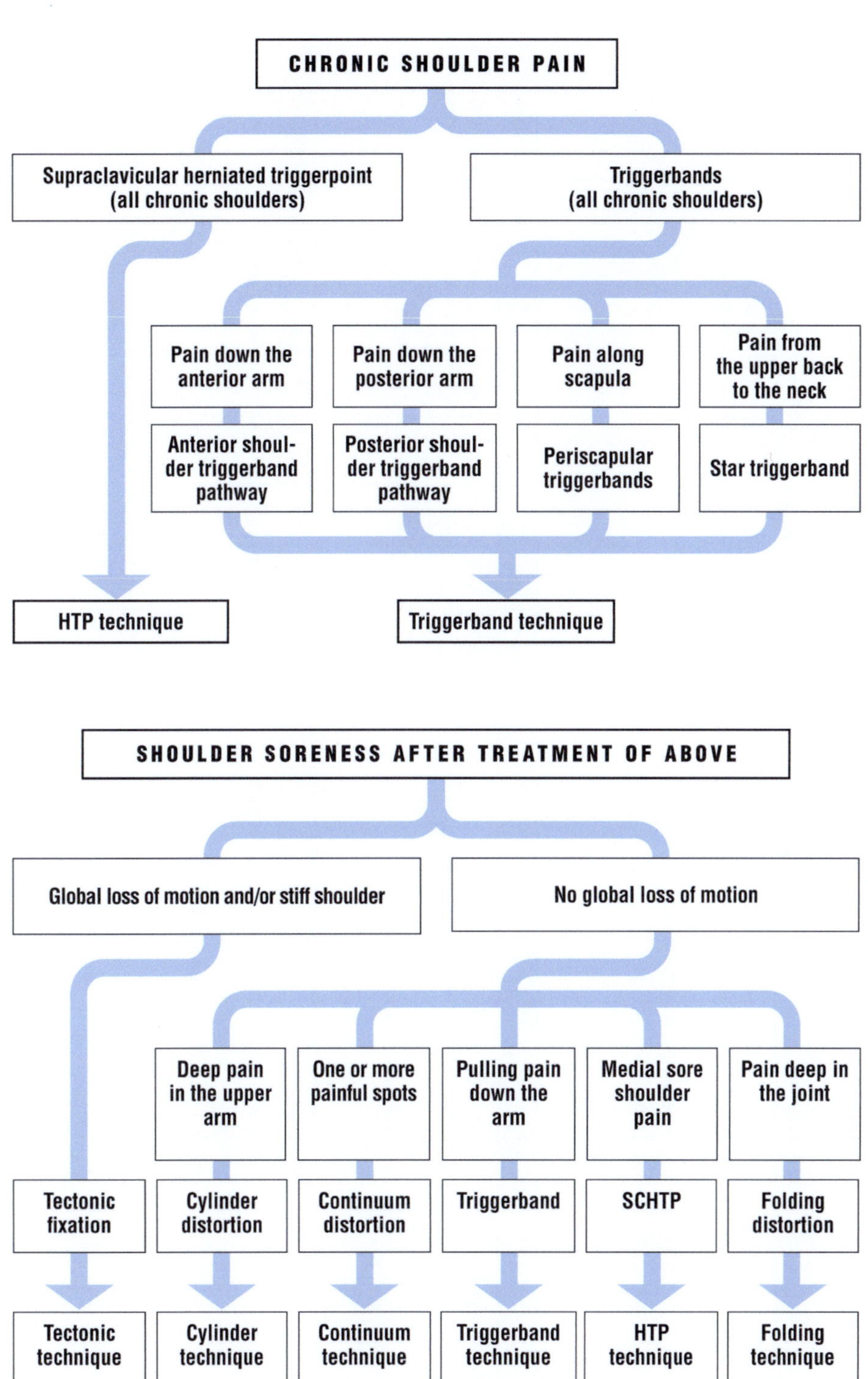

Fig. 6.2 Flowchart for the treatment of chronic shoulder pain [2]

FASCIAL DISTORTION GRID

	Anamnesis	Examination	Body language	Treatment
Triggerband (TB) 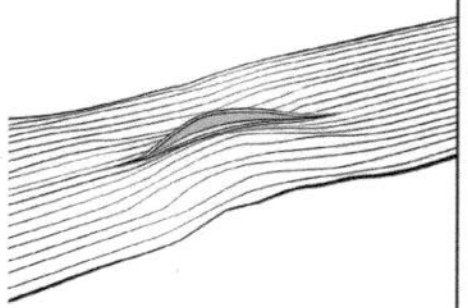	• Formation through traumatic sprain, strain or overuse; tendency for chronification • Pulling, burning pain • Mobility restriction, weakness and loss of coordination • Start-up pain • Local swelling	• Manual pressure elicits typical pain along the entire pathway • Palpable tissue change	• Dynamic stroking with fingertips along a pathway	• Triggerband technique • Active mobilization
Herniated triggerpoint (HTP) 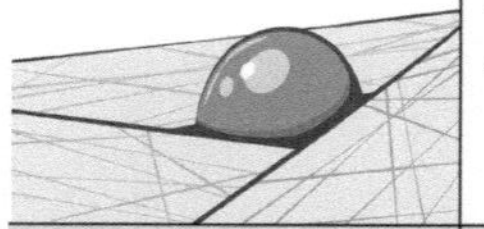	• Formation traumatically or gradually, usually due to pressure increase in the body • Mobility restriction • Dull, localized pain and tension-type pain	• Tender to manual pressure • Palpable tissue change	• Pressing with several fingers, the thumb or the knuckles into a soft tissue area	• Herniated triggerpoint technique
Continuum distortion (CD) 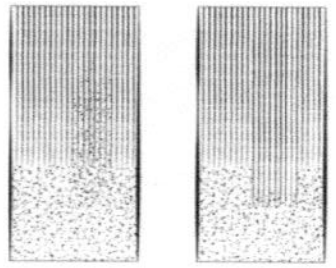	• Formation through traumatic sprain, strain or overuse • Localized pain (usually on the bone) • Mobility restriction, weakness and loss of coordination • Local swelling	• Manual pressure elicits typical pain • Palpable tissue change (usually on the bone)	• Pointing with a fingertip	• Continuum technique • Impulse manipulation (for inverted continuum distortions)

Fig. 6.3 Distortion matrix. (© Anker 2022)

	Anamnesis	Examination	Body language	Treatment
Folding distortion (FD)	• Formation traumatically through traction/shearing forces (unfolding distortion) or compression/shearing forces (refolding distortion); formation through overuse more common for folding distortions of the interosseous membranes or the muscle septa • Deep pain in the joint • Feeling of instability • Rare: major mobility restriction (except folding distortions of the interosseous membranes or the muscle septa) • Joint swelling	• No tenderness to palpation • No palpable tissue change	• Placing the hand on the affected region • Stroking horizontally across the joint (for refolding distortions) • Pressing several fingers between bones (for interosseous membrane folding distortions), between muscles (for muscle septa folding distortions)	• Mobilization or impulse manipulation according to the mechanism of injury • Automobilization according to the mechanism of injury
	Anamnesis	Examination	Body language	Treatment
Cylinder distortion (CyD)	• Formation traumatically through soft tissue contusion, constriction, overloading or without recognizable cause • Diffuse pain; night pain • Phenomenon of jumping pain • Active mobility restriction • Weakness, loss of coordination, cramps, pseudo-neurological symptoms • Local swelling	• No tenderness to palpation (except pain provocation through lifting up the skin) • No palpable tissue change	• Dynamic wiping, kneading or pinching of the affected tissue	• Manual cylinder technique • Tool-assisted cylinder technique
	Anamnesis	Examination	Body language	Treatment
Tectonic fixation (TF)	• Primary formation (blockage) or secondary formation (as a result of other fascial distortions, e.g. chronic triggerbands) • Local movement restriction or global loss of mobility • Feeling of stiffness • Pain is not the main feature	• Objectifiable movement restriction	• Attempt at automobilization	• Tectonic pump technique • Mobilization or thrust manipulation • Application of heat • Automobilization

Fig. 6.3 (continued)

The EFDMA is part of the *Fascial Distortion Model Global Organization (FDMGO),* which also includes the *American Fascial Distortion Model Association (AFDMA)* and the *Fascial Distortion Model Asian Association (FAA).* This international confederation works to protect and promote the Fascial Distortion Model in accordance with the empirical research and publications of Stephen Typaldos, and fosters exchange and collaboration among its members. To this end, the international members of the FDMGO organize a world congress every three years.

6.4   EFDMA Curriculum

The EFDMA curriculum regulates training in the "Fascial Distortion Model (FDM) and Typaldos method" in Europe. It is divided into

- basic training in three modules (FDM Basic), and
- advanced seminars and clinical training courses (FDM Advanced).

Eligible for training in the "Fascial Distortion Model and Typaldos method" are all healthcare professionals who, independently or on medical referral, are permitted by local law to perform manual techniques (including mobilization techniques) on patients within their professional scope. This includes, for example, physicians, physiotherapists, and osteopaths.

In addition, the EFDMA curriculum regulates the final examination (FDM Basic Certificate – FDM BC), international certification (FDM International Certificate – FDM IC), and training to become a certified FDM instructor.

Further information on the EFDMA curriculum can be found at:

www.FDM-europe.com

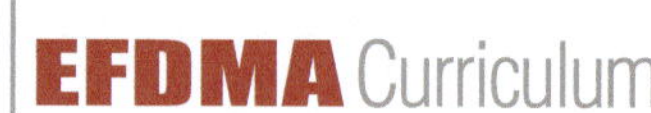

References

1. Typaldos S (2002) Clinical and theoretical application of the Fascial Distortion Model within the practice of medicine and surgery, 4th edn. Orthopathic Global Health Publications, Brewer, p 144
2. Typaldos S (2002) Clinical and theoretical application of the Fascial Distortion Model within the practice of medicine and surgery, 4th edn. Orthopathic Global Health Publications, Brewer, p 145

Glossary

Adhesions Fascial fibers (torn crosslinks) in the area of the band-like fascia that heal in a non-functional position. They lead to restrictions of the affected tissue and to subsequent chronicity.

All-or-none principle Clinical phenomenon, typically observed in the correction of a continuum distortion: there is no partial success with the continuum technique; the correction is either completely successful or not at all.

Anterior ankle continuum distortion (AACD) Continuum distortion at the anterior ankle. This everted continuum distortion typically results from an ankle sprain and restricts active dorsiflexion of the ankle.

Ball therapy A form of treatment for folding distortions and tectonic fixations, in which the rebound effect of a gymnastic ball is utilized. The round shape of the ball also allows for the application of traction or compression forces.

Band-like fascia (banded fascia) Dense, tensile tissues with a high proportion of connective tissue fibers that adapt to specific mechanical demands, found throughout the body. They play an important role in force transmission, protect tissues such as bones, muscles, and vessels, and direct the flow of interstitial fluid within the tissue.

Body language Unconscious, regularly occurring movements and postures by which patients, among other things, indicate fascial distortions.

Bullseye herniated triggerpoint Herniated triggerpoint centrally located in the gluteal region.

Chronification Clinical picture in which adhesions have formed. Chronification is characterized by the increasing spreading of pain (from local to regional) and increasing movement restriction. The goal of the treatment is to resolve the adhesion and thereby convert the chronic condition into an acute condition (i.e. without adhesions).

Clamp/Vice technique Treatment of cylinder distortions using clamps or vices.

Continuum distortion (CD) Principal fascial distortion type; the transition zone between different tissue types loses the ability to adapt to applied forces.

Continuum distortion; subtypes Everted continuum distortions (eCD) and inverted continuum distortions (iCD) can be differentiated according to their mechanism of formation and their response to specific treatment interventions.

Continuum technique (CD technique) Correction technique using the tip of the thumb, which corrects the step formation in the transition zone and thereby resolves the continuum distortion.

Continuum theory Concept that views fascia as a continuous, adaptable anatomical structure. Different tissue types merge seamlessly into one another and can adapt to internal and external mechanical forces in the area of transition zones.

Compression Cylinder Variant (CCV) A variant of the double-thumb technique, the squeegee technique, or the Indian burn technique, in which the cylinder distortion is resolved by compression instead of traction. According to experience, these techniques are particularly suitable for stuck cylinder distortions.

Comb technique Treatment used both for the correction of cylinder distortions and for the release of adhesions.

Crossband Typaldos uses this term to refer to structures that are arranged at a right angle to the course of a fascial band. These can be retinacula or aponeuroses that are located in the area of joints or at prominent bony points (for example, at the mastoid or the coccyx).

Crosslink Stabilizing cross-connections between parallel fibers of the band-like fascia.

Cumulative repetitive injury Overuse syndrome that develops over a prolonged period due to the repetition of a specific movement or load beyond the tissue's capacity. Repetitive overuse leads to increasingly complex, often chronic, patterns of strain. As a result, tissue resilience is reduced and treatment can be more prolonged. It is advantageous to initially reduce the movements and loads which trigger symptoms, and only gradually increase them again once a stable improvement in symptoms has been achieved.

Cupping with movement Treatment of cylinder distortions by applying suction cups while the patient performs active movements.

Cylinder distortion (CyD) Principal fascial distortion type; entanglement of the cylinder fascia, leading to constriction of the tissue it encloses.

Cylinder distortion; subtypes Typaldos distinguishes cylinder distortions that are caused by traction from those that are caused by compression (see compression cylinder variant—CCV).

Cylinder fascia Spirally structured fascia enveloping soft tissues such as muscles, vessels, and internal organs in multiple layers. Like the folding fascia, it has a shock-absorbing function for non-articular areas.

Double-thumb technique Cylinder technique in which the cylinder fascia is spread apart with the thumbs to resolve entanglement.

Fascia Typaldos defines fascia as primary connective tissue that surrounds muscles, bones, nerves, and organs. Fascia also forms, among other things, tendons, ligaments, fascial bands, muscle sheaths, adhesions, and retinacula.

Current definitions consider fascia as a dissectible anatomical structure that is part of a functional system. This fascial system, in turn, is part of human connective tissue.

Fascial Continuum Model This concept, introduced by Typaldos in 1992, establishes an independent perspective on anatomy in which fascia plays a central role.

Fascial distortion Deformation of fascia, which leads to dysfunction of the affected tissue and other related structures. From the perspective of the Fascial Distortion Model, fascial distortions are the primary causes of pain and functional limitations. The Fascial Distortion Model describes six different types of fascial distortions.

Fascial Distortion Model (FDM) This model represents relationships between clinical phenomena and fascial distortions. It serves as a guiding framework for the analysis and interpretation of symptoms in order to derive practice-relevant conclusions for treatment.

Folding distortion (FD) Principal fascial distortion type; deformation of the folding fascia, resulting in impaired shock-absorbing capacity of the affected tissue.

Folding distortion; subtypes Typaldos distinguishes between unfolding and refolding distortions, depending on the mechanism of injury, the symptomatology, and the response to specific treatment interventions.

Folding fascia This fascia is found in the area of joints. In addition, the interosseous membranes and muscle septa are also considered folding fascia. Due to its structure, it serves as a shock-absorber for articular regions and ensures free mobility.

Folding technique Treatment of folding distortions with and without impulse under traction or compression and additional shearing movements.

Grain-of-salt technique Variant of the triggerband technique for grain-of-salt-like triggerbands.

Headlight effect Phenomenon in the triggerband technique: the patient feels the characteristic pain along the entire course of the triggerband when the therapist corrects the distortion piece by piece.

Herniated triggerpoint (HTP) Principal fascial distortion type; tissue protrusion through a smooth fascial layer, leading to blockage in the area of the affected soft tissues and adjacent joints.

Herniated triggerpoint; banded HTP tissue protrusion through a band-like fascial layer, which is additionally deformed by a triggerband.

Herniated triggerpoint technique (HTP technique) Repositioning technique performed with the thumb; the goal is to press the tissue protrusion back into the original fascial plane.

Hit-by-a-truck effect Potential side effect that occurs as a result of releasing adhesions. It is typically characterized by soft tissue pain, fatigue, autonomic symptoms such as nausea or hypotension, as well as hematoma formation. These side effects last up to 48 hours, and in rare cases, several days.

Impulse technique Mobilization technique that uses a short acceleration impulse to break through a previously established tension barrier in the tissue. The impulse can trigger traction (to correct an unfolding distortion), produce compression (to correct a refolding distortion), or initiate a neutral gliding movement (for the treatment of tectonic fixations).

Indian burn technique Cylinder technique in which the tangled cylinder fascia is first pulled apart and then twisted in opposite directions.

Inversion therapy A treatment method for the back and legs in which the patient is placed in an upside-down position using various therapeutic devices, resulting in sustained traction.

KIWI® technique Treatment of cylinder distortions using a vacuum extractor.

Milking the release Completion of the HTP technique; to push the last remnant of the protrusion back into the appropriate fascial plane, the thumb is dynamically flexed and extended. This promotes the functional closure of the protrusion canal.

Model of continuity The FDM promotes a perspective regarding the human body that centers on the continuity of tissues. Fascial fibers traverse the entire body and form a framework for all structures of the organism.

Orthopathic medicine Term that Typaldos temporarily used to describe his concept of fascial distortions.

Phenomenon of jumping pain A typical symptom in cylinder distortions, in which the complaints change their location without any apparent reason.

Pinch technique Cylinder technique in which the cylinder fascia is locally pinned down and the patient actively moves against this resistance.

Plunger technique Pumping technique in which a suction cup is fixed to the region to be treated, and a pumping mobilization is performed by repeatedly pulling and pressing.

Pseudo-herniated triggerpoint This distortion is not a tissue protrusion, but is caused by the overlap of several triggerbands. Treatment is performed using the triggerband technique.

Posterior wrist continuum distortion (PWCD) Continuum distortion at the dorsal wrist, which often restricts extension movement.

Probability repetitive injury Overuse syndrome that occurs without warning, even though the triggering movement has ultimately been repeated a thousand times. The goal of the treatment is to correct the existing fascial distortions and to resume the originally triggering movement as soon as possible.

Release Reduction of tissue tension, which can be perceived during the treatment of herniated triggerpoints, continuum distortions, and cylinder distortions. Typaldos additionally describes a possible release during the correction of folding distortions.

Roadblock effect Phenomenon that describes the effects of fascial distortions on fluid transport along the fascial bands. All six fascial distortions can act as a mechanical obstacle to fluid dynamics, disrupting fascial metabolism in the medium and long term and consequently triggering additional symptoms.

Smooth fascia Supple, adaptable, overlapping fascial layers that lines joints, abdomen and internal organs. They are less resistant than banded fascia, but their ability to glide allows for a high degree of mobility.

Supraclavicular herniated triggerpoint (SCHTP) Shoulder HTP; this protrusion often restricts abduction or internal rotation of the shoulder, or limits the mobility of the neck (primarily its rotational movement).

Squeegee technique Cylinder technique that strips the cylinder fascia under firm hand pressure and resolves entanglement.

Star triggerband Triggerband extending from the upper back to the occiput or the mastoid. This triggerband was the first fascial distortion treated by Typaldos and marks the starting point for the development of the Fascial Distortion Model.

Starting point Palpable tissue alteration at which the course of a triggerband begins and where, consequently, the triggerband correction starts.

Tectonic fixation (TF) Principal fascial distortion type; fascial distortion characterized by the loss of gliding ability of the smooth fascia.

Tectonic fixation; subtypes Typaldos describes subjective tectonic fixations, which are characterized by a subjective feeling of stiffness. In contrast, objectively verifiable tectonic fixations can also be identified by the therapist as clear movement restrictions. Furthermore, according to the mechanism of formation, primary tectonic fixations can be distinguished from secondary tectonic fixations. The former occur as singular, acute fascial distortions (e.g. a joint blockage), while the latter arise as a consequence of other fascial distortions (e.g. due to chronic triggerbands).

Tectonic pump technique Treatment of a tectonic fixation at the limit of movement by slow, repeated, passive mobilization under compression or traction.

Triggerband (TB) Principal fascial distortion type; twist in the area of the band-like fascia. This fascial distortion causes pulling, burning pain and movement restrictions.

Triggerband; subtypes Typaldos describes six different subtypes, which differ on palpation in the shape and consistency of the deformation: the twist, the nodule, the pea, the crumb, the wave, and the grain of salt.

Triggerband technique Correction technique performed with the thumb; adhesions are released, the twist in the area of the band-like fascia is untwisted, and the band-like fibers are aligned and approximated.

Transition zone Area between adjacent tissue types within the tissue continuum (see continuum theory), which can adapt to acting forces. If the transition zone loses this adaptability, a continuum distortion occurs.

References

1. Adstrum S, Hedley G, Schleip R, Stecco C, Yucesoy C (2017) Defining the fascial system. J Bodyw Mov Ther 2:173–177
2. Anker S (2011) Interrater reliability in evaluating the body language based on the Fascial Distortion Model (FDM) [thesis]. Vienna School of Osteopathy, Danube University Krems—Centre for Traditional Chinese Medicine and Complementary Medicine, Vienna
3. Drake RL (2011) Federative international programme on anatomical terminologies FIPAT Terminologia Anatomica. International anatomical terminology, 2nd edn. Georg Thieme, Stuttgart, p 33
4. Guimberteau JC (2022) Human living microanatomy. In: Schleip R, Stecco C, Driscoll M, Huijing PA (eds) Fascia. The tensional network of the human body, 2nd edn. Elsevier, London, pp 239–248
5. Hinz B (2022) Extracellular matrix. In: Schleip R, Stecco C, Driscoll M, Huijing PA (eds) Fascia. The tensional network of the human body, 2nd edn. Elsevier, London, pp 276–285
6. Hoheisel U, Taguchi T, Mense S (2022) Nociception: the thoracolumbar and crural fascia as sensory organs. In: Schleip R, Stecco C, Driscoll M, Huijing PA (eds) Fascia. The tensional network of the human body, 2nd edn. Elsevier, London, pp 179–187
7. Huijing PA (2009) Epimuscular myofascial force transmission between antagonistic and synergistic muscles can explain movement limitation in spastic paresis. In: Huijing PA, Hollander P, Findley WT et al (eds) Fascia research II. Basic science and implications for conventional and complementary health care. Elsevier, Munich, pp 40–56
8. Huijing PA (2022) Epimuscular myofascial force transmission: an introduction. In: Schleip R, Stecco C, Driscoll M, Huijing PA (eds) Fascia. The tensional network of the human body, 2nd edn. Elsevier, London, pp 204–210
9. Levin SM (2002) The tensegrity-truss as a model for spine mechanics: biotensegrity. J Mech Med Biol 02(03–04):375–388.
10. Levin SM, Scarr G (2022) Biotensegrity and the mechanics of fascia. In: Schleip R, Stecco C, Driscoll M, Huijing PA (eds) Fascia. The tensional network of the human body, 2nd edn. Elsevier, London, pp 232–238
11. Meert GF (2022) Fluid dynamics in fascial tissues. In: Schleip R, Stecco C, Driscoll M, Huijing PA (eds) Fascia. The tensional network of the human body, 2nd edn. Elsevier, London, pp 294–298
12. Rutkokwski JM, Swartz MA (2012) A driving force for change: interstitial flow as a morphoregulator. In: Chaitow L, Findley TW, Schleip R (eds) Fascia research III. Basic science and implications for conventional and complementary health care. Kiener, Munich, pp 21–27
13. Schleip R (2003) Fascial plasticity. A new neurobiological explanation: part 1 and part II. J Bodyw Mov Ther 7(1):11–19; 7(2):104–116
14. Schleip R (2022) Fascia as an organ of communication. In: Schleip R, Stecco C, Driscoll M, Huijing PA (eds) Fascia. The tensional network of the human body, 2nd edn. Elsevier, London, pp 156–159
15. Schleip R, Calsius J, Jäger H (2022) Interoception: a new correlate for intricate connections between fascial receptors, emotion, and self-awareness. In: Schleip R, Stecco C, Driscoll M, Huijing PA (eds) Fascia. The tensional network of the human body, 2nd edn. Elsevier, London, pp 169–178
16. Schleip R, Jäger H, Klingler W (2022) Fascia is alive. How cells modulate the tonicity and architecture of fascial tissues. In: Schleip R, Stecco C, Driscoll M, Huijing PA (eds) Fascia. The tensional network of the human body, 2nd edn. Elsevier, London, pp 265–275
17. Stark J, Pöttner M (2007) Stills Faszienkonzepte. Eine Studie. Jolandos, Pähl
18. Stecco C (2015) Functional atlas of the human fascial system. Elsevier, Edinburgh
19. Stechmann K (2011) Interrater-reliability of distortion-classification using body language within the

© The Editor(s) (if applicable) and The Author(s), under exclusive license to Springer-Verlag GmbH, DE, part of Springer Nature 2026

S. Anker, *Fascial Distortion Model in Clinical Practice,* https://doi.org/10.1007/978-3-662-72081-3

fascial distortion model (FDM) [thesis]. University of Applied Science and Arts, Hildesheim

20. Typaldos S (1992) The fascial continuum model. A new philosophical and practical approach for enhancement of athletic performance and treatment of musculo-skeletal dysfunction and pain. https://www.fascialdistortion.com/the-fascial-continuum-model/

21. Typaldos S (1994) Introducing the fascial distortion model. AAO J 4(2):14–18, 30–36. https://afdma.com/articles/introducing-fascial-distortion-model/

22. Typaldos S (1994) Triggerband technique. AAO J 4(4):15–18, 30–33. https://afdma.com/articles/triggerband-technique/

23. Typaldos S (1995) Continuum technique. AAO J 5(2):15–19. https://afdma.com/articles/continuum-technique/

24. Typaldos S, Meddeb G (1997) Orthopathische Medizin. Die Verbindung von Orthopädie und Osteopathie durch das Fasziendistorsionsmodell. Verlag für Ganzheitliche Medizin Wühr, Kötzing/Bayerischer Wald

25. Typaldos S (2002) Clinical and theoretical application of the Fascial Distortion Model within the practice of medicine and surgery, 4th edn. Orthopathic Global Health Publications, Brewer

26. van den Berg F (2022) The physiology of fascia. An introduction. In: Schleip R, Stecco C, Driscoll M, Huijing PA (edn) Fascia. The tensional network of the human body, 2nd edn. Elsevier, London, pp 258–264

27. van der Wal J (2009) The architecture of the connective tissue in the musculoskeletal system. An often overlooked functional parameter as to proprioception in the locomotor apparatus. In: Huijing, PA., Hollander, P., Findley, WT et al (eds) Fascia research II. Basic science and implications for conventional and complementary health care. Elsevier, Munich, pp 21–35

28. van der Wal J (2022) Proprioception. In: Schleip R, Stecco C, Driscoll M, Huijing PA (eds) Fascia. The tensional network of the human body, 2nd edn. Elsevier, London, pp 160–168

29. Willard, FH (2022) Somatic fascia. In: Schleip R, Stecco C, Driscoll M, Huijing PA. (eds) Fascia. The tensional network of the human body, 2nd edn. Elsevier, London, pp 28–39

30. Zügel M, Maganaris CN, Wilke J, Jurkat-Rott K, Klingler W, Wearing SC, Findley T, Barbe MF, Steinacker JM, Vleeming A, Bloch W, Scheip R, Hodges PW (2018) Fascial tissue research in sports medicine: from molecules to tissue adaptation, injury and diagnostics. Br J Sports Med 52:1497. https://doi.org/10.1136/bjsports-2018-099308)

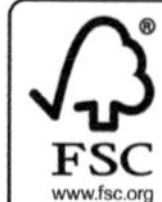